Learning Imaging

Series Editors:

P.R. Ros • A. Luna • R. Ribes

Jose Luís del Cura • Pedro Seguí
Carlos Nicolau

(Editors)

Learning Ultrasound Imaging

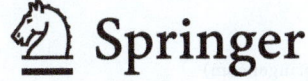 Springer

Jose Luís del Cura
Servicio de Radiodiagnóstico
Hospital de Basurto
Bilbao
Spain

Carlos Nicolau
Servicio de Radiodiagnóstico (CDIC)
Hospital Clinic
Barcelona
Spain

Pedro Seguí
Servicio de Radiodiagnóstico
Hospital Universitario Reina Sofía
Córdoba
Spain

ISBN 978-3-642-30585-6   ISBN 978-3-642-30586-3 (eBook)
DOI 10.1007/978-3-642-30586-3

Springer Heidelberg New York Dordrecht London

Library of Congress Control Number: 2012950865

Printed on acid-free paper

Springer is part of Springer Science+Business Media (www.springer.com)

Contents

5 Thorax

Rosa Zabala, Jose Luís del Cura

6 Pediatrics

Fermín Sáez, Elena Elizagaray, José Martel

7 Vascular

Blanca Paño, Pedro Seguí

8 Contrast Ultrasound

Teresa Fontanilla, Carlos Nicolau, Javier Minaya,
Rafael Pérez-Arangüena, Blanca Paño

9   Interventional Ultrasound

JOSE LUÍS DEL CURA, ROSA ZABALA, IGONE KORTA

Contributors

Xavier Bargalló
Servicio de Radiodiagnóstico
(CDIC)
Hospital Clinic
Barcelona
Spain

Angel Bueno
Diagnóstico por Imagen
Hospital Universitario Fundación
Alcorcón
Alcorcón
Spain

Jose Luís del Cura
Servicio de Radiodiagnóstico
Hospital Basurto
Bilbao
Spain

Montserrat Domingo
Servicio de Radiodiagnóstico
(CDIC)
Hospital Clinic
Barcelona
Spain

Elena Elizagaray
Servicio de Radiodiagnóstico
Hospital Basurto
Bilbao
Spain

Simona Espejo
Servicio de Radiodiagnóstico
Hospital Universitario Reina Sofía
Córdoba
Spain

Teresa Fontanilla
Servicio de Radiodiagnóstico
Hospital Universitario Puerta de
Hierro
Majadahonda
Spain

Igone Korta
Servicio de Radiodiagnóstico
Hospital Basurto
Bilbao
Spain

Carmen Kraemer
Departamento de Enfermería
Universidad de Granada
Granada
Spain

Jose Martel
Diagnóstico por Imagen
Hospital Universitario Fundación
Alcorcón
Alcorcón
Spain

Javier Minaya
Servicio de Radiodiagnóstico
Hospital Universitario Puerta de
Hierro
Majadahonda
Spain

Carlos Nicolau
Servicio de Radiodiagnóstico
(CDIC)
Hospital Clinic
Barcelona
Spain

Blanca Paño
Servicio de Radiodiagnóstico
(CDIC)
Hospital Clinic
Barcelona
Spain

Rafael Pérez-Arangüena
Servicio de Radiodiagnóstico
Hospital Universitario Puerta de
Hierro
Majadahonda
Spain

Enrique Remartínez
Departamento de Radiología
Hospital General de Melilla
Melilla
Spain

Fermín Sáez
Servicio de Radiodiagnóstico
Hospital Cruces
Baracaldo
Spain

Gorane Santamaría
Servicio de Radiodiagnóstico
(CDIC)
Hospital Clinic
Barcelona
Spain

Ana Sanz
Diagnóstico por Imagen
Hospital Universitario Fundación
Alcorcón
Alcorcón
Spain

Pedro Seguí
Servicio de Radiodiagnóstico
Hospital Universitario Reina Sofía
Cordoba
Spain

Martín Velasco
Servicio de Radiodiagnóstico
(CDIC)
Hospital Clinic
Barcelona
Spain

Ximena Wortsman
Departmento de Radiología
Clinica Servet
Facultad de Medicina
Universidad de Chile
Santiago
Chile

Rosa Zabala
Servicio de Radiodiagnóstico
Hospital Basurto
Bilbao
Spain

Abdominal Ultrasound

Carlos Nicolau, Pedro Seguí, Jose Luís del Cura, and Blanca Paño

Introduction

Although in developed countries the availability of CT and MRI equipments has made these techniques widely used, ultrasound is the most available image technique worldwide for the study of abdominal diseases. However, ultrasound is highly operator-dependent and the performance of the technique may be very variable even within the same health organization jeopardizing the confidence of the clinicians in the technique.

Following the American College of Radiology Appropriateness Citeria, ultrasound is the most appropriate technique in adults for the evaluation of blunt abdominal trauma in unstable patient (FAST scan), jaundice, right upper quadrant pain, recurrent symptoms of stone disease, renal failure, acute abdominal pain and fever in pregnant patient and to assess gallstones in acute pancreatitis.

Moreover, there are some conditions in which ultrasound is a useful alternative test: palpable abdominal mass, right lower quadrant pain, acute flank pain and hematuria. Also, it is the most used imaging technique to follow-up patients with liver cirrhosis.

A very important advantage of ultrasound is that it is a technique that does not use radiation, iodinated contrast agents or gadolinium. Therefore it is the technique of choice for children and pregnant women in most abdominal pathologies.

Thus, ultrasound has an important role in the management of abdominal diseases. New improvements like contrast ultrasound and elastography, together with the growing concern about the effects of radiation from CT scans and the rising cost of imaging tests, will probably lead to a even further increase.

J.L. del Cura et al. (eds.), *Learning Ultrasound Imaging*, Learning Imaging,
DOI 10.1007/978-3-642-30586-3_1, © Springer-Verlag Berlin Heidelberg 2012

Case 1: Cholelithiasis

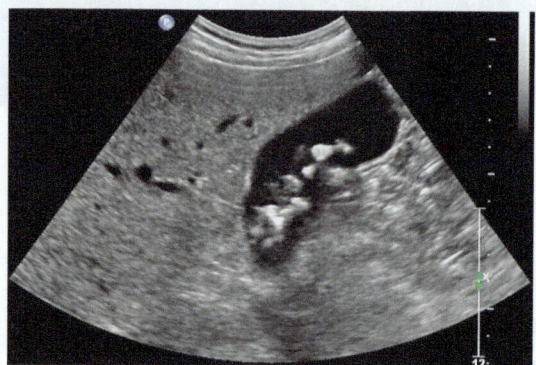

Fig. 1.1.1

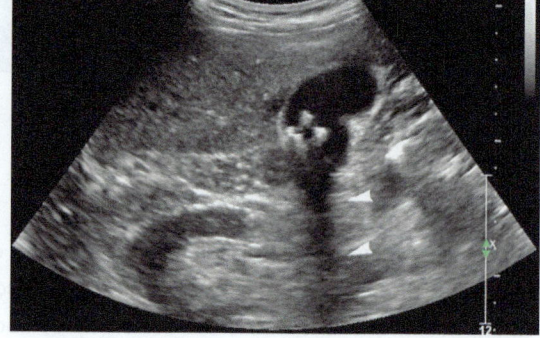

Fig. 1.1.2

A 48-year-old female complained of digestive disorders and dyspepsia. She related occasional pain in the right upper quadrant of the abdomen. An ultrasound exam was performed.

Ultrasound is the first choice technique for any pain in the upper right quadrant of the abdomen and, also, the most reliable when gallbladder pathology is suspected. Biliary pathology is very frequent with a 10 % of the population having gallstones, usually asymptomatic. Cholelithiasis is more frequent in women, and its incidence increases with age and in obese persons.

A third of the patients with cholelithiasis develop biliary colic: the painful expulsion of the biliary calculi. In some cases, the gallstone become impacted in the bile duct and obstructs it, causing obstructive jaundice. The gallstones can also obstruct the cystic duct eventually followed by inflammation and infection of the gallbladder, causing cholecystitis.

Ultrasound has a sensitivity of 95 % and a negative predictive value of 97 % for the diagnosis of cholelithiasis. The characteristic sonographic appearance of a gallstone is a mobile, usually multiple, hyperechogenic image with acoustic shadowing, within the gallbladder. When all these criteria are met, the image is pathognomonic.

When the gallbladder is full of stones or there is lithiasis occupying the entire lumen, the classic appearance may be changed into the sign of the "double-arch shadow": two echogenic curved and parallel lines separated by a thin anechoic space, with acoustic shadowing.

The differential diagnosis should be made with the biliary sludge—which does not produce an acoustic shadowing—and with cholesterolosis (concretions of cholesterol attached to the wall of the gallbladder). The lack of mobility and their location, attached to the gallbladder wall, allow differentiating this later condition from cholelithiasis.

Ultrasound exam (Figs. 1.1.1 and 1.1.2) showed multiple echogenic images with posterior acoustic shadowing (*arrowheads*) in the gallbladder. These images were mobile, moving to the most dependent portion of the gallbladder. These images are characteristic of cholelithiasis.

Case 2: Acute Cholecystitis

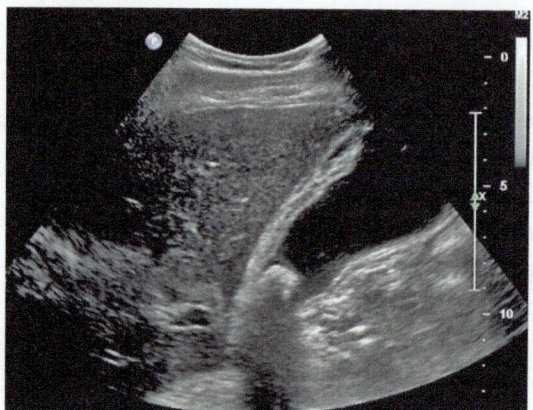

Fig. 1.2.1

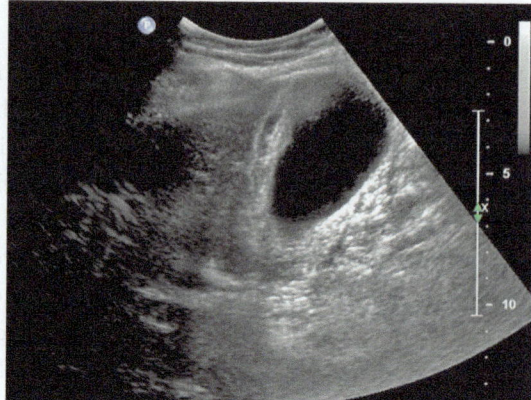

Fig. 1.2.2

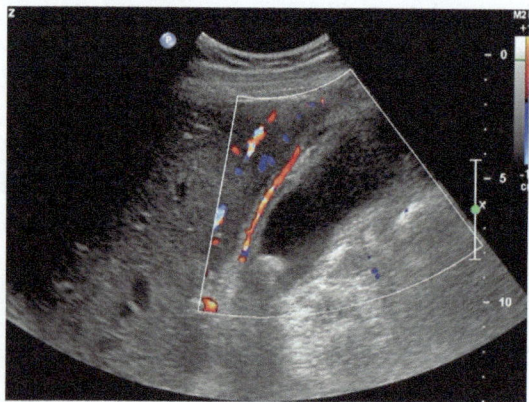

Fig. 1.2.3

Case Presentation   A 66-year-old man with a 3-day history of right upper quadrant pain was admitted to the hospital. He had severe leukocytosis but no fever.

Comments   Acute cholecystitis results from obstruction of the gallbladder neck or cystic duct with inflammation of the gallbladder wall. Approximately 95 % of the cases result from obstruction due to gallstones. Acute cholecystitis manifests as persistent right upper quadrant pain that may radiate to the right scapula. Nausea, vomiting, fever, and leukocytosis are common.

Ultrasonography is usually the initial imaging procedure of choice in a patient with suspected acute cholecystitis. In uncomplicated cases, the US findings include gallstones (often impacted in the gallbladder neck or cystic duct), positive sonographic Murphy's sign, gallbladder larger than 4×10 cm, gallbladder wall thickening greater than 3 mm, and pericholecystic fluid. Of these findings, the first two are considered the most specific. The sonographic Murphy's sign refers to localized tenderness directly over the gallbladder, and it is positive when pressure applied with the transducer elicits maximal tenderness over the gallbladder visualized at sonography. The combination of gallstones and Murphy's sign has a positive predictive value over 90 %. This sign may be absent in nonresponsive patients, when pain medication has been administered, or in cases of gangrenous cholecystitis. Thickening of the gallbladder wall occurs to some degree in most cases of acute cholecystitis. However, many causes of gallbladder wall thickening exist beyond cholecystitis, so this finding is less specific. Pericholecystic fluid is found in approximately 20 % of patients, and its presence implies a more advanced type of cholecystitis. It is usually seen as a focal collection adjacent to the gallbladder wall.

Gangrenous cholecystitis is a severe advanced form of acute cholecystitis, with increased morbidity and mortality rates. The sonographic hallmark is the presence of heterogeneous or striated thickening of the gallbladder wall, which is often irregular with localized disruptions or projections into the lumen. Murphy's sign may be absent. Intraluminal membranes and wall disruptions are more specific but less frequent findings.

Emphysematous cholecystitis is a rare complication of acute cholecystitis and is associated with gas-forming bacteria. Up to 50 % patients may have diabetes. Gas may be intraluminal or intramural. Intraluminal gas can be recognized by the antidependent gas echoes within the lumen.

Acalculous cholecystitis may occur in extremely ill patients. In these cases, US is often equivocal because these severely ill patients have distended, thick-walled gallbladder even in the absence of inflammation, and Murphy's sign is unreliable in these patients.

Imaging Findings

US image of the gallbladder in the sagittal (Fig. 1.2.1) and transverse plane (Fig. 1.2.2) demonstrated distension of the gallbladder, a gallstone impacted in the gallbladder neck, and thickened gallbladder wall with a striated appearance. There was a positive sonographic Murphy sign. Color Doppler US (Fig. 1.2.3) shows a hypervascular gallbladder wall, which is a nonspecific feature.

US examination showed signs of acute calculous cholecystitis. The patient underwent emergency open cholecystectomy. Acute inflammation and wall necrosis (gangrenous cholecystitis) without gallbladder perforation was observed at surgery and on histological examination.

Case 3: Gallbladder Carcinoma

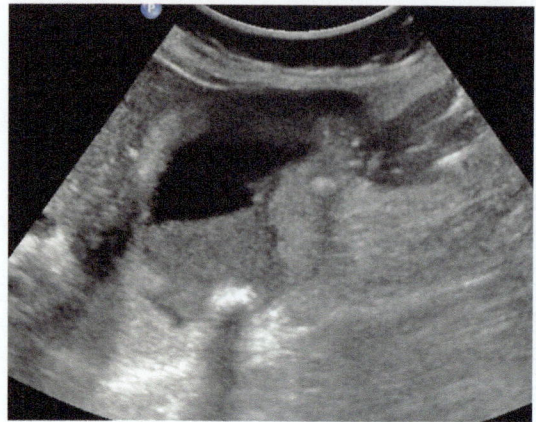

Fig. 1.3.1

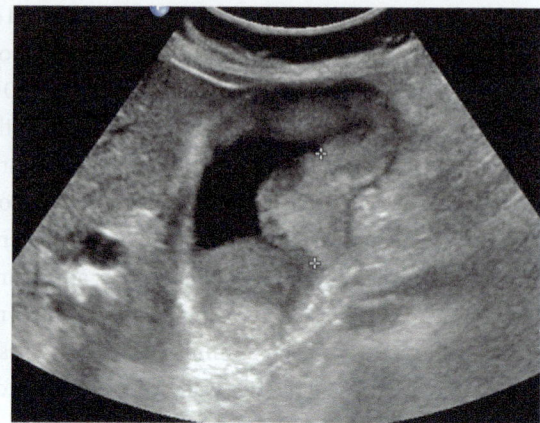

Fig. 1.3.2

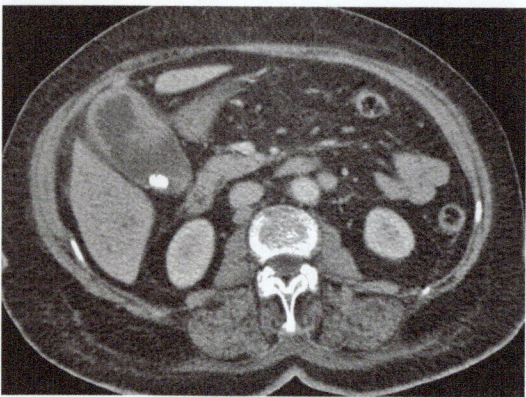

Fig. 1.3.3

Case Presentation   A 78-year-old woman was admitted with 4-day history of right upper quadrant pain and jaundice. An ultrasound exam was performed.

Comments   Primary carcinoma of the gallbladder is an aggressive malignancy that has a low overall prevalence; however, it is the most common malignant tumor of the biliary tract. It is three times more common in women than in men, and the frequency of diagnosis increases with age (mainly in postmenopausal status). Cholelithiasis is a well-established risk factor for the development of gallbladder carcinoma. Porcelain gallbladder is an uncommon condition in which there is diffuse calcification of the gallbladder wall, and 10–25 % of patients with this condition have gallbladder carcinoma. Several congenital anatomic anomalies are associated with a higher prevalence of gallbladder carcinoma. These conditions include congenital cystic dilatation of the biliary tree, choledochal cyst, anomalous junction of the pancreaticobiliary ducts, and low insertion of the cystic duct. Primary sclerosing cholangitis is thought to be a precursor to gallbladder carcinoma. Cigarette smoking has also been related to this malignancy.

The diagnosis of gallbladder carcinoma is usually unsuspected. Early stage carcinoma is typically diagnosed incidentally because of inflammatory symptoms related to coexistent cholelithiasis or cholecystitis. Most patients with gallbladder carcinoma present with advanced disease, and the clinical features include chronic abdominal pain, anorexia, weight loss, and jaundice.

Three sonographic patterns of gallbladder carcinoma have been described:
1. *Mass Replacing the Gallbladder*
It is the most common form of gallbladder cancer. The mass occupies the entire lumen of the gallbladder. It appears as a heterogeneous mass located in the subhepatic space, and a normal gallbladder is not visualized. However, the inability to visualize the normal gallbladder has also been described in other conditions, such as chronic cholecystitis, normally contracted gallbladder, perforation of the gallbladder, and congenital absence. Echogenic foci and acoustic shadowing associated with the tumor may be related to coexisting gallstones, gallbladder wall calcification, tumoral calcification, intraluminal air, or necrotic debris.
2. *Thickening of the Gallbladder Wall*
This pattern is seen in 20–30 % of cases of this malignancy. Thickening of the gallbladder wall may be diffuse or focal. Diffuse thickening of the wall in tumor infiltration can be similar in appearance to chronic cholecystitis. However, it has been suggested that the wall infiltrated by cancer is thicker and more irregular than the wall thickened from inflammation. Focal thickening of the wall may represent an early stage of the tumor.
3. *Intraluminal Mass Within the Gallbladder*
The mass has usually irregular borders. This presentation is not completely specific: an intraluminal mass may also represent either a cholesterol or inflammatory polyp or a benign tumor. Also, it can be confused with a nonshadowing stone, blood clot, biliary sludge, or pus. The demonstration of changes in shape and position of the "mass" after changes in the position of the patient will usually identify these other lesions.

Imaging Findings

Longitudinal US image of the gallbladder (Figs. 1.3.1 and 1.3.2) shows an asymmetric and irregular thickening of the gallbladder wall. There is a shadowing gallstone and biliary sludge along the dependent wall of the gallbladder.

A CT of the abdomen revealed a nodular thickening of the gallbladder wall highly suggestive of malignancy. In Fig. 1.3.3, an axial contrast-enhanced CT image shows thickening and nodular enhancement of the gallbladder wall and a gallstone within the gallbladder lumen.

The pathological study of the cholecystectomy specimen confirmed the diagnosis of adenocarcinoma of the gallbladder.

Case 4: Gallbladder Adenomyomatosis

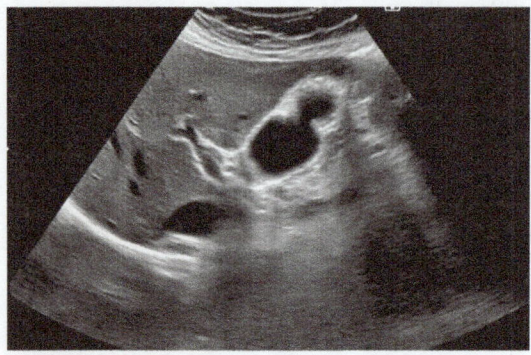

Fig. 1.4.1

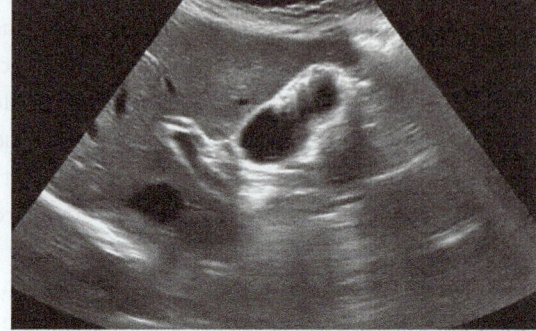

Fig. 1.4.2

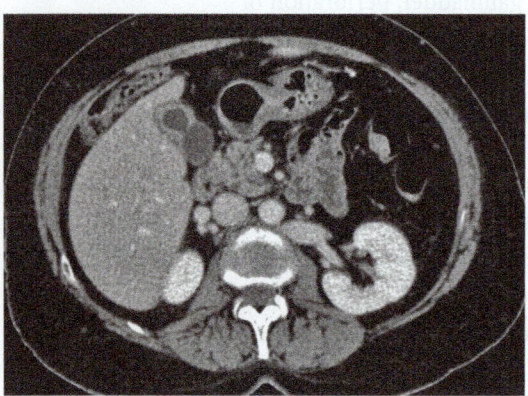

Fig. 1.4.3

Case Presentation

Ultrasound and CT exams were performed on a 60-year-old female with pain in hypogastrium.

Comments

It is also called adenomatous hyperplasia. It deals with a frequent hyperplastic lesion (up to 5 % of the cholecystectomies), that occasionally are classified as a subtype of chronic cholecystitis. It can appear at any age, it is frequently, an incidental finding in imaging that does not require treatment. It often coexists with cholelithiasis. In this entity, the gallbladder presents mural thickening secondary to hyperplasia of the mucous and muscularis propia and some intramural diverticula (Rokitansky-Aschoff sinuses) with cholesterol in their interior. The adenomyomatosis can be diffuse or, more frequently, focal, with the fundus being in this case the most commonly involved area. An infrequent form is the focal involvement of the mean portion of the gallbladder giving a so-called hour-glass appearance.

Ultrasound is usually the imaging method with which this entity is initially detected, often incidentally in examinations performed for other reasons. The appearance on ultrasound is quite variable depending on whether it deals with a focal or diffuse form. The gallbladder presents thickening of the wall (focal or diffuse, depending on the type), although this feature is non-specific. The most specific feature is the visualization of intramural hyperechogenic foci with comet-tail artifact in B-mode or with "twinkling" artifact in the Doppler register, corresponding to the cholesterol crystals in the interior of the Rokitansky-Aschoff sinuses. Also specific, although less frequent, is the visualization of the sinuses as intramural cystic spaces. In both the lumen of the gallbladder and in the interior of the intramural diverticula, biliary sludge or lithiasis can be found.

In focal or segmentary cases, the lesion can be visualized as a mass (called in these cases adenomyoma). If the cystic spaces and the typical findings of cholesterol crystals are not visualized, differentiation with a tumor can be difficult or impossible. In these cases, PET can be useful to rule out malignancy. On rare occasions, comet-tail artifact of the cholesterol crystals can make it difficult the differential diagnosis with the reverberation artifact or "dirty shadow" of the gas in the emphysematous cholecystitis. The very distinct clinical context and the movement of the gas bubbles after the compression of the gallbladder or the mobilization of the patient help to differentiate them.

Imaging Findings

Sonography of the gallbladder showed focal wall thickening in the fundus (Fig. 1.4.1) and echogenic intramural foci with comet-tail reverberation artifacts (Fig. 1.4.2) indicative of cholesterol crystals within Rokitansky-Aschoff sinuses. This finding is diagnostic of adenomyomatosis of the gallbladder. CT (Fig. 1.4.3) also showed focal wall thickening in the fundus of the gallbladder.

Case 5: Hepatic Metastases of Breast Carcinoma in Hepatic Steatosis

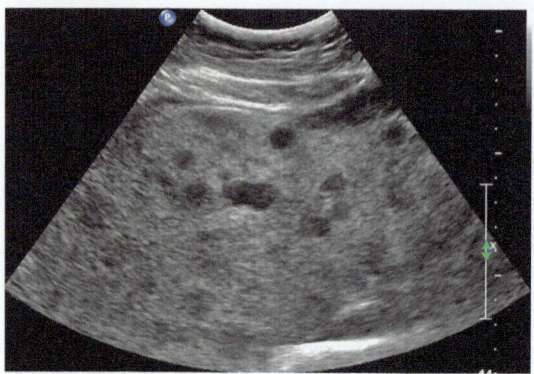

Fig. 1.5.1

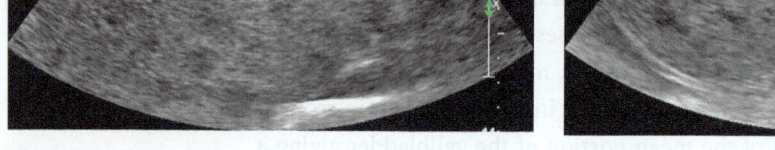

Fig. 1.5.2

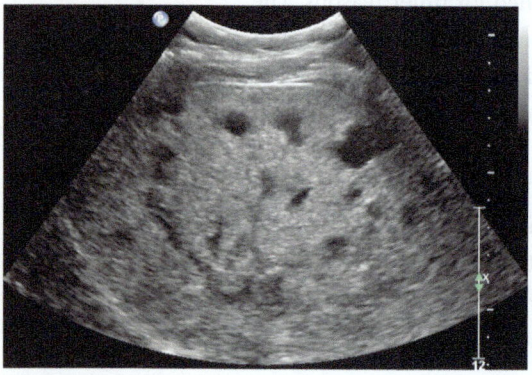

Fig. 1.5.3

Female, 52-years-old, with history of breast carcinoma 7 years ago. She was treated with mastectomy, radiotherapy, and chemotherapy. In the yearly follow-up, an abdominal ultrasound was performed.

In oncological patients, the search for possible hepatic metastases is a part of the routine diagnosis. Ultrasound, due to its low cost and lack of ionizing radiations, is one of the most used techniques in the follow-up of these patients. This is also the usual practice in breast carcinoma given that the liver is one of the most usual target organs of the metastases.

Hepatic metastases usually appear as hypoechoic lesions, sometimes with a more echogenic peripheral halo, which gives them a "bull's-eye" appearance. Larger metastases can have internal necrosis and, when they are of slow growth, a peripheral pseudocapsule. Occasionally, metastases can be hyperechoic (especially those of neuroendocrine or carcinoid tumors) or present calcifications (typically in colon mucinous carcinoma).

The number of metastases is variable, ranging from few isolated lesions to multiple nodules extended throughout the entire liver. In oncological patients, the appearance of these lesions is usually enough to characterize them as metastatic. So, a biopsy is only indicated in patients without a known primary tumor or with several ones.

Hepatic steatosis is an acquired metabolic disease that results from the deposit of triglycerides within the hepatocytes. It is very frequent, being found in 1–9 % of the hepatic biopsies. It can be due to many causes, among which is the treatment with tamoxifen, used in the treatment of breast cancer. Therefore, it is frequently observed it in the follow-up of patients who have suffered this disease.

On ultrasound, steatosis causes an increase of the echogenicity because of the high sonic reflectivity of the fat. In more advanced cases, it can cause an increase in the attenuation of the signal making it difficult the visualization of the deepest regions of the liver. It can be diffuse, nodular, or geographic. In the diffuse forms, preserved focal areas of fat can be found, that will appear hypoechoic. The focal forms are characterized by not presenting a mass effect (they do not deform the boundaries or displace the vessels).

Abdominal ultrasound (Figs. 1.5.1, 1.5.2 and 1.5.3) detected multiple rounded hypoechoic solid nodules throughout the liver. The liver presented a diffusely increased echogenicity and a loss of definition of the deepest structures, those farthest from the transducer, due to the loss of ultrasound signal in these areas because of the increased sonic attenuation of the liver. The findings are characteristic of a hepatic metastatic dissemination on a hepatic steatosis secondary to the treatment with tamoxifen.

Case 6: Hepatic Hydatid Cyst

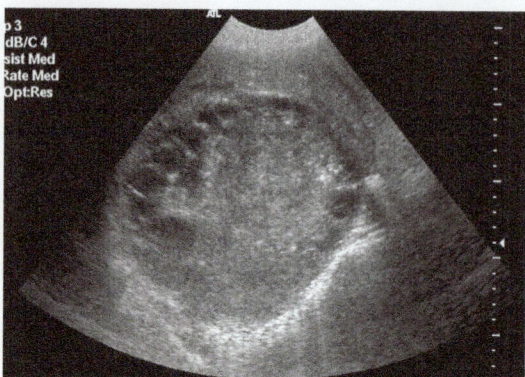

Fig. 1.6.1

An abdominal ultrasound was performed on a 28-year-old North African male, with pain in the right upper quadrant of the abdomen and alterations in liver function tests.

The hydatid cyst is a zoonosis caused by the larval state of the taeniae, *Echinococcus granulosus* and *Echinococcus multilocularis*. This infection appears in many parts of the world, especially in South America, Africa, and Middle East. Man, who is an intermediary host, like sheep, acquires the parasite by drinking water or vegetables contaminated by dog feces. The dog is the final host. The dog is contaminated by ingesting contaminated viscera of sheep or any other intermediate host.

After the parasite crosses the intestine, the liver acts as the first defensive filter, thus being the most frequently involved organ (75 % of the cases). There, the parasite forms the hydatid cyst. These cysts have a peripheral pseudocapsule, the pericystic membrane, which is the fibrous reaction of the liver to contain the growth of the cyst, and a cystic content, surrounded by the membrane of the cyst. Within the cyst, small vesicles can be formed that appear as cysts within the cyst. These vesicles can break and collapse, forming magma composed of the wall of the small vesicles in the center of the cyst. Calcification of the pericystic membrane is frequent.

Ultrasound is the most sensitive technique for the detection of the hepatic hydatid cyst and its complications. The appearance of the hepatic hydatid cyst is variable.

- Simple cyst. It is a unilocular cyst, similar to the biliary cysts.
- Cyst with small vesicles. It presents a multiloculated pattern, with a honeycomb appearance. Occasionally, an echogenic matrix can be seen in the center caused by the broken membranes of the small vesicles, giving the lesion the appearance of a cartwheel.
- Echogenic mass. When all the small vesicles have broken and collapsed.
- Calcified cyst. Usually the exterior wall of the cyst becomes calcified, but the internal matrix can also be calcified. On ultrasound an echogenic wall with acoustic shadowing can be seen. When the calcification is complete, the hydatid cyst is considered to be dead.

The cyst can break, leading to:

- Contained breakage, which appears as fluid between the cyst and the pericystic membrane. Sometimes the membranes of the cyst appear folded inside the cyst (the "water lily sign").
- Communicating breakage, in which the content of the cyst opens to the exterior or the biliary channel.

Ultrasound (Fig. 1.6.1) showed a spherical, well-delimited liver lesion with a central echogenic area surrounded by a ring of smaller cystic vesicles.

Case 7: Littoral-Cell Angioma of the Spleen

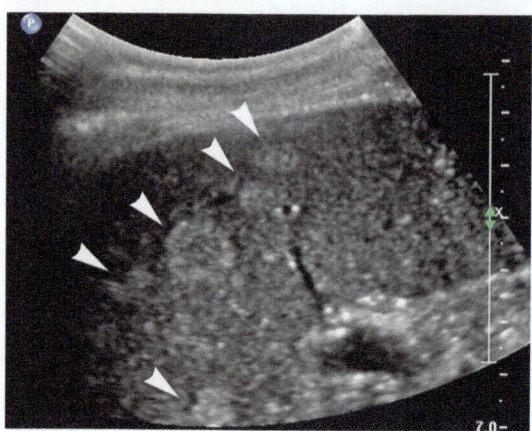

Fig. 1.7.1

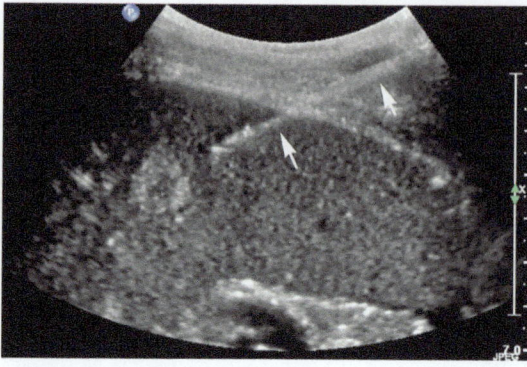

Fig. 1.7.2

An ultrasound study was carried out in a 63-year-old female for suspicion of biliary pathology.

The littoral-cell angioma is an infrequent splenic vascular tumor derived from the cells that surround the splenic red pulp sinuses (littoral cells). It is usually detected as an incidental finding. Given its rarity, there is no consensus on its nature, and, although it is considered benign, some cases of malignant tumors have been described. It is usually managed by splenectomy, with a diagnostic and, at the same time, therapeutic intention. The ultrasound features are variable, appearing as hypoechoic, heterogeneous, or, more frequently, as echogenic nodules.

Splenic focal lesions detected on ultrasound can correspond to benign as well as to malignant lesions. Among the benign lesions are hemangiomas, hamartomas, lymphangiomas, littoral-cell angiomas, splenic infarctions, and abscesses. The most frequent malignant lesions are lymphoma, metastasis, and angiosarcoma.

When single or multiple splenic focal lesions are detected on ultrasound, several factors such as clinical manifestations, presence of concomitant pathology, or known malignant tumors should be considered for differential diagnosis. In the presence of signs of infection, an abscess is the most probable diagnosis. In patients with a malignant tumor or known lymphoma, a metastatic involvement should be considered in the first place.

Ultrasound features are also useful in suggesting the diagnosis. A triangular, subcapsular morphology is typical of splenic infarction. When the lesions are echogenic, hemangioma, hamartoma, or littoral-cell angioma should be considered. MRI can be useful in the differential diagnosis among these entities; for example, the littoral-cell angiomas are usually hypointense on T1 and T2. Other possible causes of echogenic lesions are Gaucher's disease or lymphoma. When the lesion is hypoechoic, the diagnostic possibilities to consider are lymphoma, abscess, metastasis, or atypical hemangioma.

In case of diagnostic doubt, absence of infectious clinical manifestations or significant medical history and especially in hypoechoic lesions, an ultrasound-guided biopsy can be performed. This specialized technique has scarcely been used due to the fear of complications, specifically bleeding (5 % of the published cases). In our experience, and given that the alternative is the diagnostic splenectomy, the percutaneous biopsy can avoid splenectomy in many cases, limiting it to that carried out for therapeutic purposes. It is especially useful in compromised patients.

Ultrasound showed several splenic lesions (Fig. 1.7.1). These lesions were variable in size hyperechoic nodules, most of them with hypoechoic center (*arrowheads*). The MRI was nonconclusive, and an ultrasound-guided core biopsy was performed on one of the lesions (Fig. 1.7.2). The images show the biopsy needle (*arrows*) being directed toward one of the lesions. The diagnosis of the biopsy was littoral-cell angioma, which was confirmed in the splenectomy.

Case 8: Mesenteric Lymphoma

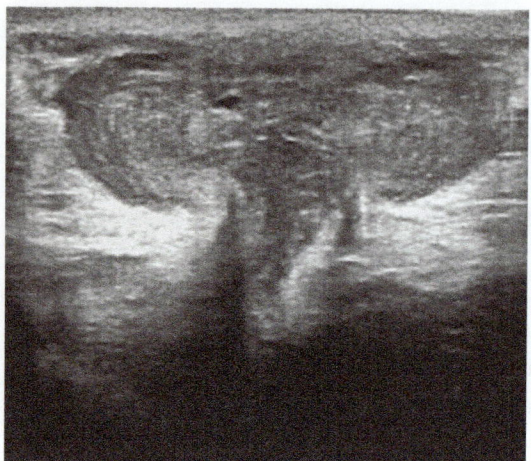

Fig. 1.8.1

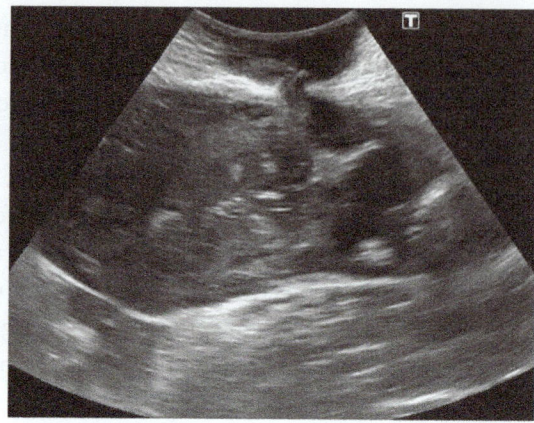

Fig. 1.8.2

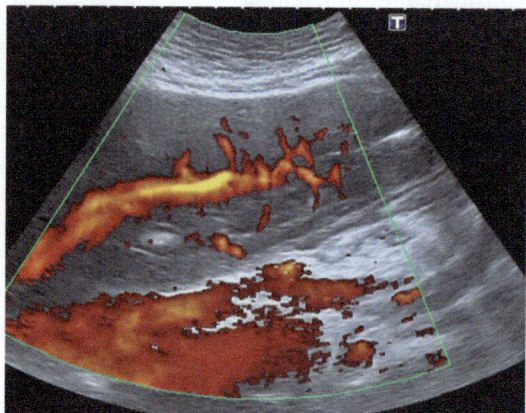

Fig. 1.8.3

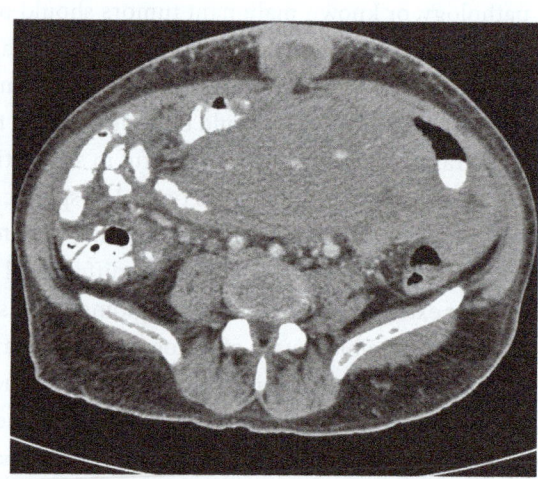

Fig. 1.8.4

Case Presentation   A 60-year-old male presented with a palpable painless umbilical nodule of 2 months of evolution. An ultrasound was performed.

Comments   Most of the non-Hodgkin's lymphomas (NHL) and less than half of Hodgkin's lymphomas (HL) have abdominal involvement. The most frequent findings are the para-aortic lymphadenopathy, but they can be present in any place or organ of the abdomen as a single mass, multiple masses, lymphadenopathy, or diffuse infiltration. Lymphomatous masses have a tendency to displace structures, rather than invade them, and this characteristic can help distinguish them from carcinomas and sarcomas. Although ultrasound can detect abdominal lesions related to the lymphoma and can be useful as a guide in performing the biopsies, the initial staging and the monitoring of the response to treatment is generally performed with CT and PET.

Lymphoma is the most frequent cause of mesenteric masses. Other causes of mesenteric lymphadenopathy are metastatic lymph nodes of carcinoma, sarcoma, or carcinoid tumor of the small intestine, and nonneoplastic pathologies such as tuberculosis, intestinal inflammatory diseases, and the polyadenopathy syndrome associated with AIDS. When the lymph nodes are multiple and large sized, the diagnosis is, almost invariably, lymphoma. When the lesion is a single mesenteric mass, the differential diagnosis includes principally lymphoma, desmoid tumor (mesenteric fibromatosis), gastrointestinal stromal tumors (GIST), and sarcomas.

The masses and adenopathy related to the lymphoma are usually quite homogeneous and hypoechogenic, due to the hypercellularity of these lesions. Classically, some of these adenopathies were described with a "cystic" or anechoic appearance, although this appearance is infrequent with the modern ultrasound equipment. The size of the lesions can go from very small to large bulky masses and can be rounded-oval or irregular, or else appear as multiple rounded masses surrounding and encompassing the mesenteric vessels (without causing ischemia). A characteristic form of presentation of the lymphoma is the "sandwich sign" consisting of soft lobular and confluent tissue that encompasses the mesenteric vessels between them (sandwich filler). The lymphoma can also be disseminated in sheets throughout the peritoneal surfaces and show an image of multiple thickened and stacked mesenteric sheets (the peritoneal involvement can also produce nodular implants, omental caking, and ascites, all similar to the peritoneal carcinomatosis). With less frequency, it can be presented as "misty mesentery," with this being more common after treatment. The larger-sized masses can be heterogeneous because of the presence of central necrosis. Calcifications are very rare prior to treatment.

Imaging Findings

Transverse US of the palpable nodule (Fig. 1.8.1) showed a solid subcutaneous umbilical nodule communicated through a neck to a large solid mesenteric mass.

Transverse abdominal US image showed (Fig. 1.8.2) an 18-cm soft tissue mass in the mesentery. Umbilical nodule appeared communicated with the mesenteric mass via a neck. On power Doppler US (Fig. 1.8.3), the mesenteric vessels were seen in the middle of the mass (sandwich sign).

On contrast-enhanced CT scan (Fig. 1.8.4), a large homogeneous soft tissue mesenteric mass displacing the small intestine and encasing the vessels were observed.

The histological analysis of the surgical biopsy of the mass resulted in infiltration by low-grade B cell lymphoma.

Case 9: Mesenteric Metastases of Seminoma

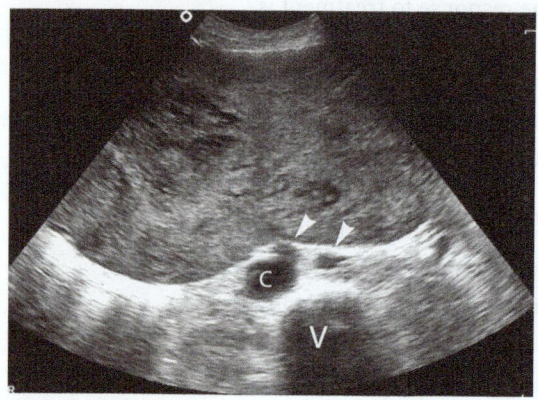

Fig. 1.9.1

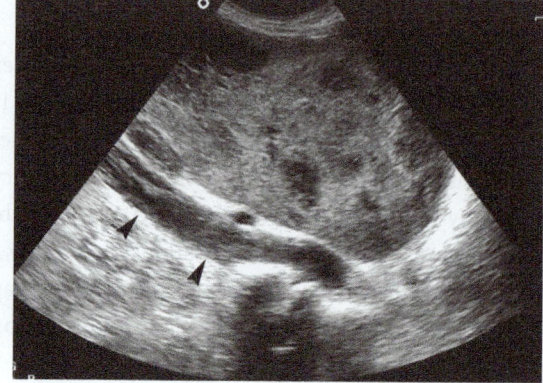

Fig. 1.9.2

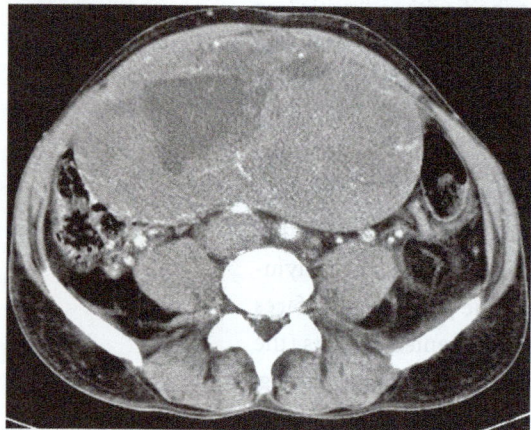

Fig. 1.9.3

A 28-year-old male has been noticing a gradual increase in his abdominal diameter in recent months, despite having followed a strict diet and maintain regular physical activity. In recent days, he has experienced abdominal discomfort accompanied by nausea.

A palpable abdominal mass always requires an examination by imaging techniques. Although CT is the most specific technique to achieve a specific topographic location of the lesion, ultrasound is often the first exploration in these patients. It is also the most useful technique for guiding the biopsy of these masses, when this is necessary for diagnosis.

Peritoneal cavity is lined by the peritoneum, which is folded upon it forming the mesentery. This mesentery serves both to attach the jejunum and the ileum to the retroperitoneum as to bring to the bowel the vessels, lymphatics, and nerves. Because of its relationship with these structures, the mesentery may have different pathological processes such as tumors (primary or metastatic), infections, cysts,…. Almost all of them manifest with nonspecific clinical symptoms (abdominal pain, weight loss, diarrhea, palpable mass).

Primary neoplasms of the mesentery are rare. The most common are desmoid tumor, lipoma, lymphoma, and carcinoid. Secondary tumors can spread to the mesentery by various routes: direct from the small intestine, lymphatic, hematogenous, or by peritoneal seeding. The tumors that most frequently metastasize in the mesentery are carcinoid, lymphoma, melanoma, and cancers of the stomach, small intestine, colon, pancreas, ovary, breast, and lung.

Seminoma is the most common testicular tumor. It appears as a pure seminoma or, more frequently, associated to other tumors. It is generally found in patients between 30 and 40 years old. A third of them have metastases at diagnosis. The spread of seminoma is exclusively lymphatic initially, but at advanced stages of the disease, visceral metastases may occur. So, pure seminomas only rarely spread to other organs without evidence of disease in the retroperitoneum. An exclusive spread to the mesentery, as in this case, is exceptional.

Ultrasound showed a large mass that occupies most of the abdominal cavity. Figure 1.9.1 is an axial image in which a solid mass is seen before a widened vena cava (*C*), the two common iliac arteries (*arrowheads*), and the vertebral column (*V*). Figure 1.9.2 corresponds to a sagittal image, in which the mass is seen before the cava (*arrows*). Figure 1.9.3 is the CT section corresponding to the ultrasound image in Fig. 1.9.1. It shows the huge mass displacing bowel loops laterally. The biopsy of the mass, performed with ultrasound guidance, showed a metastatic seminoma.

Case 10: Appendicitis

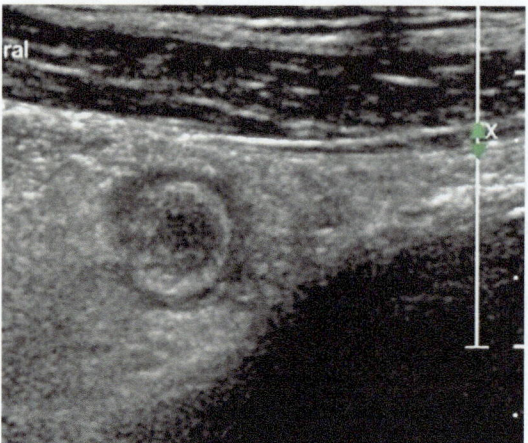

Fig. 1.10.1

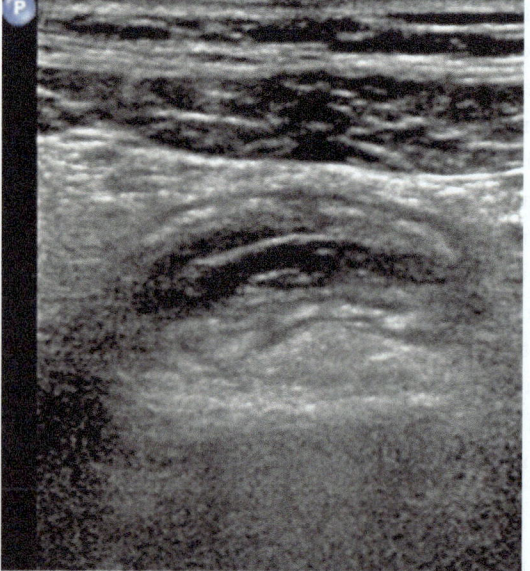

Fig. 1.10.2

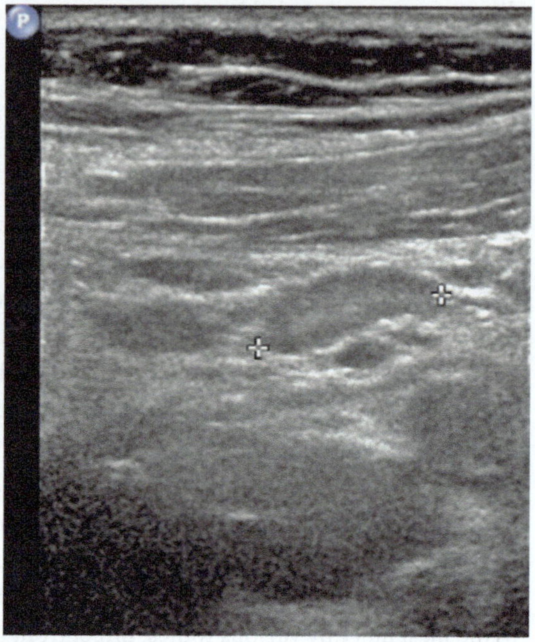

Fig. 1.10.3

Case Presentation A 12-year-old female patient was admitted to the hospital with a 1-day history of epigastric and right lower quadrant pain, fever, and vomiting. Physical examination revealed tenderness in right lower quadrant. Laboratory studies yielded leukocytosis with neutrophilia. An US examination of the right lower quadrant was performed.

Comments Acute appendicitis is the most common abdominal surgical emergency in the western world. The overall accuracy of clinical diagnosing of appendicitis is approximately 80 %, with a mean false-negative appendectomy rate of 20 %

and a mean overall incidence of perforation of 20 %. New imaging technology (helical CT, graded-compression US) has the potential to improve these clinical outcomes. US examination of the patient with suspected appendicitis usually starts with a curvilinear 3.5–5-MHz transducer. The linear transducer is used later for more detailed images.

The typical appearance of an inflamed appendix is a thick-walled, noncompressible sausage-like and blind-ended structure in a fixed position at the point of maximal tenderness. The appendix is considered enlarged when its outer anteroposterior diameter under compression measured in the transverse plane is 6 mm or larger. The average maximum diameter is 9 mm. Appendicoliths are found in 30 % of inflamed appendices and appear as bright, echogenic foci with clean distal acoustic shadowing. The adjacent fat of the mesoappendix may become larger, hyperechoic, and less compressible, and, if inflammation progresses, this fatty tissue tends to increase in volume around the appendix. With perforation of the appendix, the distended appendix may no longer be visualized at US examination, and the inflammatory changes in the perienteric fat are more obvious. Patients evaluated with a considerable delay from the onset of the appendicitis may show a large mass of noncompressible fat around the appendix, interspersed with poorly marginated hypoechoic zones (appendiceal phlegmon) or a fluid collection (appendiceal abscess). A small amount of free intraperitoneal fluid in nonspecific and may be present in both nonperforated and perforated appendicitis as well as in many other conditions. A large amount of peritoneal fluid in the presence of an inflamed appendix usually represents pus from perforated appendix.

Color Doppler US is also useful. Circumferential color in the wall of the inflamed appendix is strongly supportive evidence of active inflammation. With gangrene, color Doppler may show decreased perfusion or none at all.

US and CT have similar positive and negative predictive values (both over 90 %) for appendicitis. The choice between US and CT is largely dependent on institutional preference and on available expertise. Operator skill has particular importance in the US evaluation of the patient with right lower quadrant pain, and the learning curve required is considerable. Patient sex, age, and body habitus are important factors. US is usually the recommended initial imaging study in children, in young women, and during pregnancy. In patients with equivocal US findings, most of which are obese, CT scan is indicated.

Imaging Findings

Cross-sectional (Fig. 1.10.1) and long-axis (Fig. 1.10.2) US images obtained with a linear transducer show a blind, tubular structure measuring 10 mm in diameter with a layered wall. This structure was not compressible and corresponds to an inflamed appendix. Some oval, reactive lymph nodes were also demonstrated near the terminal ileum, a common finding in the context of acute appendicitis (Fig. 1.10.3).

An inflamed nonperforated appendix was found at surgery. Histologic examination demonstrated acute phlegmonous appendicitis.

Case 11: Acute Colonic Diverticulitis

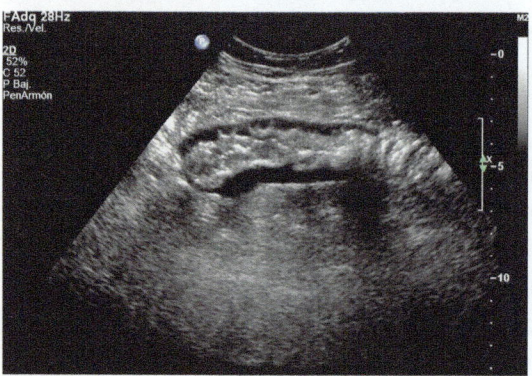

Fig. 1.11.1

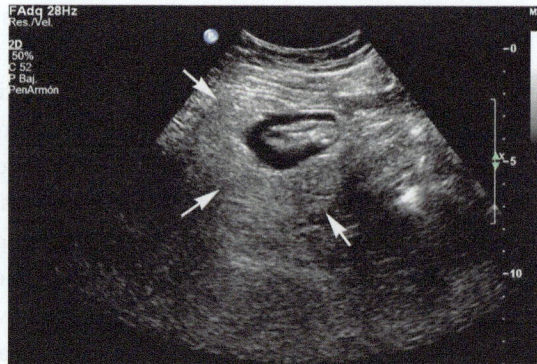

Fig. 1.11.2

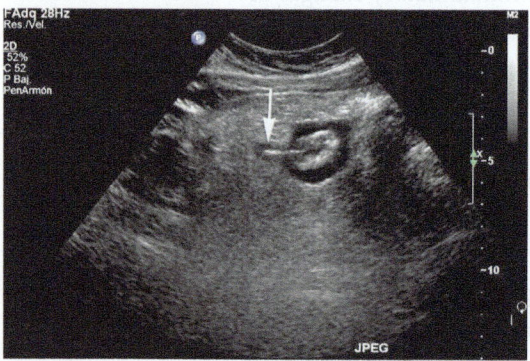

Fig. 1.11.3

Case Presentation

A 43-year-old man was admitted with left lower quadrant pain and fever of one day´s duration. Physical examination revealed tenderness and guarding in the left lower abdomen. Laboratory tests showed leukocytosis with neutrophilia.

Comments

Diverticulitis is a common cause of left-sided abdominal pain in the adult population. It is related to inflammatory changes involving acquired diverticula, most often in the descending and the sigmoid colon. Diverticulitis occurs in up to 25% of patients with known diverticulosis. The classic presentation is localized pain and guarding in the left lower abdomen, fever, and leukocytosis.

A differential diagnosis includes urinary tract infection, renal colic, adnexitis, sigmoid carcinoma, and epiploic appendagitis. Diverticulitis is considered uncomplicated (simple) in the presence of peridiverticulitis or phlegmon and complicated when associated with obstruction, perforation, fistula, or abscess formation. This information can help in deciding whether medical or surgical management is indicated. Many authors recommend radiological evaluation of all patients with clinically suspected diverticulitis, both to confirm the diagnosis and to assess the location and extent of the inflammatory processes.

The normal descending colon and upper part of the sigmoid can be reliably identified on ultrasound in virtually all patients because of its consistent location in the left paracolic gutter. In diverticulosis the muscularis layer is often thickened, and fecalith-containing diverticula can be easily recognized as large, strongly hyperechoic, round-ovoid structures with acoustic shadow located on the outside contour of the colon.

In acute diverticulitis there is usually local thickening (> 3 mm) of the intestinal wall. The inflammatory pericolic fat that surrounds the fecalith is seen as hyperechoic, non-compressible halo, and shows local tenderness induced by graded compression. This inflamed fat must be present to diagnose diverticulitis. In about 20-30% of patients, diverticulitis takes a complicated course with a > 2.5 cm diverticular abscess, fistula or free perforation; these patients are less likely to respond to conservative treatment.

Right-sided diverticulitis is much less common. It involves congenital or true diverticula and occurs more commonly in young women. The differentiation between diverticulitis and perforated colonic neoplasm can be very difficult with any imaging technique. Once the inflammatory changes have solved, a colonoscopy is warranted to exclude carcinoma.

Although CT is the preferred image technique for acute diverticulitis, US might as well be initially performed in patients referred for lower quadrant or pelvis pain, with CT reserved for initial imaging of patients with clinical suspicion of free intraperitoneal perforation or for reassessment of patients with a non-diagnostic US.

Imaging Findings

Longitudinal (Fig. 1.11.1) and transverse (Fig. 1.11.2) sonograms demonstrate hypoechoic mural thickening of the sigmoid colon. Note the surrounding hyperechoic, non-compressible tissue representing the inflammatory fat (*arrows*). Transverse sonogram at a different level (Fig. 1.11.3) reveals an inflamed diverticulum (*arrow*), also with surrounding inflamed fat.

US findings were suggestive of uncomplicated sigmoid diverticulitis.

Case 12: Anal Abscess and Fistula

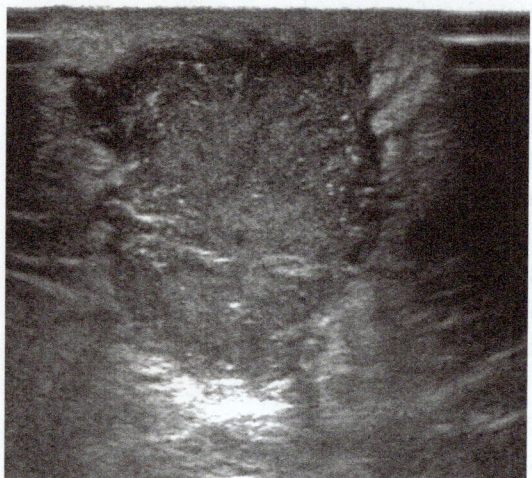

Fig. 1.12.1

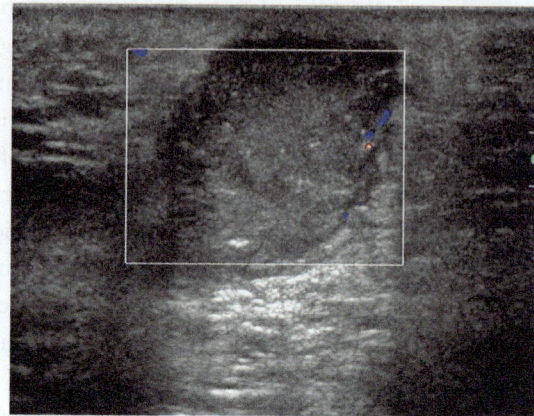

Fig. 1.12.2

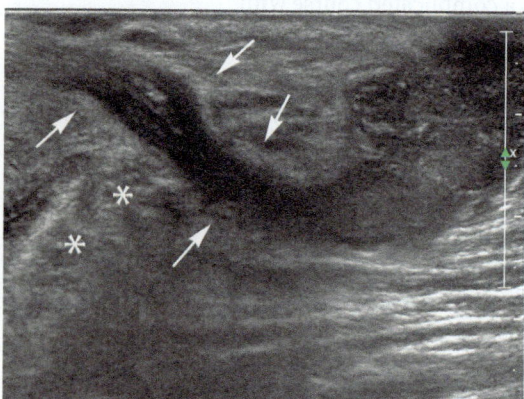

Fig. 1.12.3

Case Presentation   A 52-year-old male consults his doctor for a palpable lump in the perineal region. On palpation, the lesion was hard, firm, and slightly painful. No external signs of inflammation were observed. With the suspicion of a perineal tumor, an ultrasound of the mass was scheduled.

Comments   Masses are rare in the perineum, and it is also unusual to think of ultrasound as a method for their study. However, most lesions in this area are very accessible to the ultrasound examination using the standard technique of soft tissue examination. Ultrasound can usually precisely determine their location and, in many cases, diagnose them. If necessary, ultrasound can be also used to guide diagnostic procedures such as biopsy.

In addition to inflammatory diseases, the perineal region can present traumatic pathology (hematomas) or tumors originated both from mesenchymal tissue of the anus and from perianal glands. In the case presented here, the absence of vascularization in color Doppler makes it unlikely to be a tumor. The demonstration of a fistula on the contrary, shows that it is an abscess secondary to a perianal fistula.

While abscesses are fluid collections, they often have dense content, including fibrin, particles, or sphacelus. This sometimes makes them not to show the typical anechoic appearance on ultrasound, or even appear echogenic, making them difficult to differentiate from a solid tumor. A sign that helps, when present, to differentiate between both is to observe mobility in the echoes from inside the lesion. While in the abscess, it is usual to observe small movements or oscillations, in different kind of lesions, this is not observed.

Perianal abscesses and anal fistulas are the result of the infection of the glands of the anus. In most cases, they are caused by inflammation and infection of the glands of the anal canal, although there are also a smaller number of fistulas secondary to Crohn's disease, radiation, malignancy, and pelvic infections. Perianal fistulas are a communication between the digestive tract and skin and appear in 1/10,000 of the population and in 17–43 % of patients with Crohn's disease.

The imaging techniques indicated for the study of anal fistulas are endoanal ultrasound and MRI, which can identify trajects, extent, type of fistula, and integrity of the sphincters, information that is critical for surgical treatment.

Fistulas can be intersphincteric (crossing the internal sphincter without affecting external), transsphincteric (the fistulous tract crosses both sphincters), and extrasphincteric (an extension appears outside the external sphincter or levator ani). The one presented here correspond to the latter. Surgical management depends on the type of fistula and secondary route, as well as the presence or absence of abscess.

Imaging Findings

Ultrasound (Fig. 1.12.1) showed a well-circumscribed lesion, with irregular contours and fine internal echoes. Doppler ultrasound (Fig. 1.12.2) showed that the lesion showed no vascularity. When the lesion was explored in transverse planes (Fig. 1.12.3), it appeared as continued with a linear structure (*arrows*) that crossed the external rectal sphincter muscle (*asterisks*) to reach the anus. The mass was diagnosed as a perianal abscess with associated anal fistula.

Case 13: Ascites and Peritoneal Metastases of Colon Carcinoma

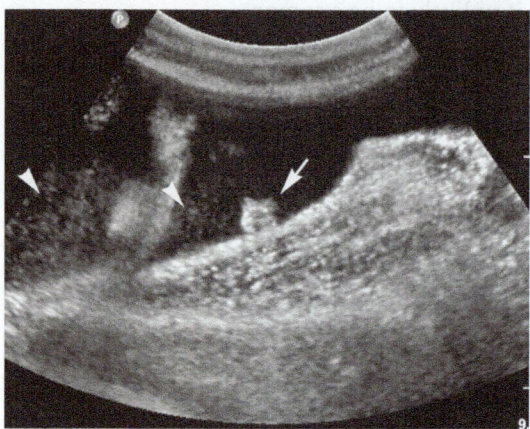

Fig. 1.13.1

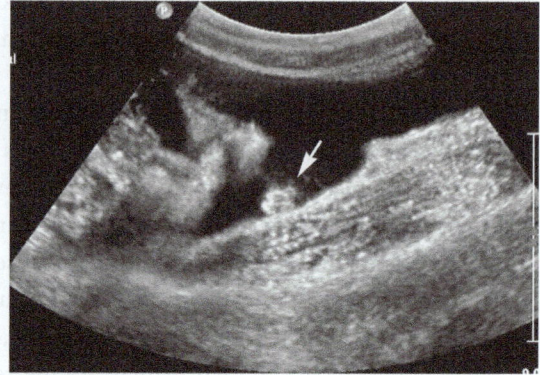

Fig. 1.13.2

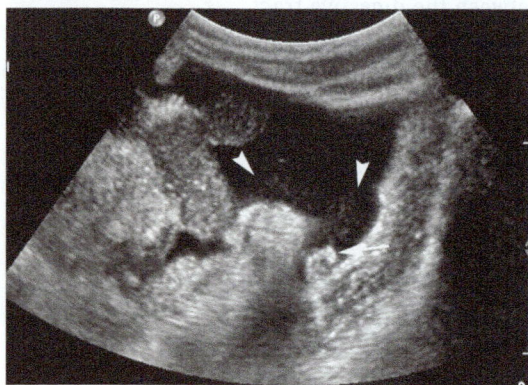

Fig. 1.13.3

Case Presentation   A 42-year-old female consulted for a recent and progressive increase in her abdominal volume. An abdominal ultrasound exam was performed.

Comments   The most usual causes of ascites are cirrhosis, cardiac failure, and neoplasm. They are responsible of 90 % of the ascites. Other rarer causes are hemoperitoneum, biliary ascites, and chylous ascites. Ultrasound is the most sensitive technique for detecting peritoneal fluid. The ascites appears in form of collections with acute angles among intestinal loops or mesenteric folds, or in the peritoneal recesses. Loculation and the presence of echoes in the fluid suggest that the ascites is an exudate. Moreover, ultrasound is the best technique for guiding the paracentesis.

Peritoneal carcinomatosis can appear in neoplasms of any intra- or extra-peritoneal abdominal organ and even in an extra-abdominal organ (lung, breast, melanoma), sometimes years after the diagnosis of the primary tumor. The ovary is the most frequent origin (70 % with peritoneal carcinomatosis at diagnosis), followed by colon and stomach.

The peritoneal fluid moves freely through the right peritoneal spaces and recesses. However, its circulation is more difficult between the left supra- and inframesocolic spaces or between the lesser and greater sacs. It tends to accumulate in the pelvic recesses, the Morrison's pouch, the right iliac fossa, the mesosigmoid, the subphrenic spaces, and the right gutter. Thus, it is in these areas where neoplastic implants are more frequent in peritoneal metastatic dissemination.

The greater omentum is another frequent place for the implants, due to its larger surface. Pelvic deposits can cause ovarian masses (Krukenberg tumor) that can mimic ovarian carcinoma.

Ultrasound is usually the first examination performed on these patients, and it has excellent diagnostic reliability in experienced hands. The findings in peritoneal carcinomatosis are:

- Ascites, usually forming collections and showing fine internal echoes.
- Thickening and/or nodular implants in the peritoneum. The ascites makes them easier to detect. Implants can be detected down to 2 mm.
- Infiltration of the omentum. It appears as nodules or thickening of the omentum. Frequently these nodules are ill-defined and appear as "dirty" areas in omental fat.
- Calcifications. In serous papillary carcinoma implants of the ovary and mucinous carcinomas.

Imaging Findings

Abdominal ultrasound showed high amounts of peritoneal fluid. In the images obtained in the right (Figs. 1.13.1 and 1.13.2) and in the left (Fig. 1.13.3) lower quadrants of the abdomen, a high amount of peritoneal fluid can be observed, with fine echoes in suspension in the most dependent areas (*arrowheads*). These fine echoes suggest the exudative nature of the ascites. Also, some small nodules were observed attached to the surface of the peritoneum (*arrows*) revealing the presence of metastatic implants. A later investigation demonstrated a colonic carcinoma with extensive peritoneal metastatic implants.

Case 14: Abdominal Wall Endometriosis

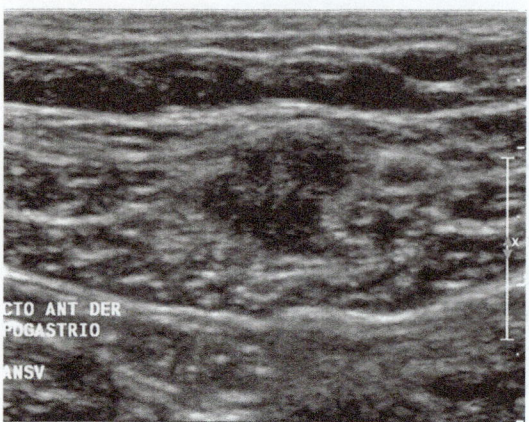

Fig. 1.14.1

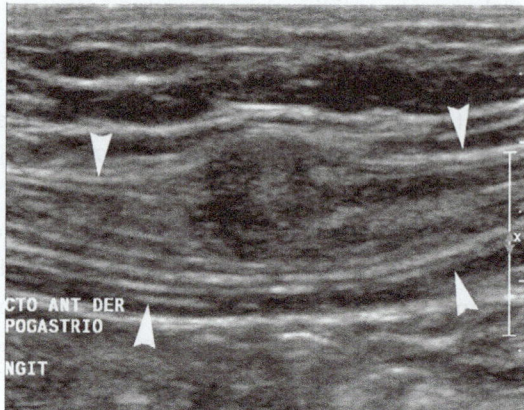

Fig. 1.14.2

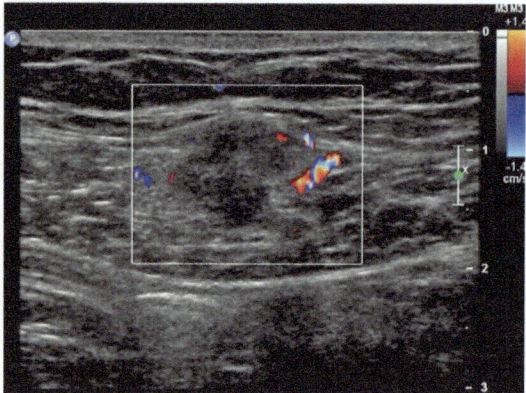

Fig. 1.14.3

Case Presentation   A 37-year-old woman presented with right lower quadrant pain of 2-month duration. Pain was cyclic, increasing during menses. She had a history of a cesarean section with Pfannenstiel's incision 2 years before. Physical examination found no palpable masses. An US exam of the pelvis was performed.

Comments   Endometriosis is classically defined as the presence of functional endometrial glands and stroma outside the uterine cavity. Endometriosis is a common and important clinical problem in women, predominantly affecting those in the reproductive age group. The most common site of involvement is the ovary, but virtually all pelvic organs can be affected and endometriosis can also occur in nongynecologic sites.

Endometriosis can occur within surgical scars, generally from prior gynecologic operations. Abdominal wall endometriosis may occur after pelvic surgery that violates the uterine cavity, such as a cesarean section, allowing endometrial tissue to be transplanted, and this usually occurs in the absence of any history of pelvic endometriosis. Other lesions, such as those of the umbilicus, are thought to occur spontaneously. Endometriosis of the abdominal wall may be difficult to diagnose, both clinically and with diagnostic imaging, and is often confused with other abnormal conditions such as a suture granuloma, incisional hernia, abscess, hematoma, sebaceous cyst, or malignant tumor.

Abdominal wall endometriosis can manifest clinically weeks to years after surgery as a palpable mass or focal cyclic pain associated with menses, both located near or under the surgery scar. However, many patients present with constant pain not associated with the menstrual cycle, and a palpable mass is not always present.

US features of abdominal wall endometriomas are variable. The most common appearance of these masses is solid, hypoechoic lesions with internal vascularity on color or power Doppler examination. An inflammatory reaction to the endometrial implant may be seen as a hyperechoic border. Cystic masses and complex cystic and solid masses have also been described, but these are uncommon. Lesions may be confined to the rectus sheath, located in the subcutaneous fat, or infiltrating both of these layers. Sonographic findings are nonspecific, but hernia, hematoma, and abscess can be excluded in view of the solid appearance of Doppler-detected internal flow.

US-guided fine-needle aspiration (FNA) is a rapid and accurate diagnostic procedure, enabling malignancy to be excluded. If FNA results are inconclusive, as may occur because endometriomas are often fibrous in nature, an additional histological biopsy may be considered. Therapeutic options for abdominal wall endometriosis are pharmacologic therapy or surgical excision.

Imaging Findings

US showed a focal solid nodule into the rectus abdominis muscle. Transverse (Fig. 1.14.1) and longitudinal (Fig. 1.14.2) sonograms of the nodule show a 13 × 7-mm hypoechoic solid mass with irregular margins confined to the rectus abdominis sheath (*arrowheads*). A hyperechoic rim partially circumscribes the nodule. Color Doppler sonogram (Fig. 1.14.3) shows some vessels within the peripheral rim.

US-guided core biopsy was inconclusive, showing fibrosis. The nodule was surgically excised. Histologic examination disclosed endometrial tissue infiltrating muscular tissue.

Case 15: Abdominal Wall Hernia

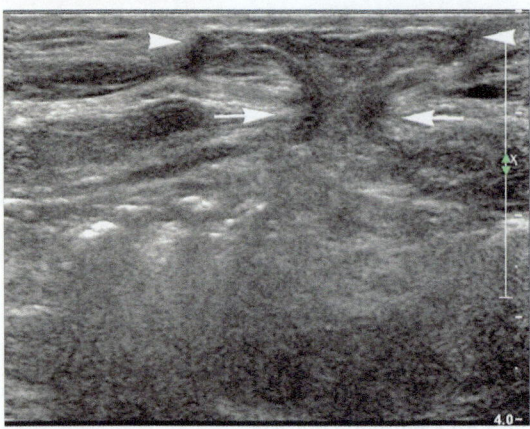

Fig. 1.15.1

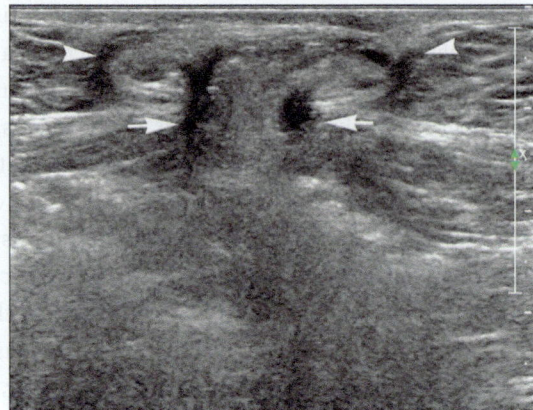

Fig. 1.15.2

A 62-year-old man has noticed a few months ago a lump in his abdomen. At palpation, the lump is superficial, not painful, and is located in the midline of the abdomen, just above the umbilicus. An ultrasound was performed.

Abdominal wall hernias are frequent and include a variety of types: inguinal (femoral inguinal, direct inguinal, or indirect inguinal), umbilical and paraumbilical, epigastric, and spigelian. Also, incisional hernias may occur after surgery through the anterior abdominal wall. Epigastric hernias appear between the xiphoid process and the umbilicus, umbilical hernias occur through a weak umbilical scar, and a paraumbilical hernia occurs through the linea alba just above or, less commonly, just below the umbilicus.

In some cases, clinical diagnosis of hernia may be difficult. Several pathologies like abdominal wall tumors, or hematomas, or enlarged lymph nodes may be difficult to differentiate from a hernia. Sonography is an excellent tool to confidently diagnose a hernia. But even when a hernia is confidently diagnosed, sonography is useful to characterize its contents and determine the extent of reducibility of the hernia contents. This information is critical for surgery.

Abdominal wall hernias are diagnosed on sonography by visualizing abdominal contents moving through an abdominal wall defect. Also they can appear as bulging abdominal contents due to abnormal thinning of the anterior abdominal wall. The contents of the hernia usually appear echogenic because they are fatty tissue or bowel. The presence of peristalsis, fluid, or gas indicates the latter. Fluid may be seen in the hernial sac and surrounding the herniated contents.

Abdominal wall hernias are confined to the anterior abdominal wall. Thus, using a high-frequency linear transducer is optimal for exploration. Any hernia that is found should be compressed with the ultrasound probe to determine if it is reducible or tender. In reducible hernias, the content can be seen moving in and out during dynamic maneuvers. The patient should be scanned in the supine position and also in the upright position. Upright scanning is particularly important for evaluation of a femoral hernia. Sometimes ultrasound can identify hernias that are completely reducible when the patient is lying down but become nonreducible when the patient is standing. The Valsalva maneuver is very useful also.

Longitudinal (Fig. 1.15.1) and transverse (Fig.1.15.2) sonograms show defect (*arrows*) in abdominal wall through which peritoneal fat herniates (*arrowheads*). The lesion showed no changes during Valsalva maneuver. The findings are characteristic of a paraumbilical hernia.

Case 16: Renal Angiomyolipoma

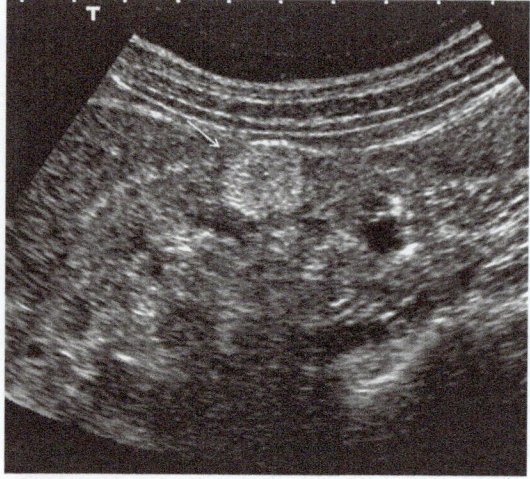

Fig. 1.16.1

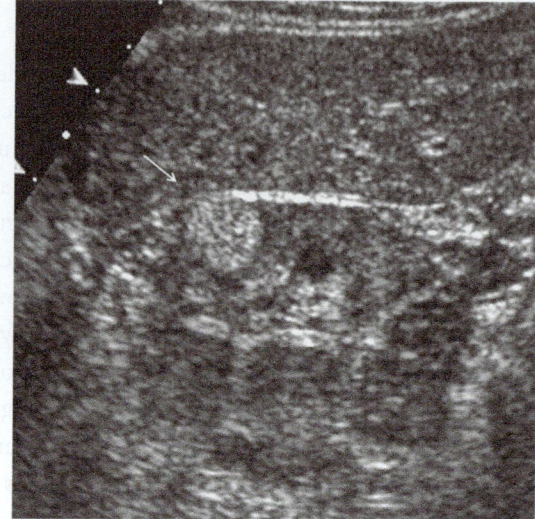

Fig. 1.16.2

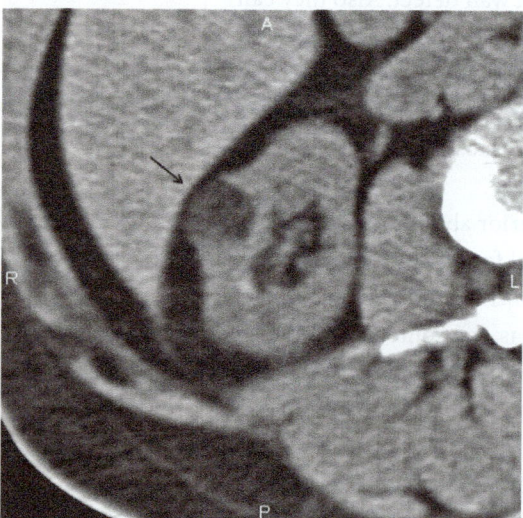

Fig. 1.16.3

A 42-year-old woman with a history of nonspecific abdominal pain was referred to the ultrasound (US) department to undergo an abdominal US study.

Angiomyolipomas (AMLs) are benign hamartomatous renal lesions. They contain blood vessels, smooth muscle, and fatty tissue in varying proportions. They are usually found incidentally at US examinations performed for unrelated reasons (more frequently in middle-age women) and are usually small and asymptomatic. However, AMLs can also be seen in patients with tuberous sclerosis. In these patients, AMLs are usually multiple and bilateral and can reach a large size and be symptomatic (pain, gross hematuria, anemia). The US features are characteristic but nonspecific. AMLs are usually well defined, homogeneous, and hyperechoic relative to renal parenchyma and show no calcifications. The degree of echogenicity of AMLs depends on the relative proportion of its components, with a higher percentage of fatty portion in more echogenic lesions. AMLs can also present as heterogeneous, but predominantly echogenic masses, but this feature is more common in large AMLs and generally related to the presence of intratumoral hemorrhage. There is an increased risk of bleeding in angiomyolipomas >4 cm, thus nephron-sparing surgery or even percutaneous embolization of the tumor should be considered in these tumors.

   The detection of a homogeneous echogenic renal lesion cannot rule out other tumors such as small renal cell carcinomas (RCC) may present with similar US appearance. Some features can help in the differentiation since the presence of posterior acoustic shadowing has been described in some angiomyolipomas. The presence of fat and nonfat interfaces and the relatively large acoustic impedance differences at these interfaces are believed to be responsible for the shadowing. On the contrary, the presence of a hypoechoic rim has been described in some RCCs, but not in AML. The presence of intratumoral cysts is another typical feature of RCCs. However, these findings are detected in few cases.

   There is controversy about the imaging management of small (<1.5 cm) hyperechoic homogeneous cortical lesions. It is advisable to perform a CT or MR imaging examination to confirm the presence of fat that allows the diagnosis of angiomyolipoma. However, as the US detection of small lesions with typical features of angiomyolipomas is very common, some authors consider the possibility of performing US monitoring instead of further CT or MR imaging examinations. In these cases, US monitoring is recommended every 6 months during at least 2 years to rule out the small possibility of the lesion being an echogenic RCC. On the contrary, if the lesion is higher than 1.5 cm, further investigation using CT or MR to rule out RCC is mandatory.

Longitudinal (Fig. 1.16.1) and transverse (Fig. 1.16.2) In the US scan of the right kidney a cortical homogeneous hyperechoic lesion of 17 mm was detected within the lower pole of the kidney cortex (*arrow*). Corresponding CT (Fig. 1.16.3) confirmed the presence of a kidney lesion with containing predominantly fat (*arrow*) compatible with angiomyolipoma.

Case 17: Renal Cortical Necrosis

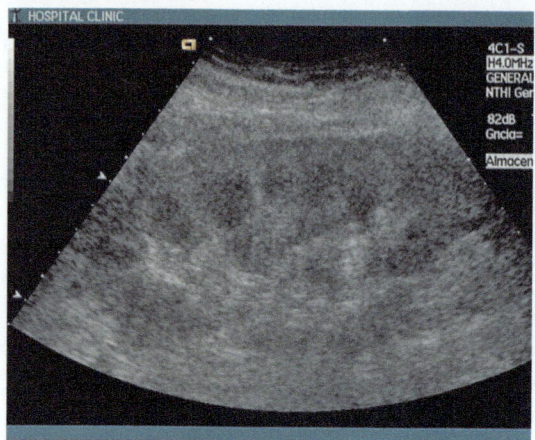

Fig. 1.17.1

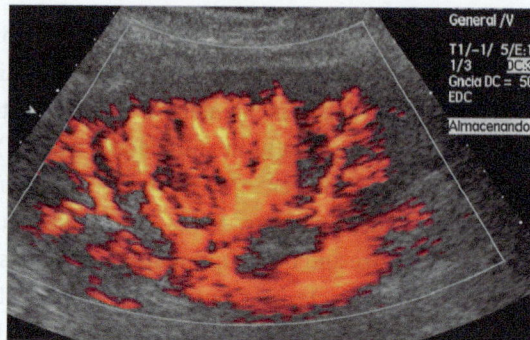

Fig. 1.17.2

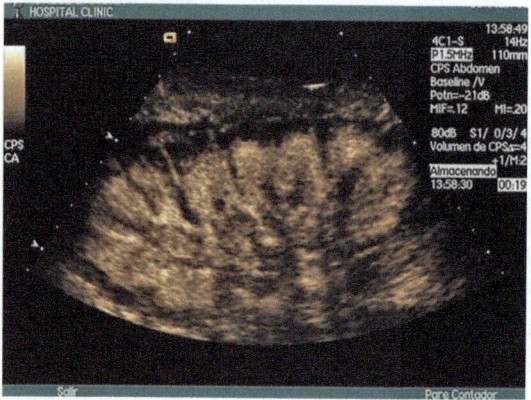

Fig. 1.17.3

A 38-year-old man who received his second kidney transplantation underwent Doppler ultrasound 48 h after kidney transplantation due to oligoanuria.

Ultrasound is the main imaging technique used in the diagnosis and management of complications arising in renal transplants. It allows a global assessment of the renal transplant arterial and venous system, renal parenchyma, urinary excretory tract, and peritransplant region, and it is very useful to differentiate among vascular, urological, and parenchymal complications. The vascular group of complications includes acute renal vein or artery thrombosis, renal acute cortical necrosis (ACN), renal arterial infarction, and renal artery stenosis. ACN is a rare cause of acute renal failure characterized by ischemic necrosis of the renal cortex with sparing of the renal medulla. In some cases, a subcapsular rim of cortex is also spared, and this fact can be explained due to the presence of collateral circulation to the subcapsular cortex from capsular vessels. Diagnosis of ACN can be suggested on gray-scale US when a hypoechoic cortical tissue adjacent to the renal capsule is detected. However, this finding is not always present, and in some cases, there is also loss of corticomedullary differentiation, making the diagnosis more difficult. Color Doppler US is usually the imaging technique able to provide an accurate diagnosis demonstrating the absence of cortical flow with preservation of the medullary vascularization. In doubtful cases, the diagnosis can be confirmed after the administration of a contrast agent using CT, MR imaging, or contrast-enhanced US (CEUS). One of the advantages of CEUS is that, unlike CT or MR imaging, it can be performed in patients with impaired renal function. CEUS increases the diagnostic confidence of color Doppler US demonstrating medullary enhancement and lack of cortical rim enhancement that correlates to the histologic zone of cortical necrosis. The rim-like peripheral location of the ischemic area allows the differentiation of ACN from other renal transplant vascular complications. These include hypoperfused cortical areas that manifest as wedge-shaped areas of decreased parenchymal enhancement usually secondary to arterial complications related to surgery and segmentary avascular areas usually in the upper or lower pole when a polar artery has been "sacrificed" during surgery.

Gray-scale US (Fig. 1.17.1) showed a very tiny hypoechoic rim in the peripheral part of the cortex. There was no dilation of the urinary excretory tract or perinephric fluid collections. Power Doppler US (Fig. 1.17.2) showed absence of flow in this peripheral part of the cortex. Flow was detected in the interlobar arteries as well as in the main renal artery and vein. The absence of peripheral cortical flow was confirmed using contrast-enhanced US (Fig. 1.17.3). After 48 h without improvement of the renal function, a transplantectomy was indicated, and cortical necrosis was confirmed histologically.

Case 18: Nephrocalcinosis

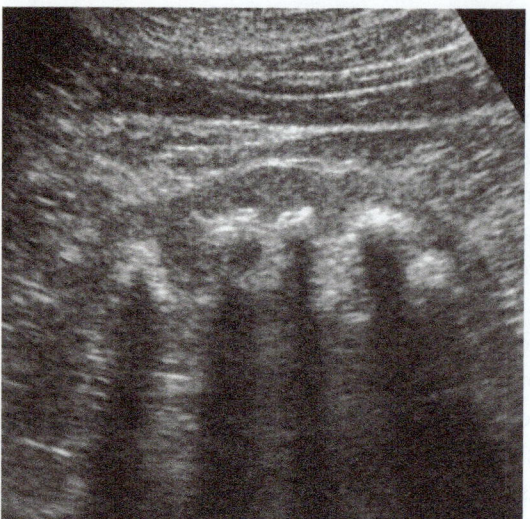

Fig. 1.18.1

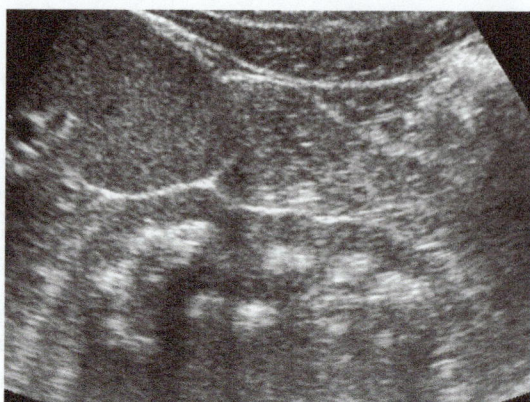

Fig. 1.18.2

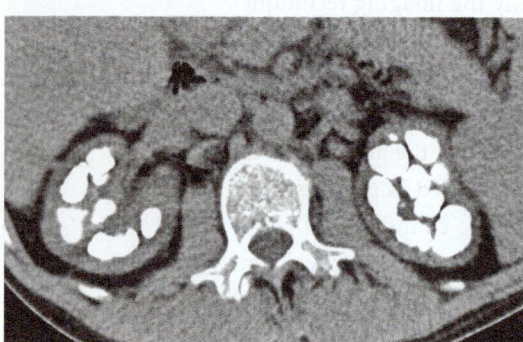

Fig. 1.18.3

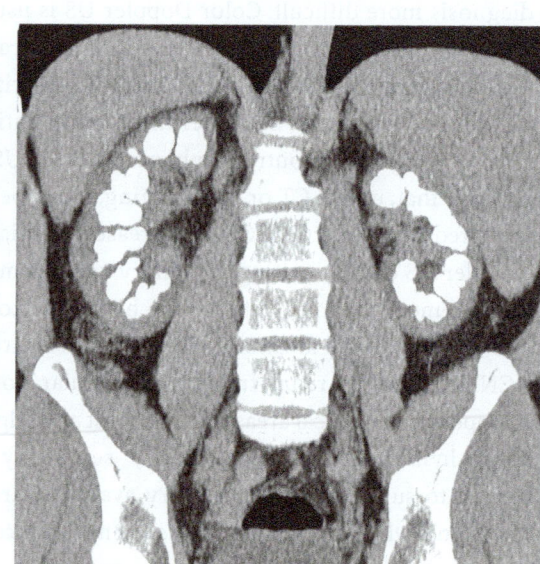

Fig. 1.18.4

Case Presentation

A 40-year-old male presented with a several-month history of nonspecific symptoms including asthenia, anorexia, nausea, and vomiting. Lab tests showed hypercalcemia, elevated levels of parathyrine (PTH), and hypercalciuria. Glomerular filtration rate was 40 ml/min.

Nephrocalcinosis is a pathologic deposition of calcium salts in the renal parenchyma in contradistinction to nephrolitiasis, where the deposit is in the renal collecting system. Nephrocalcinosis is classified according to the anatomical area involved. The most common form is medullary nephrocalcinosis (95 %) that involves the renal pyramids, specifically the distal convoluted tubules. Cortical nephrocalcinosis (5 %) refers to calcium deposition in the renal cortex.

Medullary nephrocalcinosis may be attributable to a variety of causes and commonly results from hypercalcemic states. The most common cause in adults is hyperparathyroidism followed by distal renal tubular acidosis (type 1) and medullary sponge kidney. This condition is relatively common in premature infants.

At ultrasonography (US), in the very early stages of calcium deposition, medullary nephrocalcinosis causes increased echogenicity and asymmetric involvement at the periphery of the medullary pyramid; however, nephrocalcinosis may eventually progress and involve most of the pyramids in both kidneys. Moreover, uniform deposition of calcium salts in medullary nephrocalcinosis is most commonly seen in hyperparathyroidism or distal renal tubular acidosis, whereas medullary sponge kidney causes asymmetric medullary nephrocalcinosis with clumped calcifications within the renal papillae.

In nephrocalcinosis, acoustic shadowing is rarely seen; nevertheless, it may be seen only in rare cases of extreme involvement of the pyramids or in association with calculi in the adjacent calices. In fact, most of the conditions that cause nephrocalcinosis can also result in nephrolithiasis.

For the detection and monitoring of nephrocalcinosis, ultrasonography is the optimal imaging method. An US and CT comparison of induced nephrocalcinosis in a rabbit model demonstrated a higher sensitivity for US (96 % vs. 64 %) but a better specificity for CT (96 % vs. 85 %). Renal ultrasonography is still the first diagnostic imaging modality in suspected nephrocalcinosis.

Plain film radiography of the abdomen is less helpful, as only gross calcifications can be diagnosed.

Comments

Gray-scale US images of both kidneys (Figs. 1.18.1 and 1.18.2) show diffuse increased echogenicity of the renal medulla (pyramids are normally hypoechoic in relation to the cortex) with acoustic shadowing. The renal cortex is thinned with normal echogenicity. In this instance, it may be difficult to determine how much of the increased echogenicity is related to hyperechogenicity of the pyramids and how much is due to the presence of a stone in the adjacent calyx. There is no evidence of hydronephrosis. This appearance is suggestive of late medullary nephrocalcinosis.

Axial (Fig. 1.18.3) and coronal unenhanced CT images (Fig. 1.18.4) show multiple, uniform, and symmetric deposition of calcium involving the renal pyramids of both kidneys.

Imaging Findings

Case 19: Ureteral Lithiasis

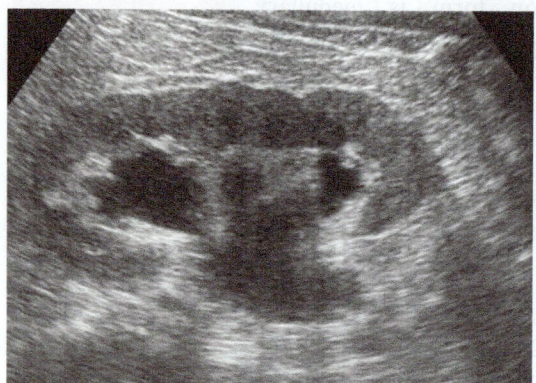

Fig. 1.19.1

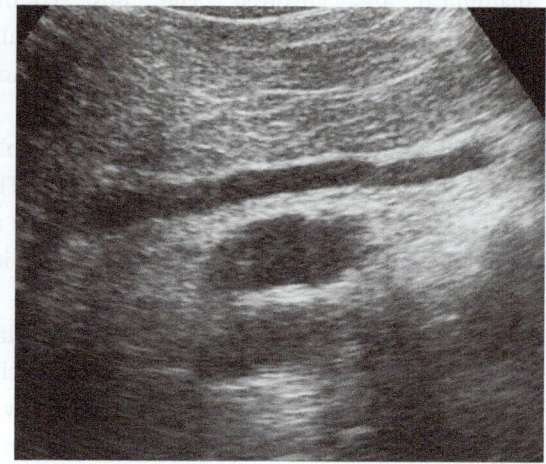

Fig. 1.19.2

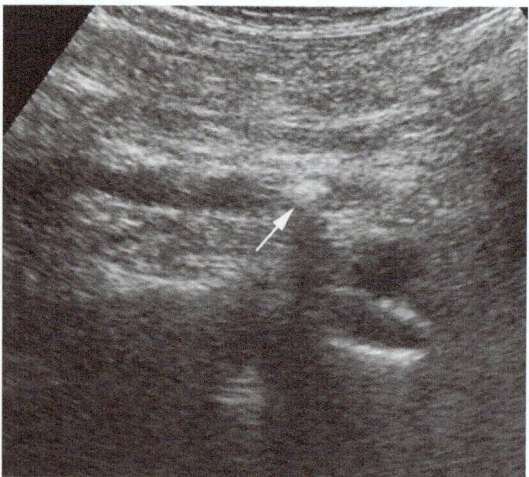

Fig. 1.19.3

A 44-year-old man presented to the emergency department with acute and severe left flank pain.

Case Presentation

Flank pain secondary to urolithiasis is a frequent problem in patients presenting to emergency departments. Acute ureteral obstruction often manifests as renal colic, with severe pain that is often spasmodic; this pain peaks and then decreases before increasing again. The pain may radiate to the groin or testicle with or without nausea, vomiting, dysuria, or hematuria. It needs quick diagnosis and prompt treatment. Radiologic imaging has a primary role in the work-up of these patients. US is recommended as the first-line modality to diagnose urinary tract obstruction from calculi and to rule out other abdominal emergencies. In addition, the lack of ionizing radiation makes US the method of choice for evaluating pediatric and pregnant patients. However, this technique has limited value in demonstrating pathological conditions of the ureter.

Comments

The US diagnosis of urinary obstruction from calculi is achieved by visualizing the ureteral calculi with proximal dilatation of the ureter and pelvicalyceal system. A ureteral calculus is identified as an intraluminal echogenic focus with acoustic shadowing within the distal portion of a dilated ureter.

Sensitivity of US in diagnosing ureteric stones in the setting of acute flank pain has been reported to be 37–64 %. This is directly related to the anatomic nature of the examination, which relies mainly on the presence of hydronephrosis to make the diagnosis. When urinary tract calculi cause obstruction, US is very effective in demonstrating hydronephrosis (these rates rise to 74–95 %). Moreover, as the grade of hydronephrosis rises, the detection rate of ureteral stones with US also rises. Nevertheless, renal sinus cysts may mimic hydronephrosis. Furthermore, early in the course of ureteral obstruction (up to 36 h after onset), in partial obstructions, or in insufficiently hydrated patients, no dilatation (or minimal dilatation) of the collecting system is observed. However, there are many causes of nonobstructive pyelocaliectasis, including those due to reflux, which may be mistaken for dilatation of the collecting system secondary to obstruction. It has been suggested that the determination of intrarenal resistive index (RI) with duplex Doppler US helps distinguish between obstructive and nonobstructive causes of dilatation of the collecting system. Several authors have suggested that RI > 0.7 is indicative of obstruction. However, determination of the RI has not been adopted into widespread clinical use for acute obstruction because partial obstruction may not result in elevated RI and mainly because most pathologic processes decrease renal perfusion and thus increase the RI. In addition, ureteral stones located in the middle third or in distal ureter (between the iliac crossing and the ureterovesical junction) are the most difficult to visualize by US because of intestinal overlying.

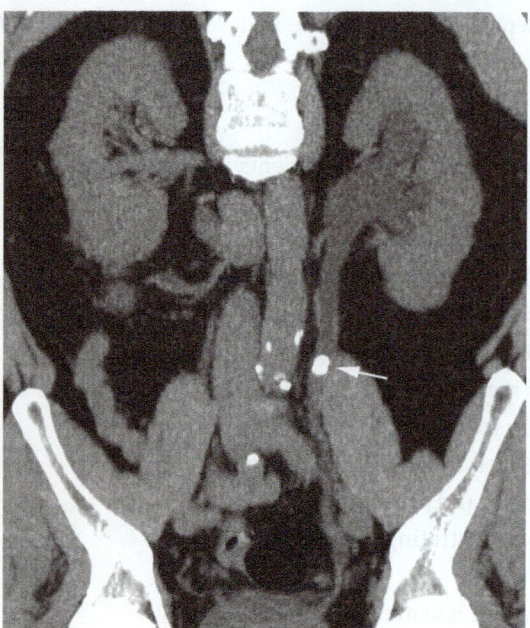

Fig. 1.19.4

The assessment of ureteral jet is another US parameter that is helpful in the evaluation of urinary obstruction. The ability to detect jets is improved by color Doppler and with a well-hydrated patient. In the absence of obstruction, intermittent and bilateral ureteral jets can be observed. Obstruction manifests as either complete absence of ureteral jet on the affected side or as continuous low-level flow on the affected side.

Major disadvantages of US are the inability to accurately measure the size of the stones, the poor detection of calculi, and the fact that this technique requires an experienced operator. Nonenhanced CT has a higher sensitivity for the detection of ureteral calculi (96 %) compared with US and provides additional knowledge of calculus size and location that can be helpful in making prospective patient care decisions. However, one disadvantage of non-enhanced CT is the use of ionizing radiation.

Imaging Findings

Longitudinal gray-scale US image of the left kidney (Fig. 1.19.1) and upper and middle third of the left ureter (Fig. 1.19.2) shows moderate hydronephrosis. Longitudinal gray-scale US of the middle third of the left ureter (Fig. 1.19.3) shows an echogenic focus with acoustic shadowing (8 mm), located before the iliac bifurcation, and lying in a dilated proximal ureter (*arrow*). Axial nonenhanced CT MIP curved reconstruction (Fig. 1.19.4) also depicts well the 8-mm obstructing calculus with adjacent periureteral stranding (*arrow*).

Case 20: Ureterocele

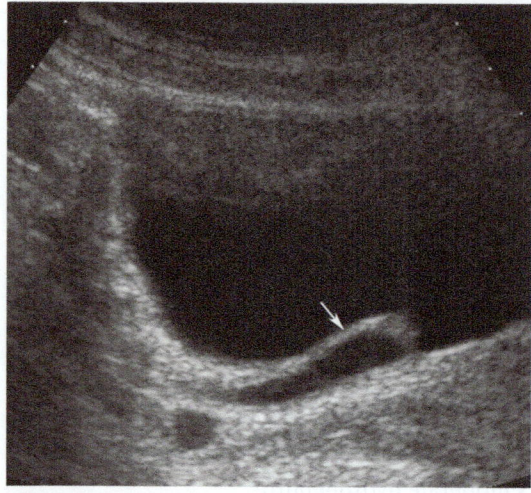

Fig. 1.20.1

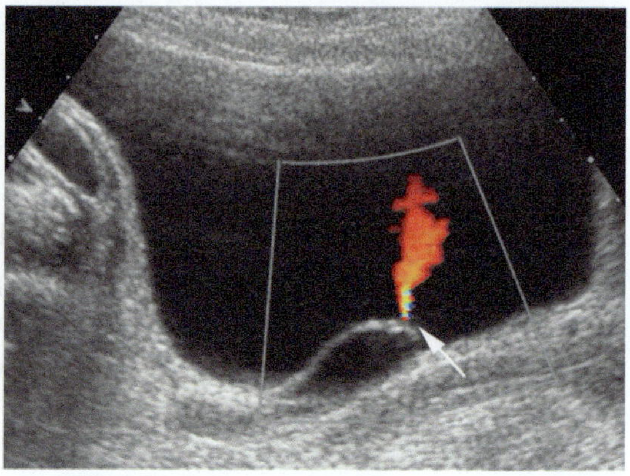

Fig. 1.20.2

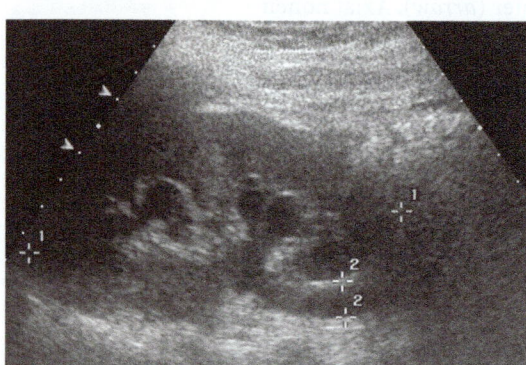

Fig. 1.20.3

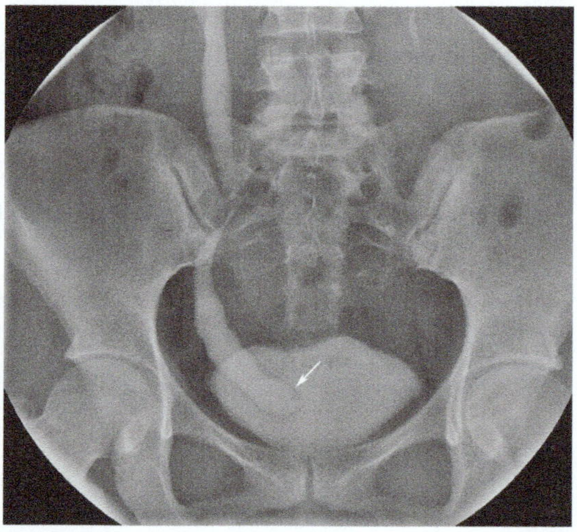

Fig. 1.20.4

Case Presentation   A 27-year-old female presented with recurrent urinary tract infection and right flank pain.

Comments   Ureterocele is a congenital cystic dilatation of the intravesical segment of the ureter. The congenital defect is the obstruction of the meatus, and the ureterocele is a response to this obstruction. Ureterocele occurs in one in every 4,000 children with a 4–7:1 female to male ratio. Approximately 10 % of ureteroceles are bilateral. Patients may be asymptomatic, but in adult population, ureteroceles are usually diagnosed during an investigation for dysuria, urinary sepsis, voiding difficulty, flank colics, or hematuria.

A simplified classification subdivides ureteroceles based on:
1. The number of ureters that drain the ipsilateral kidney
2. The location and extent of the ureterocele
3. Additional anatomic distortions resulting from ureterocele eversion, pro-lapse, or secondary incompetence or obstruction of the other ureteral orifice(s) or the bladder neck

In adults, ureteroceles commonly occur in normal ureteric (intravesical) loca-tions and are called simple or orthotopic as opposed to heterotopic uretero-celes that generally accompany an ectopic ureteric orifice or an ectopic-du-plex renal system, seen in pediatric population. While ureteroceles are more common in women, stones in ureteroceles tend to be more common in men. Stones in ureteroceles are believed to be due to associated ureteral atony with urinary stasis that may contribute to urolithiasis.

The diagnostic work-up relies on the use of an US, a cystourethrogram, and a renal isotope scan.

Ultrasound of the urinary tract is the first imaging modality to be per-formed. The classic appearance at US of ureterocele is a sonolucent round image that sits on the bladder base and occupies a portion of the bladder. An associated ureteral jet helps confirm diagnosis.

Ultrasound also provides valuable information on the presence of unilateral or bilateral renal duplicity and on the dilatation of the collecting systems. Cortical cysts and renal tissue hyperechogenicity may suggest renal dysplasia.

A voiding cystourethrogram is an important part of an ureterocele evalua-tion. The ureterocele is seen in the first films as a negative shadow in the blad-der, with a surrounding contrast rim. This technique may also show vesicoureteral reflux and is useful to evaluate the degree of detrusor backing of the ureterocele. Eversion of the inner wall of the ureterocele upward into its ureter causes an appearance indistinguishable from paraureteral bladder diverticulum. During voiding, the ureterocele may also be seen prolapsing through the urethra and obstructing urinary flow.

A 99 m-technetium dimercaptosuccinic acid (DMSA) renal scan may quan-tify the amount of functioning renal tissue.

Differential diagnosis should be made with pseudoureterocele (secondary to obstructive lesions), such as bladder tumors.

Imaging Findings

Longitudinal gray-scale US image of the bladder (Fig. 1.20.1) shows an an-echoic cystic structure at the right ureteral orifice and right dilated distal ure-ter (*arrow*). Color Doppler imaging (Fig. 1.20.2) shows a ureteral jet arising from fluid-filled intraluminal wall bladder lesion (*arrow*), a finding that confirms ureterocele. Longitudinal gray-scale US image of the right kidney (Fig. 1.20.3) demonstrates mild dilatation of ureteropelvicaliceal system.

Intravenous pyelography demonstrated mild dilatation of ureteropelvical-iceal system and, on late excretory urogram (Fig. 1.20.4), dilatation of the dis-tal ureter, surrounded by a thin lucent line ("cobra sign") (*arrow*), which is seen in patients with orthotopic ureterocele.

Case 21: Bladder Neoplasm

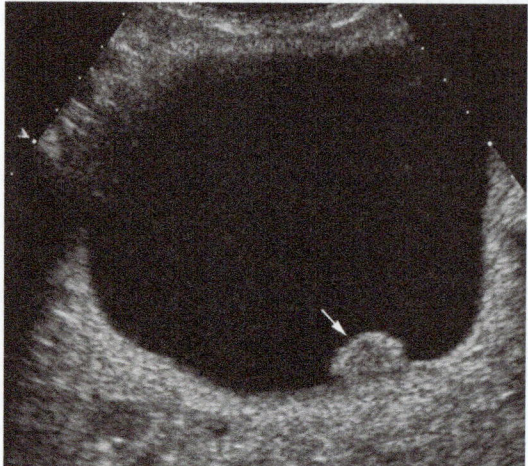

Fig. 1.21.1

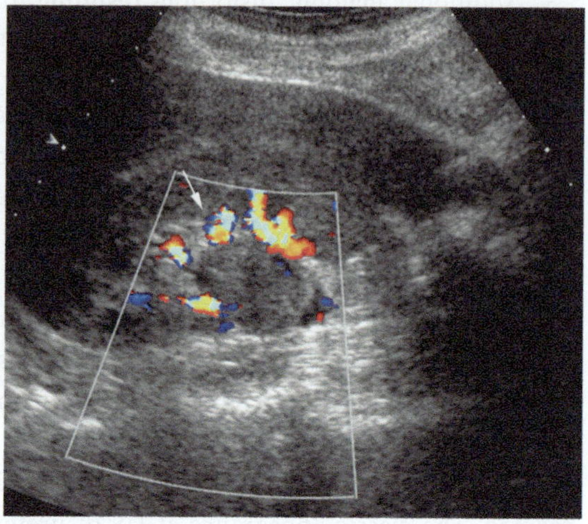

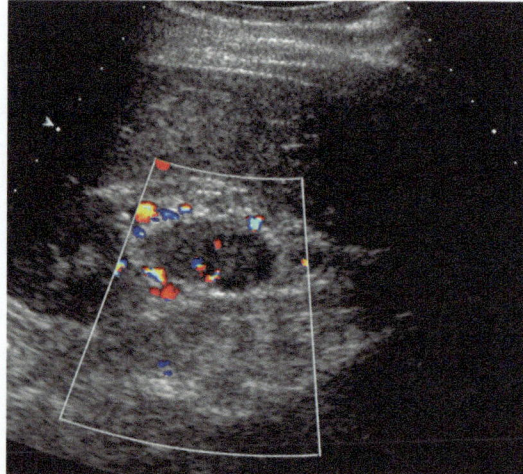

Fig. 1.21.3

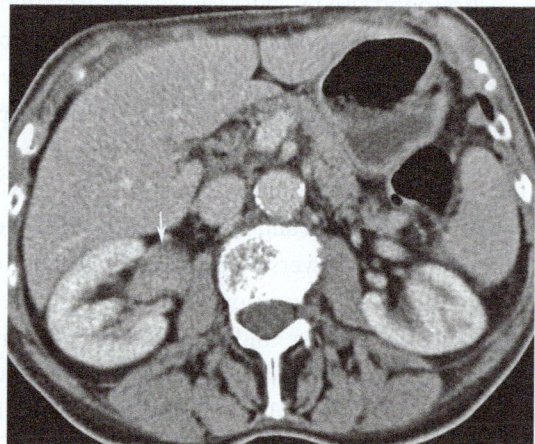

Fig. 1.21.2

Fig. 1.21.4

Case Presentation

An 80-year-old smoker male presented with a 7-month history of macroscopic hematuria.

Comments

Tumors of the bladder are among the most common neoplasm of the urinary tract and the fourth most common malignancy. The most frequent subtype is the urothelial cell carcinoma (95 % of cases). Bladder cancer generally occurs in older patients (usually >65 years) and is more common in men with a male-to-female ratio of 3–4:1. The most common presenting symptom is gross hematuria, although microscopic hematuria may be detected through urinalysis. Cigarette smoking is the main risk factor for bladder cancer. Smokers have four times more likely to develop bladder cancer. Other risk factors are a variety of occupational and environmental chemicals including beta-naphthylamines. Chronic bladder infection, bladder stones, and drugs such as cyclophosphamide are also related to bladder cancer.

Seventy percent of patients have superficial low-grade papillary tumors, which tend to be multifocal and often recur after surgery but have a relatively good prognosis. The remaining 30 % of high-grade invasive tumors have a much poorer prognosis.

Although it is a disease of the entire transitional epithelium, most urothelial tumors (80 %) are located at the bladder in the initial diagnosis. An important fact is that urothelial carcinoma tends to be multicentric with synchronous and metachronous bladder and upper tract tumors. Multicentric bladder tumors occur in up to 30–40 % of cases. Upper tract tumors occur in 2.5–4.5 % of bladder tumor cases and most frequently are seen when multiple bladder lesions are present.

Ultrasonography (US) is the first examination to be performed in the clinical evaluation of hematuria for detection of bladder tumors because it is simple and safe for the patient. On US, bladder appears as an intraluminal smooth or papillary hypoechoic soft tissue mass or as focal mural thickening. Clots and hydronephrosis may also be associated. Doppler flow should be employed to establish flow within the mass and for differentiation from clots. US examination is particularly useful for neoplasm arising from diverticula, sometimes difficult to evaluate by cystoscopy.

However, its success in detection depends on the size, morphology, and location of the neoplasm and on the experience of the radiologist. Bladder tumors <0.5 cm in size and tumors located in the bladder neck, or in dome areas, are difficult to detect. Flat, plaque-like tumors can also be difficult to detect, even when large. Moreover, columnar hypertrophy of the bladder in association with benign prostatic hypertrophy can hide or mimic urothelial polypoid lesions, and acoustic shadowing of calcifications can mask bladder wall behind a lesion.

On the other hand, diagnostic accuracy may approach 95%for tumors >0.5 cm located on the posterior or lateral walls of the bladder.

Optimum bladder filling is of primary importance. Although insufficient filling prevents lesion identification, excessive bladder distention results in bladder wall thinning and reduces the conspicuity of the wall layers. Overdistension of the urinary bladder also increases patient discomfort, resulting in a difficult examination, and an increase in artifacts.

It is important to know that the extent of invasion of the bladder wall and extravesical extension cannot be assessed accurately by US which does not

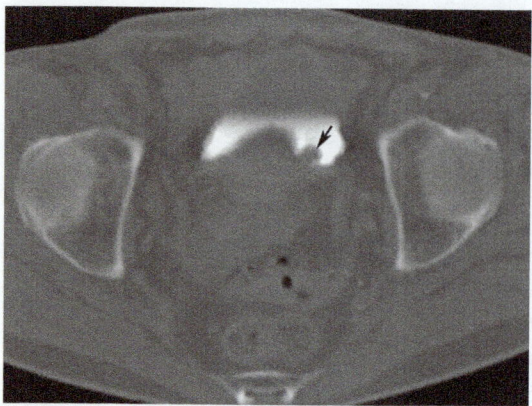

Fig. 1.21.5

allow evaluation of the entire genitourinary tract. When US identifies a bladder cancer, computed tomography is usually employed to study the whole urinary tract, detect lymphadenopathy and liver lesions.

Cystoscopy and biopsy remain the standard of reference for bladder evaluation, but imaging is important for accurate staging and treatment planning.

Imaging Findings

Gray-scale US image of the bladder (Fig. 1.21.1) shows a papillary hypoechoic soft tissue lesion of 1.5 cm within the base of the bladder (*arrow*).

Color Doppler US image of the right kidney (Fig. 1.21.2) demonstrates a well-defined mass (3 cm) located at the renal pelvis that is hypoechoic relative to the renal sinus fat (*arrow*). The mass shows tumoral vascularity on power Doppler sonography (Fig. 1.21.3), thus excluding blood clot. This lesion is suggestive of a synchronous tumor.

Contrast-enhanced CT (Figs. 1.21.4 and 1.21.5) demonstrated the same findings than US (*arrows*). Additionally, the whole urinary tract was explored, and no further lesions were found.

Further Reading

Abbott RM, Levy AD, Aguilera NS, Gorospe L, Thompson WM (2004) From the archives of the AFIP: primary vascular neoplasms of the spleen: radiologic-pathologic correlation. Radiographics 24:1137–1163

Albrecht T, Hohmann J, Oldenburg A, Skrok J, Wolf KJ (2004) Detection and characterization of liver metastases. Eur Radiol 14(Suppl 8):P25–P33

Bennett GL, Balthazar EJ (2003) Ultrasound and CT evaluation of emergent gallbladder pathology. Radiol Clin North Am 41:1203–1216

Bennett GL, Slywotzky CM, Cantera M (2010) Unusual manifestations and complications of endometriosis – spectrum of imaging findings: pictorial review. Am J Roentgenol 194(6 Suppl):WS34–WS46

Benter T, Klühs L, Teichgräber U (2011) Sonography of the spleen. J Ultrasound Med 30:1281–1293

Berrocal T, Lopez-Pereira P, Arjonilla A et al (2002) Anomalies of the distal ureter, bladder, and urethra in children: embryologic, radiologic and pathologic features. Radiographics 22:1139–1164

Berton F, Gola G, Wilson SR (2007) Sonography of benign conditions of the anal canal: an update. AJR Am J Roentgenol 189:765–773

Bortoff GA, Chen MY, Ott DJ, Wolfman NT, Routh WD (2000) Gallbladder stones: imaging and intervention. Radiographics 20:751–766

Boscak AR, Al-Hawary M (2006) Best cases from the AFIP: adenomyomatosis of the gallbladder. Radiographics 26:941–946

Chan L, Shin LK, Pai RK (2011) Pathologic continuum of acute appendicitis: sonographic findings and clinical management implications. Ultrasound Q 27:71–79

Daneman A, Navarro OM, Somers GR (2010) Renal pyramids: focused sonography of normal and pathologic processes. Radiographics 30:1287–1307

Dyer RB, Chean MYM, Zagoria RJ (1998) Abnormal calcifications in the urinary tract. Radiographics 18:1405–1424

Farrelly C, Delaney H, McDermott R, Malone D (2008) Do all non-calcified echogenic renal lesions found on ultrasound need further evaluation with CT? Abdom Imaging 33:44–47

Francois M, Tostirint I, Mercadal L et al (2000) MR imaging features of acute bilateral renal cortical necrosis. Am J Kidney Dis 35:745–748

Hanbidge AE, Lynch D, Wilson SR (2003) US of the peritoneum. Radiographics 23:663–684

Hensen JH, Van Breda AC, Puylaert JB (2006) Abdominal wall endometriosis: clinical presentation and imaging features with emphasis on sonography. AJR Am J Roentgenol 186:616–620

Jamadar DA, Jacobson JA, Morag Y et al (2006) Sonography of inguinal region hernias. AJR Am J Roentgenol 187:185–190

Jamadar DA, Jacobson JA, Morag Y, Girish G, Dong Q, Al-Hawary M, Franz MG (2007) Characteristic locations of inguinal region and anterior abdominal wall hernias: sonographic appearances and identification of clinical pitfalls. AJR Am J Roentgenol 188:1356–1364

Jeong JY, Kim SH, Sim JS et al (2002) MR findings of renal cortical necrosis. J Comput Assist Tomogr 26:232–236

Karcaaltincaba M, Akhan O (2007) Imaging of hepatic steatosis and fatty sparing. Eur J Radiol 61:33–43

Kessler N, Cyteval C, Gallix B et al (2004) Appendicitis: evaluation of sensitivity, specificity, and predictive values of US, Doppler US, and laboratory findings. Radiology 230:472–478

Kim KW, Kim MJ, Lee SS, Kim HJ, Shin YM, Kim PN, Lee MG (2008) Sparing of fatty infiltration around focal hepatic lesions in patients with hepatic steatosis: sonographic appearance with CT and MRI correlation. AJR Am J Roentgenol 190:1018–1027

Kinoshita LL, Yee J, Nash SR (2000) Littoral cell angioma of the spleen: imaging features. AJR Am J Roentgenol 174:467–469

Lee EK, Dickstein RJ, Kamat AM (2011) Imaging of urothelial cancers: what the urologist needs to know. AJR Am J Roentgenol 196:1249–1254

Levy AD, Murakata LA, Rohrmann CA Jr (2001) Gallbladder carcinoma: radiologic-pathologic correlation. Radiographics 21:295–314

Lucey BC, Stuhlfaut JW, Soto JA (2005) Mesenteric lymph nodes seen at imaging: causes and significance. Radiographics 25:351–365

Madeb R, Shapiro I, Rothschild E et al (2000) Evaluation of ureterocele with Doppler sonography. J Clin Ultrasound 28:425–429

Merlini E, Lelli Chiesa P (2004) Obstructive ureterocele – an ongoing challenge. World J Urol 22:107–114

O'Connor OJ, Maher NM (2011) Imaging of cholecystitis. Am J Roentgenol 196:W367–W374

Patlas M, Farkas A, Fisher D et al (2001) Ultrasound vs CT for the detection of ureteric stones in patients with renal colic. Br J Radiol 74:901–904

Pedrosa I, Saíz A, Arrazola J, Ferreirós J, Pedrosa CS (2000) Hydatid disease: radiologic and pathologic features and complications. Radiographics 20(3):795–817

Puylaert JB (2003) Ultrasonography of the acute abdomen: gastrointestinal conditions. Radiol Clin North Am 41:1227–1242

Ripollés T, Agramunt M, Martínez MJ et al (2003) The role of ultrasound in the diagnosis, management and evolutive prognosis of acute left-sided colonic diverticulitis: a review of 208 patients. Eur Radiol 13:2587–2595

Rooholamini SA, Tehrani NS, Razavi MK (1994) Imaging of gallbladder carcinoma. Radiographics 14:291–306

Rybkin AV, Thoeni RF (2007) Current concepts in imaging of appendicitis. Radiol Clin North Am 45:411–422

Sefzzek RJ, Beckman I, Lupentin AR, Dash N (1984) Sonography of acute cortical necrosis. AJR Am J Roentgenol 142:553–554

Sheafor DH, Hertzberg BS, Freed KS et al (2000) Nonenhanced helical CT and US in the emergency evaluation of patients with renal colic: prospective comparison. Radiology 217:792–797

Sheth S, Horton KM, Garland MR (2003) Mesenteric neoplasms: CT appearances of primary and secondary tumors and differential diagnosis. Radiographics 23:457–473

Shuman WP, Mack LA, Rogers JV (1981) Diffuse nephro-calcinosis: hyperechoic sonographic appearance. AJR Am J Roentgenol 136:830–832

Siegel CL, Middleton WD, Teefey SA, McClennan BL (1996) Angiomyolipoma and renal cell carcinoma: US differentiation. Radiology 198:789–793

Sohaib SA, Koh DM, Husband JE (2008) The role of imaging in the diagnosis, staging, and management of testicular cancer. AJR Am J Roentgenol 191:387–395

Suh JM, Cronan JJ, Monchik JM (2008) Primary hyperparathyroidism: is there an increased prevalence of renal stone disease? AJR Am J Roentgenol 191:908–911

Tamm EP, Silverman PM, Shuman WP (2003) Evaluation of the patient with flank pain and possible ureteral calculus. Radiology 228:319–329

Totaro A, Pinto F, Brescia A et al (2010) Imaging in bladder cancer: present role and future perspectives. Urol Int 85:373–380

Ünsal A, Çaliskan E, Erol H et al (2011) The diagnostic efficiency of ultrasound guided imaging algorithm in evaluation of patients with hematuria. Eur J Radiol 79:7–11

van Breda Vriesman AC, Engelbrecht MR, Smithuis RH, Puylaert JB (2007) Diffuse gallbladder wall thickening: differential diagnosis. AJR Am J Roentgenol 188:495–501

Wong-You-Cheong J, Woodward P, Manning M et al (2006) Neoplasms of the urinary bladder: radiologic-pathologic correlation. Radiographics 26:553–580

Yilmaz S, Sindel T, Arslan G et al (1998) Renal colic: comparison of spiral CT, US and IVU in the detection of ureteral calculi. Eur Radiol 8:212–217

Yoon JH, Cha SS, Han SS (2006) Gallbladder adenomyomatosis: imaging findings. Abdom Imaging 31:555–563

Zerin JM, Baker DR, Casale JA (2000) Single-system ureteroceles in infants and children: imaging features. Pediatr Radiol 30:139–146

Woman's Imaging

2

Jose Luís del Cura, Pedro Seguí, Rosa Zabala, Martín Velasco, Gorane Santamaría, Xavier Bargalló, Enrique Remartínez, and Carmen Kraemer

Introduction

The most traditional use of ultrasound, and the most popular also, has been the exploration of women and especially women of reproductive age. Childbearing-age women and the fetus share a special sensitivity to ionizing radiation and also a greater potential harm to the side effects produced by them. Therefore, imaging techniques that do not use ionizing radiation are the alternatives of choice in the study of childbearing-age women. Among these techniques, ultrasound is the most available.

The most popular application of ultrasound has undoubtedly been the monitoring of pregnancy and fetal examination. The fetus has indeed many characteristics that make it particularly suitable for evaluation by ultrasound: it is completely surrounded by fluid, it is readily accessible to exploration, and ultrasound transmits well as it has almost no ossified bone and no air.

The exploration of the genital tract of women is also performed using ultrasound with excellent reliability and resolution. The excellent acoustic window provided by the bladder or, alternatively, the possibility of placing the scanning probe very close to the organs explored using transvaginal approach has made ultrasound the basis of imaging and clinical follow-up in women of reproductive age.

Finally, breast ultrasound has emerged as an excellent complementary test to mammography for the study of breast disease. The breast consists of soft tissue, easily accessible to the ultrasound examination. Ultrasound is excellent for classifying focal lesions as solid or cystic and also is the most commonly used technique to guide interventional procedures, both diagnostic and therapeutic.

J.L. del Cura et al. (eds.), *Learning Ultrasound Imaging*, Learning Imaging,
DOI 10.1007/978-3-642-30586-3_2, © Springer-Verlag Berlin Heidelberg 2012

Female Pelvis

Pedro Seguí, Jose Luís del Cura, and Rosa Zabala

Case 1: Ovarian Functional Cysts

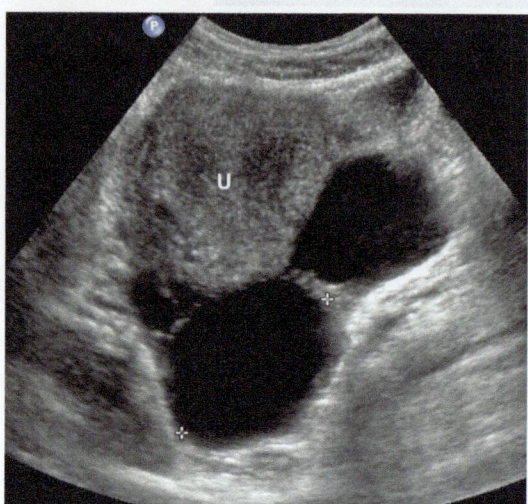

Fig. 2.1.1

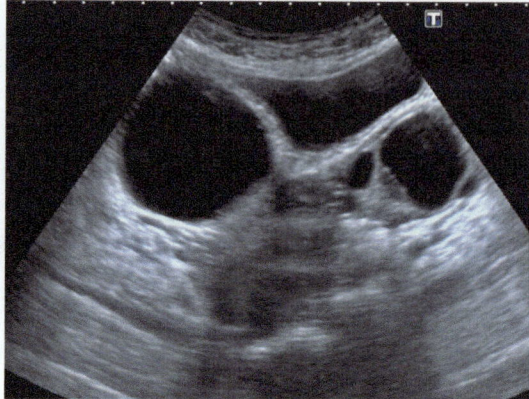

Fig. 2.1.2

An ultrasound exam was performed to a 28-year-old woman as part of her scheduled follow-up after a renal transplantation (Fig. 2.1.1). Incidentally, two anechoic, thin-walled, 5 cm in diameter lesions with posterior acoustic enhancement were detected behind the uterus (*U*). No inner walls or solid components were seen. With the diagnostic of ovarian functional cysts, a sonographic follow-up was scheduled. In the follow-up, performed 7 months after the diagnosis, the lesions had slightly decreased in size, although the sonographic features remained unchanged (Fig. 2.1.2).

Case Presentation and Imaging Findings

Ultrasound is the first-choice technique in the evaluation of suspect adnexal masses. Transabdominal and endovaginal ultrasound can be used for the evaluation of adnexal masses. Both are relatively inexpensive, noninvasive, and widely available. Ovarian cysts are the most frequent adnexal condition. Most of them are functional (follicular cysts that result from a failure of a follicle to rupture or regress and corpus luteum cysts). Functional cysts are generally anechoic, smooth, thin-walled, less than 3 cm in diameter, unilocular, and with posterior acoustic enhancement. However, similar ultrasound characteristics may be seen in benign ovarian neoplasms such as serous cystadenomas and in ovarian cancer also. Although a simple unilocular cyst without solid components is highly unlikely to be malignant, the management of adnexal masses in women of reproductive age is a common clinical gynecologic problem.

Comments

Ultrasound – whether transabdominal or endovaginal – uses morphologic features of the cyst to distinguish between benign and malignant disease. Features like thick, irregular walls and septa, papillary projections, and solid, moderately echogenic loculi suggest malignancy. The most helpful of them to diagnose ovarian neoplasms is the presence of papillary projections and nodular septa. The sensitivity of sonographic morphologic analysis in predicting malignancy in ovarian tumors is 85–97 %, whereas the specificity is 56–95 %. Some morphologic scoring systems based on the wall thickness, inner wall structure, septal characteristics, and echogenicity of the lesion have also been proposed to help distinguish benign from malignant ovarian lesions.

Color Doppler ultrasound of ovarian masses has been used also to help identify vascularized tissue and differentiate solid tumor from nonvascularized structures. However, the blood flow detection rate in functional cysts has ranged from 19 to 61 %; therefore, blood flow assessment at color Doppler ultrasound is not useful in distinguishing functional ovarian cysts from ovarian neoplasms. Follow-up sonography in benign-appearing ovarian cysts to assess for cyst resolution is the best approach for identifying functional cysts and is appropriate in both premenopausal and postmenopausal women.

Case 2: Ovarian Teratoma

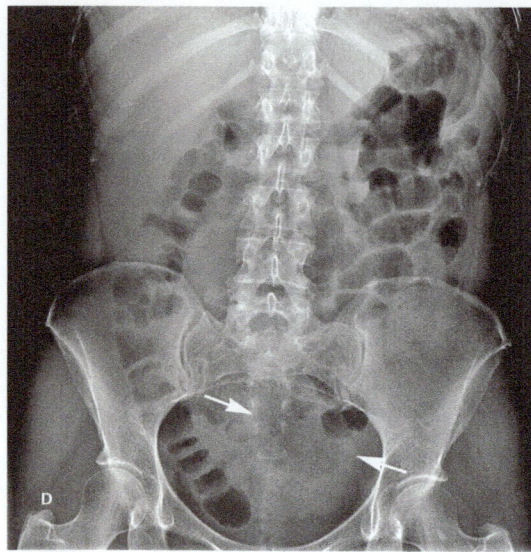

Fig. 2.2.1

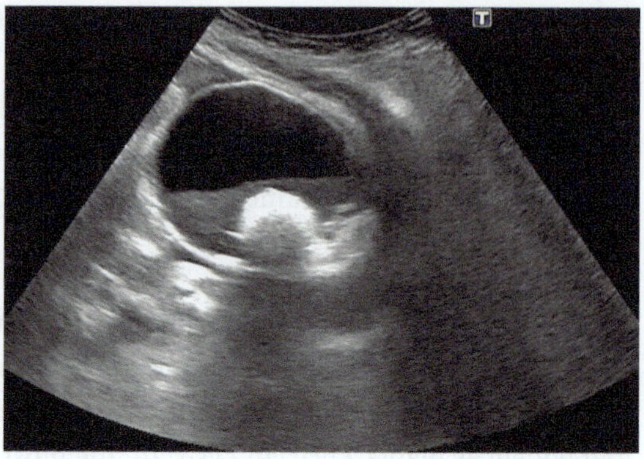

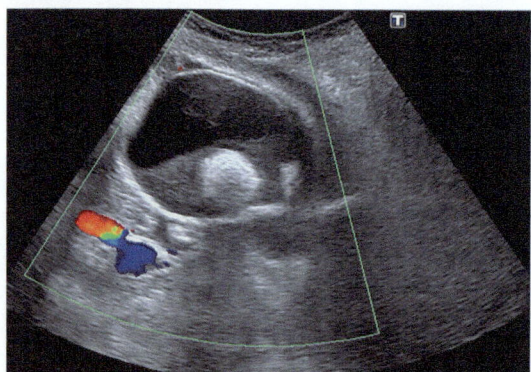

Fig. 2.2.2

Fig. 2.2.3

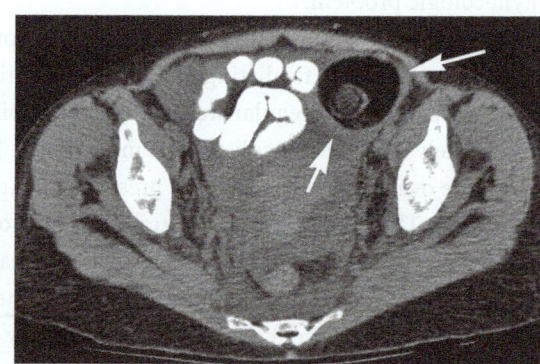

Fig. 2.2.4

Case Presentation and Imaging Findings

Female 43-year-old. An abdominal X-ray (Fig. 2.2.1) performed because unrelated reasons showed a rounded fat-density mass in pelvis (*arrows*).

A pelvic sonogram was performed (Fig. 2.2.2) showing a mass with fat-fluid level and a dependent highly echogenic nodule (dermoid plug) with shadowing. Color Doppler sonography (Fig. 2.2.3) showed no detectable flow in the mass.

A CT confirmed the diagnosis of left ovarian teratoma. Un-enhanced CT (Fig. 2.2.4) shows left ovary cyst with fat content (*arrows*) and a round Rokitansky nodule. Ascites of unrelated origin is also present.

Mature teratomas or benign cystic teratomas constitute 95 % of all the germ cell tumors and are the most frequent ovarian tumor (20 % of ovarian neoplasms) along with the cystadenoma. They can be found at any age but are usually diagnosed in the reproductive age. The most frequent form of presentation is as a casual finding in an ultrasound or CT performed for other reasons. Their size is quite variable. They contain solid or cystic components also in variable proportions and are formed by mature tissue coming from the three germ layers, being the ectodermal component usually predominant; thus, they are also called "dermoid cysts." Immature teratomas are rare (1 % of the teratomas) and are rapid-growth malignant tumors that appear in girls and teenagers. They can be solid (more frequently) or cystic, usually with thick calcifications, and contain immature tissue coming from any germ layer mixed with mature tissue. A third type of teratoma is the struma ovarii, predominantly composed of thyroid tissue. Other infrequent germ cell tumors are the dysgerminomas (similar to the testicular seminomas), endodermal sinus tumors, embryonal carcinoma, choriocarcinoma, mixed germ cell tumors, and primary carcinoid tumors.

The ultrasound appearance of mature teratomas is rather specific but quite variable. The most frequent form of presentation is as a cystic lesion with a densely echogenic nodule (dermoid plug or Rokitansky nodule). This echogenic nodule usually contains hair, teeth, or fat and generally presents a posterior dirty shadow. Another frequent form of presentation is as a predominantly echogenic mass with posterior dirty shadowing that makes it difficult visualizing part of the lesion (tip of the iceberg sign). Another less frequent presentation form is as a cystic lesion with multiple thin inner echogenic bands composed of hair (dermoid mesh). The cystic content of these lesions corresponds totally or partially to sebum (of liquid consistency at body temperature) and can be anechoic or hypoechoic. On occasions, a liquid-liquid level is visualized, with a superficial anechoic sebaceous layer and a sloped layer of more echogenic aqueous liquid (it is less frequent for the superficial layer to be echogenic). With the color Doppler, the mature teratomas do not usually have detectable vascular signs in their interior, except in the infrequent cases of struma ovarii, which are presented as solid masses with Doppler flow-signals inside, and that upon occasion can be presented with hyperthyroidism.

Differential diagnosis should be made with an acute hemorrhage in an ovarian cyst or in an endometrioma, which can simulate the dermoid plug. Also, a completely echogenic teratoma can be confused with gas in an intestinal loop. In CT, the finding of a cystic lesion with content of fat density is diagnostic. In MR, the sebaceous component is easily demonstrated using fat saturation sequences.

Comments

Case 3: Ovarian Torsion

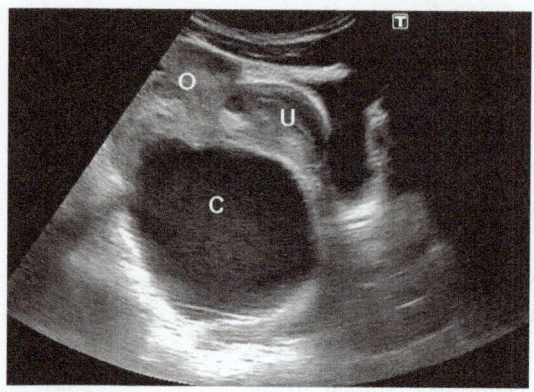

Fig. 2.3.1

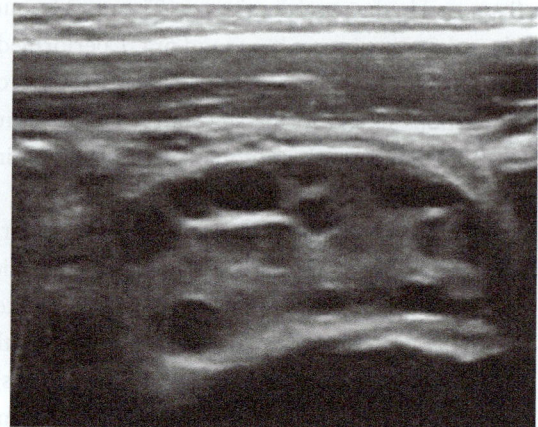

Fig. 2.3.2

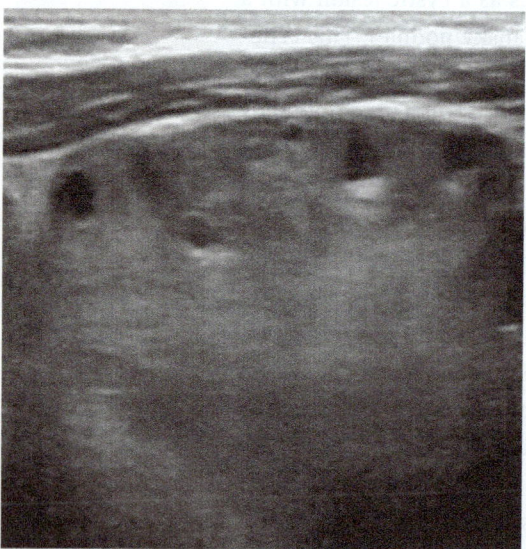

Fig. 2.3.3

A 14-year-old female consulted for progressive pain in hypogastrium of sudden onset and 2 days of evolution. She presented with fever and generalized pain in abdominal palpation. Blood tests showed leukocytosis. An emergency ultrasound was performed.

Sagittal pelvic sonogram (Fig. 2.3.1) shows an enlarged 6-cm ovary (*O*) with an adjacent 8-cm cyst (*C*), cranial to uterine fundus (*U*).

Figure 2.3.2 shows a longitudinal view of the right normal ovary and Fig. 2.3.3 a longitudinal view of the left enlarged ovary. Some peripheral small cysts can be seen in the left ovary.

Power Doppler sonogram (Fig. 2.3.4) shows normal flow in right ovary (*left side*) and absolute absence of blood flow in left enlarged ovary (*right side*).

Ultrasound diagnosis was 8-cm left adnexal cyst with associated ovarian torsion. A left adnexectomy was immediately performed. The exam of the surgical specimen confirmed an ovarian torsion with hemorrhagic necrosis and a benign simple hemorrhagic cyst.

Ovarian torsion is the rotation of the ovarian pedicle on its axis, resulting in vascular compromise. Clinically, it presents as acute abdominal pain, generally intense, and emergency surgery is indicated to try to avoid hemorrhagic infarction of the ovary and peritonitis. In most cases, it occurs in an ovary with a preexisting neoplastic mass (generally benign) or a cyst, although it can also occur in normal ovaries. It is more frequent in infancy or in reproductive ages, with an increased risk existing in pregnancy and in ovarian hyperstimulation. Ultrasound is usually the first test performed in this clinical context, and torsion should be always considered in the differential diagnosis when an ovarian mass is discovered in an acute abdomen setting. When torsion is only partial or intermittent, the symptoms could be subacute. The ovarian disease most often associated with torsion is the benign cystic teratoma. Hemorrhagic cysts and cystadenomas are also frequent causes of torsion.

Ultrasound findings are variable depending on the degree of vascular compromise and of the presence of an adnexal mass. The most constant finding is the increase in the ovarian size (>4 cm). The involved ovary is usually visible in the midline and cranial to the uterine fundus. A specific characteristic, but not always present, is the presence of multiple aligned uniform follicles in the periphery of the increased ovary (string of pearls sign). This later appearance can also be seen in the polycystic ovary, but in this case, it is bilateral and not linked to pain. Free fluid in the cul-de-sac and a solid or cystic adnexal mass are also very frequent associated features.

Doppler findings are quite variable and should be carefully interpreted. The most frequent finding is the absence of flow, but almost half of the patients present normal flow. The diagnosis of torsion should be considered

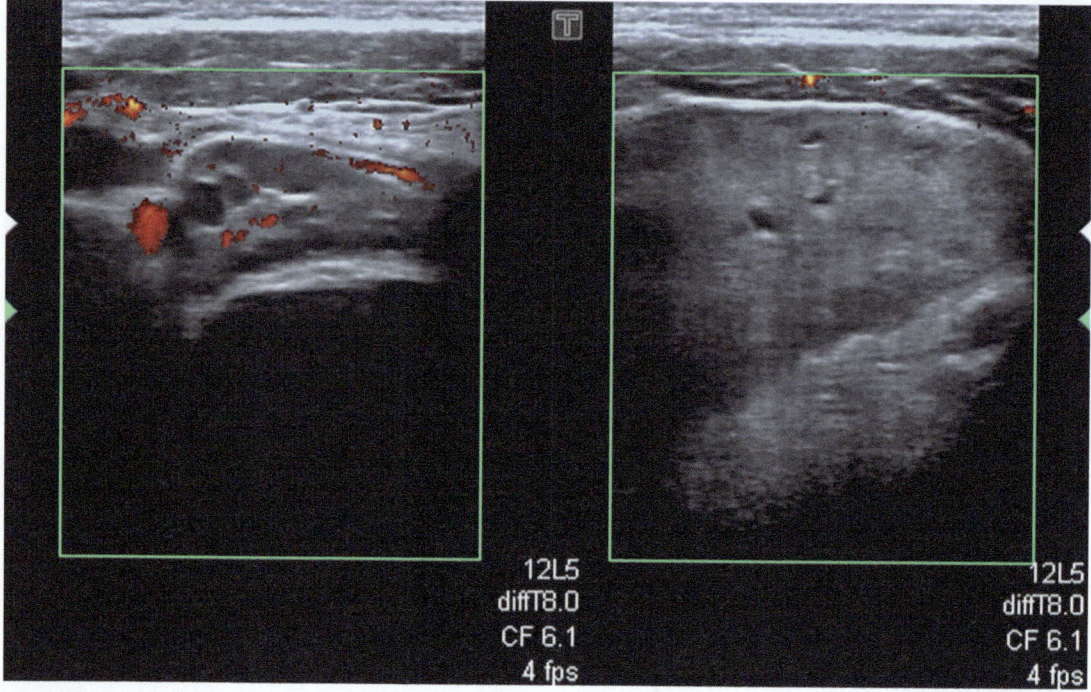

Fig. 2.3.4

when an increased in size of the ovary is detected in the context of acute intense pain, even visualizing vascularization in the ovary with color Doppler. A more specific finding is the visualization of vascular pedicle torsion, consisting of a rounded or tubular hyperechogenic structure with multiple hypoechogenic concentric bands. With the color Doppler, this pedicle torsion can show absence of flow or spiral (whirlpool sign) vascular signals. Absent flow in the vascular pedicle is correlated in surgery with necrotic or infarcted, nonviable ovaries.

Case 4: Uterine Leiomyoma

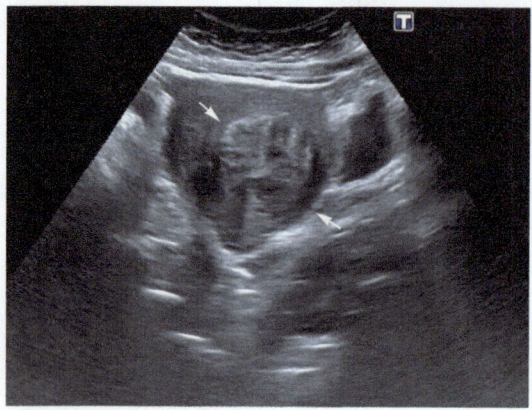

Fig. 2.4.1

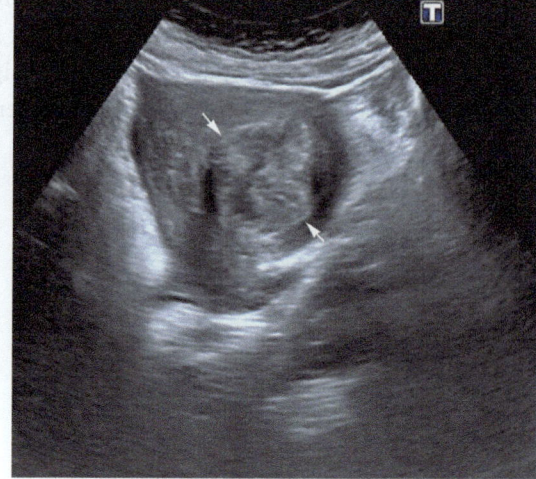

Fig. 2.4.2

A 45-year-old woman is being studied as a result of an incidental microhematuria in blood analysis. As part of the standard management of this finding, an abdominal and pelvic ultrasound is performed. Images show two sagittal (Fig. 2.4.1) and transverse (Fig. 2.4.2) sonograms of the body of the uterus. A discrete solitary hyperechoic heterogeneous lesion of 53 mm (*arrows*) can be seen in the uterine wall. A leiomyoma was diagnosed. The lesion has remained unchanged for years in follow-up studies.

Case Presentation and Imaging Findings

Leiomyomas occur in 20–40 % of women and are the most common gynecologic tumor. Although they can appear in all women, leiomyomas are more frequent at a younger age. They are benign tumors that usually arise from the smooth muscle of the uterine wall. Also, they can be ectopic, appearing in fallopian tubes, cervix, vagina, or pelvic ligaments.

Comments

Leiomyomas are masses of smooth muscle cells and fibrous tissue. They are encapsulated with a pseudocapsule and may present necrosis, hemorrhage, or calcification. Although they may be unique, they usually present as multiple lesions.

When occurring in the wall of the uterus, leiomyomas may be either submucosal, intramural, or subserosal. The symptoms depend largely on their location: submucosal lesions are associated with bleeding, while intramural and subserosal tumors can affect fertility.

Ultrasound is the primary modality to study gynecological conditions and is also the first technique used to image leiomyomas. Although usually they are easy to detect and to diagnose, sonographic appearance of leiomyomas is highly variable. They may present either as discrete masses, solitary or multiple, or as a diffuse enlargement of the uterus, caused by multiple diffuse small leiomyomas. Leiomyomas may be seen as homogeneous or heterogeneous, and hyperechoic or hypoechoic. Fibrosis and calcification of leiomyomas can cause acoustic shadowing. The uterine origin of exophytic or pedunculated leiomyomas can be difficult to trace. Such diverse sonographic presentations may lead in some cases to diagnostic confusion.

Case 5: Leiomyoma of the Fallopian Tube

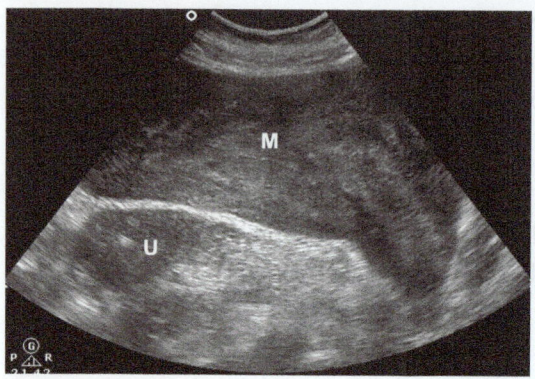

Fig. 2.5.1

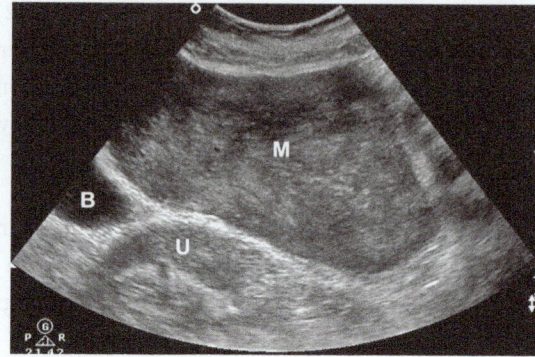

Fig. 2.5.2

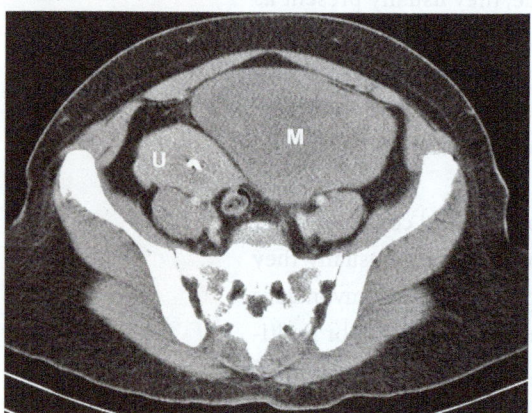

Fig. 2.5.3

In a routine health exam, a palpable pelvic mass is detected in a 41-year-old woman. On pelvic sonography, a homogeneous 14 cm in diameter big mass was seen. Figures 2.5.1 and 2.5.2 show two axial sonographic views of the mass (*M*). A CT was also performed (Fig. 2.5.3). The mass appears before the uterus (*U*) and displaces the bladder (*B*).

The origin of the mass could not be established in the explorations. A percutaneous biopsy was performed, and a leiomyoma was demonstrated. On surgery, a tubal origin of the mass was confirmed.

Case Presentation and Imaging Findings

Sonographic diagnosis of fallopian tube disease masses is frequently difficult. Normal fallopian tubes are not easily distinguishable, and thus, they are not surveyed in routine pelvic ultrasound. Moreover, diseases of the fallopian tubes, and especially neoplasms, are uncommon, and when a pelvic mass is detected, a tubal origin is not usually considered as the first option. In the case presented here, only the surgery was able to discover the tubal origin of the tumor.

Tubal diseases that can be detected on ultrasound include ectopic pregnancy, hydrosalpinx, tubo-ovarian abscess, malignant tumors, and benign neoplasms such as leiomyoma, teratoma, or fibromas. Tumors are usually distinguished on ultrasound due to its solid appearance. Although ultrasound cannot make differential diagnosis between malignancy and benignity, it should be taken on account that tubal malignancies are more frequent than benign tumors.

Leiomyoma is extremely rare in the fallopian tube compared to the uterus. It is asymptomatic, but after excessive growth, torsion or degenerative changes may cause symptoms. Its sonographic appearance is similar to that of uterine tumor: usually solitary, discrete mass, homogeneous or heterogeneous, hyperechoic or hypoechoic, and sometimes with acoustic shadowing. Given its lack of symptoms, some tumors can slowly grow to become huge masses, as in the case presented here.

Comments

Breast

Martín Velasco, Gorane Santamaría, and Xavier Bargalló

Case 6: Diabetic Mastopathy

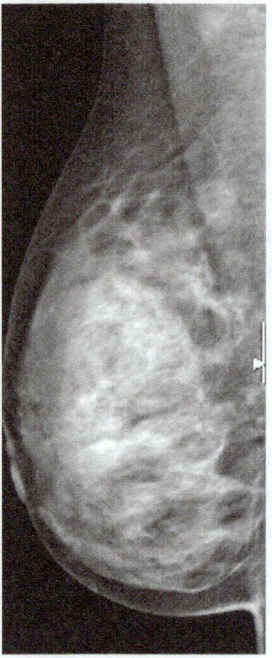

Fig. 2.6.1

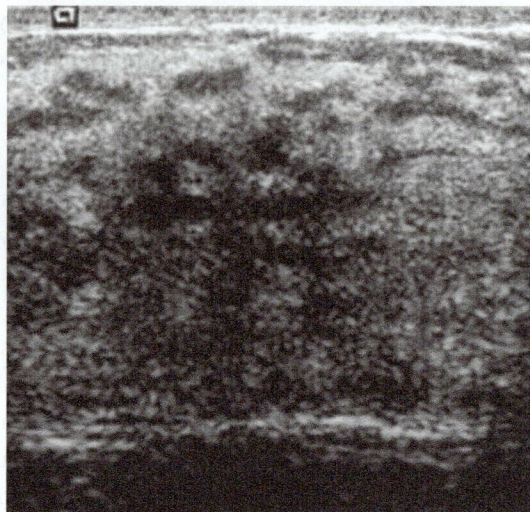

Fig. 2.6.2

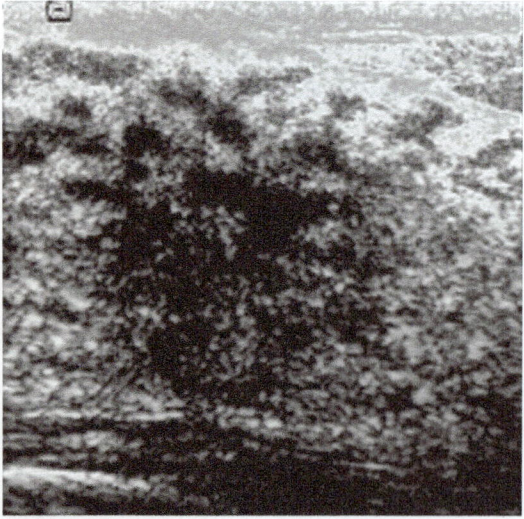

Fig. 2.6.3

A 38-year-old female presented with a 10-month history of painless right breast mass in the union of the outer quadrants. She had been suffering from diabetes mellitus type I since she was 18. Mammography (Fig. 2.6.1) shows a focal dense asymmetry in outer quadrants of the right breast with no evidence of carcinoma. Sonographic images of focal dense asymmetry (Figs. 2.6.2 and 2.6.3). Note the strong ultrasound acoustic shadow mimicking a breast carcinoma. Biopsy showed intense stromal lymphocytic infiltrate and perilobular fibrosis. A diabetic mastopathy was diagnosed.

Case Presentation and Imaging Findings

Diabetic mastopathy (DMP) is a collection of clinical, radiological, and histological features found in dense fibrous masses of the breast, initially described by Soler and Khardori in 1984. The disease is associated with long-standing type 1 diabetes mellitus but has been reported in other autoimmune disorders. The clinical and imaging findings are inconclusive, and these lesions are often misdiagnosed as breast carcinomas. The recognition of this rare but benign disease is crucial to avoid surgical biopsies.

Comments

Women between 30 and 50 years of age with long history of insulin-dependent diabetes are more likely to be affected by diabetic mastopathy. It is usually associated with chronic complications of diabetes, such as nephropathy, neuropathy, and retinopathy. The pathogenesis of diabetic mastopathy is not still well known.

Patients with diabetic mastopathy present with a palpable, hard, painless, irregular mass solitarily in one breast or in both breasts. On mammography, a very dense breast parenchyma is usually found, although, sometimes, a discrete asymmetric density between both breasts is observed. On ultrasonography, a hypoechoic solid mass with ill-defined margins, posterior acoustic shadow, and absence of Doppler signal is shown. Diabetic mastopathy may be confused with breast carcinoma because of the difficulty to distinguish between these two entities both physically and by imaging. However, there is no evidence to suggest that diabetic mastopathy predisposes to breast cancer. In cases with an appropriate clinical history and high index of suspicion, an ultrasound-guided core biopsy may be useful for the primary diagnosis of diabetic mastopathy.

Some researchers also reported similar features in autoimmune diseases, like thyroiditis and systemic lupus erythematosus, where they described the condition as lymphocytic mastopathy. On gross examination, diabetic mastopathy shows ill-defined areas of firm fibrous tissue with no evident cysts, unlike fibrocystic mastopathy. Histopathological findings demonstrate marked stromal sclerosis and B lymphocyte infiltration in the perivascular and perilobular areas which is known as sclerosing lymphocytic lobulitis.

Even though many reports have been published on diabetic mastopathy in radiological, pathologic, and surgical literature, this clinical condition is poorly recognized since breast examination is not routinely performed in young diabetic patients. Surgical treatment is not recommended, since local relapse is very likely to happen.

Case 7: Intracystic Papillary Carcinoma of the Breast

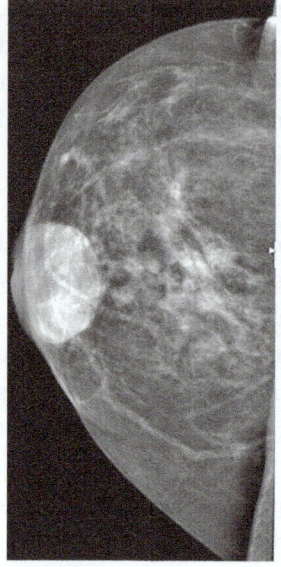

Fig. 2.7.1

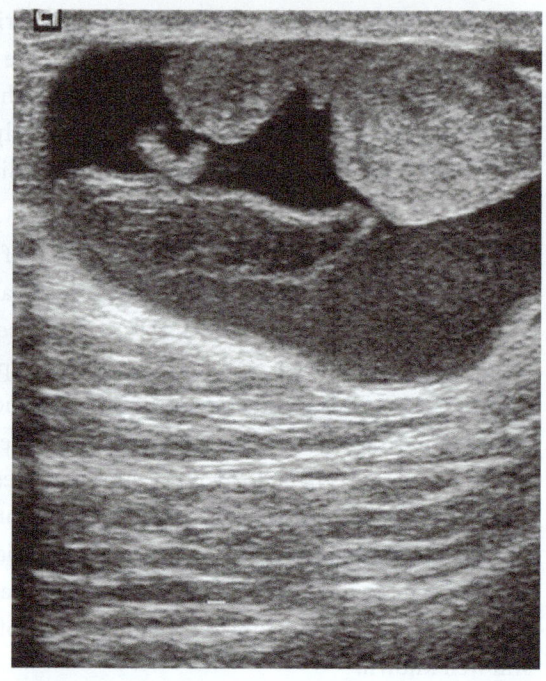

Fig. 2.7.2

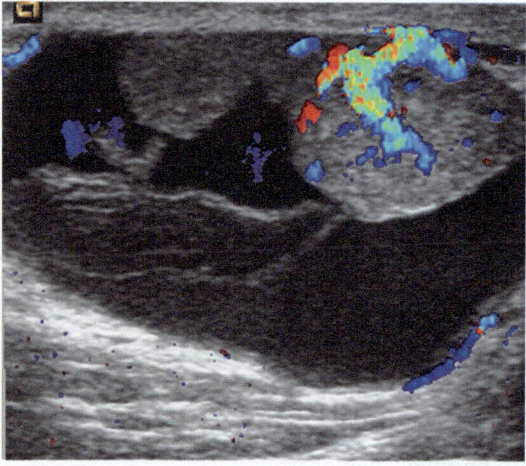

Fig. 2.7.3

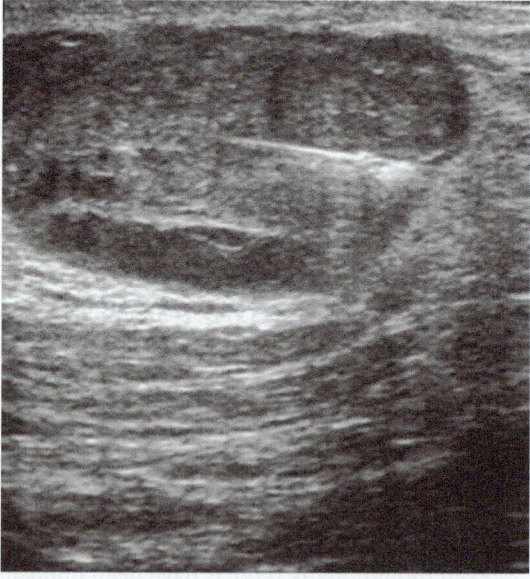

Fig. 2.7.4

A 74-year-old woman presented with a palpable mass in the retroareolar region of the left breast. Physical examination revealed a 4×2-cm subareolar breast mass with associated retraction of the skin and nipple. Mammography (Fig. 2.7.1) showed a 4-cm dense mass with retraction of the skin and nipple in the subareolar region of the left breast. Ultrasonography (Fig. 2.7.2) revealed a 3.8-cm, oval, well-circumscribed complex mass. It was predominantly cystic and contained internal septa and a 1.5-cm solid mural nodule which projected into the lumen. Color Doppler sonography (Fig. 2.7.3) showed a vascular pedicle with evident blood flow in the mural nodule. Ultrasound-guided core biopsy of the mural nodule was performed (Fig. 2.7.4). Final histologic diagnosis was invasive intracystic papillary carcinoma of the breast.

Case Presentation and Imaging Findings

Intracystic papillary carcinoma of the breast is a rare malignant tumor that accounts for 1–2 % of all breast carcinomas. Tumors of this type usually arise in dilated ducts, not in cysts, and are called intracystic only when the cystic component is relatively large, as in this case.

Comments

The tumor usually does not demonstrate invasive growth. It may be uni-or multifocal and can be found as a pure form or associated with ductal carcinoma in situ or invasive carcinoma. Usually appears in postmenopausal women, as a slowly enlarging palpable mass or as bloody nipple discharge. Retraction of the nipple and skin may be an associated clinical finding, especially in tumours large enough to be palpable.

On mammography, intracystic papillary carcinoma is usually seen as a round, oval, or lobulated circumscribed mass, generally located retroareolar. Spiculation is also a common feature, and nipple retraction may be detected. The later findings are not always due to invasion and can be related to sclerosis and inflammation of the surrounding tissue. The cyst wall is typically thickened and fibrotic.

On sonography, intracystic papillary carcinoma appears as single or multiple predominantly cystic masses, with or without septa, with solid papillary masses projecting into the cystic lumen. A posterior acoustic enhancement is frequently associated. Visualization of fluid-debris levels in the cyst is usually due to bleeding. Color Doppler sonography shows an irregular branching pattern in the solid papillary components of the tumor. Vascularization help differentiate it from a blood clot. Intracystic papillomas or carcinomas may be diagnosed with sonography when they do not fill the entire cyst lumen. Otherwise, a completely solid intracystic papillary carcinoma is not distinguishable from other solid masses.

Core needle biopsy may be unable to differentiate between in situ and invasive lesions because invasion is often identified at the periphery of the tumor. Therefore, surgical excision must be always performed.

Case 8: Borderline Phyllodes Tumor

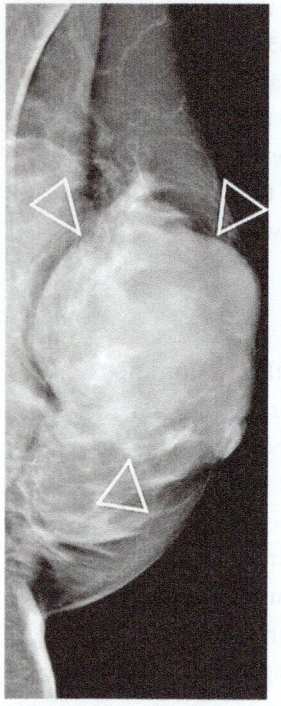

Fig. 2.8.1

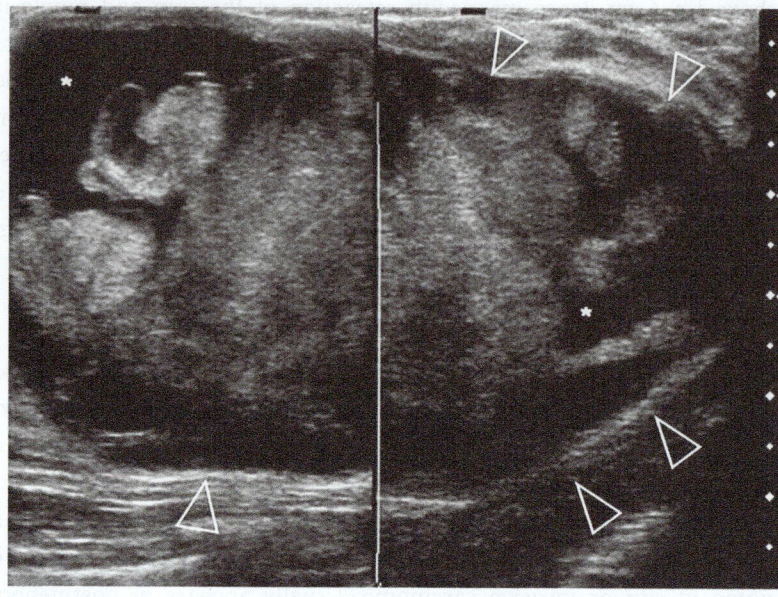

Fig. 2.8.2

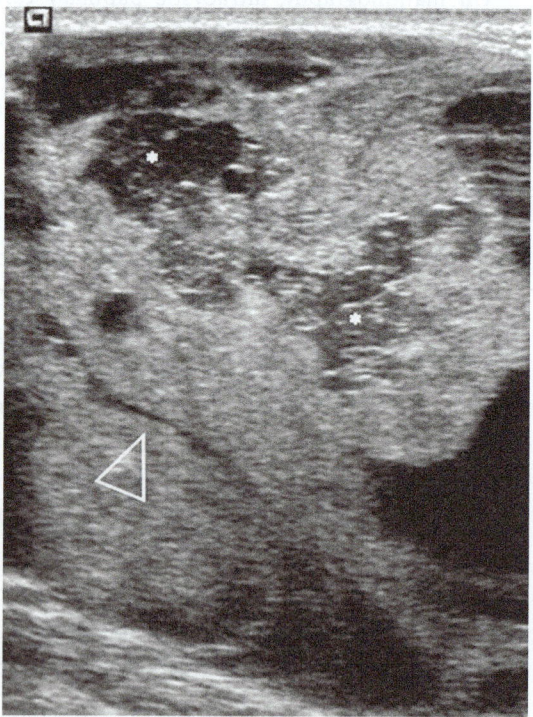

Fig. 2.8.3

A 37-year-old woman presented with a palpable mass in left breast.

Left oblique mediolateral mammography (Fig. 2.8.1) shows a large, high density, well-defined mass (*arrowheads*).

Ultrasound image shows the whole circumference of the mass (Fig. 2.8.2). The margins are well delimitated (*arrowheads*). Note anechoic, cystic-like spaces (*asterisks*) in relation to hemorrhagic or necrotic changes which are common in phyllodes tumor.

Ultrasound image (Fig. 2.8.3) shows a papillary projection with cystic-like areas (*asterisks*). Note a hypoechoic linear cleft-like structure (*arrowhead*) which has been described in phyllodes tumors.

Power Doppler image (Fig. 2.8.4) shows several vascular pedicles indicating a highly vascularized mass.

Axial T2-weighted MRI (Fig. 2.8.5) shows a heterogeneous composition with cystic-like spaces (*asterisks*). Note hypointense lines which likely reflect septations (*arrowheads*).

Contrast-enhanced T1-weighted MR imaging (Fig. 2.8.6) shows intense enhancement of the solid parts. Non-enhancing areas (*asterisks*) represent cystic, necrotic, or hemorrhagic spaces.

Case Presentation and Imaging Findings

Phyllodes tumor of the breast is a rare fibroepithelial tumor that accounts for less than 1 % of all breast neoplasms and 2–3 % of fibroepithelial neoplasms.

Phyllodes tumor arises predominantly in women between ages 35 and 55 years. It presents clinically as a well-circumscribed mobile mass, which may grow fast, becoming huge or may be eventually found after biopsy for small breast masses.

Phyllodes tumor is histologically characterized by large leaflike projections of stroma with increased stromal cellularity. This overgrowth can cause elongation and distortion of the ducts that produce slit-like, epithelium-lined clefts and cystic spaces that contributed to the older term cystosarcoma.

According to its margins, stromal cellularity, and number of mitoses, it will be classified as benign, borderline (5–9 mitoses at 10 high-power fields), or malignant (10 or more mitoses at 10 high-power fields). Approximately 20–50 % of phyllodes tumors are found to be malignant.

Surgical treatment should be performed since the distinction between benign and malignant cannot be made by radiologic means. However, the extent of the procedure is controversial. Enucleation alone is considered to be insufficient, and margins from 1 to 2 cm have been recommended. Other authors recommend simple mastectomy in tumors larger than 5 cm or in those borderline or malignant no matter what size they are.

Benign phyllodes can resemble fibroadenoma or papilloma. Sonography shows a variety of findings from well-defined, homogeneous masses to ill-defined, heterogeneous, solid-cystic masses more commonly seen in

Comments

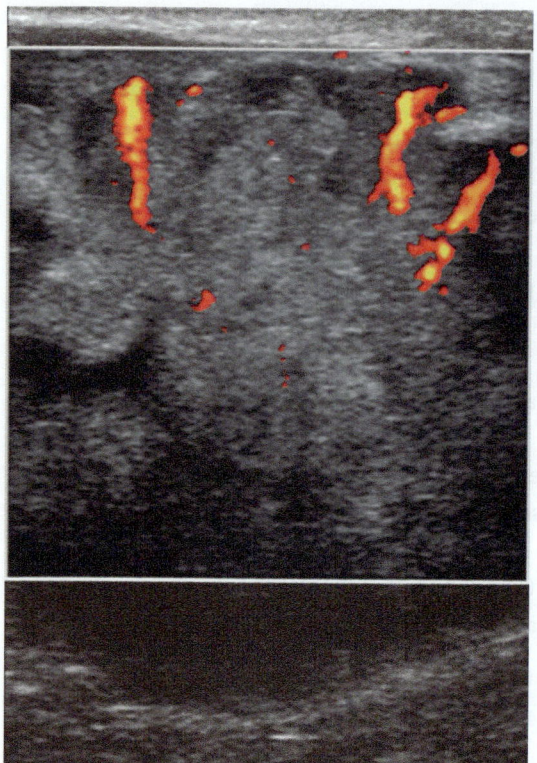

Fig. 2.8.4

Fig. 2.8.5

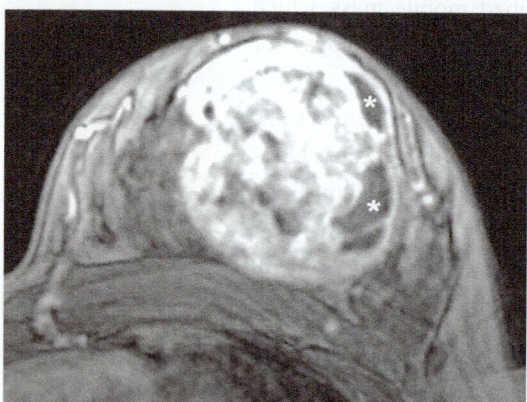

Fig. 2.8.6

borderline or malignant tumors. However, even small tumors tend to show cystic spaces. Thin, hypoechoic lines reflecting fluid-filled slits are also common, and both cystic spaces and hypoechoic lines can lead to suspect the diagnosis.

The differential diagnosis in borderline or malignant tumors should include breast abscesses, intracystic carcinoma, and metaplastic carcinoma. Breast abscesses are typically thick-walled and elongated in an axis parallel to the subareolar ducts in a clinical setting of pain and tenderness.

Metaplastic carcinomas are large solid lobulated masses that frequently have areas of cystic or hemorrhagic necrosis. The border can be circumscribed or microlobulated and angular, indicating infiltration of surrounding tissue.

Case 9: Nonpuerperal Breast Abscess

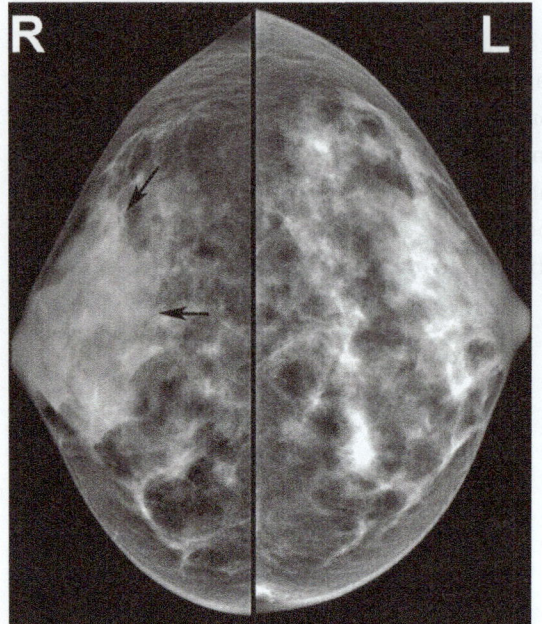

Fig. 2.9.1

Fig. 2.9.2

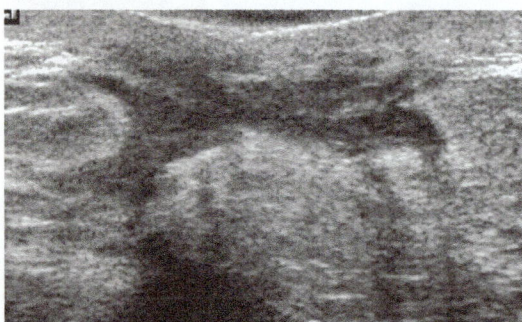

Fig. 2.9.3

A nonlactating 31-year-old woman presented with a 2-cm periareolar mass in the right breast associated with focal breast skin erythema.

Note the diffuse density increase of the periareolar parenchyma in the right breast (*arrows*) compared to the left breast on bilateral mammography, craniocaudal projection (Fig. 2.9.1).

Axial sonographic image of the right breast (Fig. 2.9.2) shows a well-defined, thick-walled, hypoechoic cavity in a periareolar location. Note the echogenic debris inside the abscess.

After abscess drainage, ultrasound (Fig. 2.9.3) shows an ill-defined collapsed residual cavity. One month later, the patient came with a draining fistulous tract to the skin which required surgical treatment.

Case Presentation and Imaging Findings

Mastitis is inflammation of the breast that may be either infectious or noninfectious in origin. Infectious mastitis most commonly is acute, occurs during lactation (puerperal mastitis), and may progress to tissue necrosis and abscess formation. Patients with acute puerperal mastitis have localized or general edema and erythema of the breast, along with fever, pain, and tenderness. Acute mastitis may also occur in nonlactating patients who usually have underlying ductal ectasia or, less commonly, breast cysts. Such cases probably begin as chemical inflammation due to rupture of ectatic ducts or cysts. The inflammation in such patients is chemical rather than infectious in origin, but secondary bacterial infection may occur. Mastitis with or without abscess, whether puerperal or nonpuerperal, must be distinguished from inflammatory carcinoma. Both cause severe edema and inflammation. Both can have masses that appear markedly hypoechoic and have enhanced acoustic through transmission.

Abscesses in association of ductal ectasia are termed nonpuerperal abscesses and are most typically periareolar in location, reflecting the underlying location of the inflamed central ducts from which they arise.

Ultrasonographically, nonpuerperal breast abscesses tend to be oval, parallel to the subareolar ducts, and unilocular with echogenic necrotic debris within the central cavity. Additionally, there are some specific signs depending on the patient age. Thus, periareolar abscess in perimenopausal women is typically thick-walled and subareolar in location and more likely to involve the areola and base of the nipple. However, in patients in their late teens and 20s, abscesses are usually thin-walled, oval or lobulated, and periareolar in location, not directly involving the areola and the nipple. The differential diagnosis should include other nonmalignant breast lesions such as seroma, hematoma, or focal fat necrosis.

It is important to drain these abscesses because they are prone to forming periareolar skin fistulas that are very difficult to cure by antibiotic treatment, percutaneous aspiration, or even open incision and drainage. In most cases, surgical excision of the entire fistula complex is required for effective treatment. Nonpuerperal abscesses are far more likely to recur and become chronic than puerperal abscesses because of the underlying chronic ductal inflammation or obstruction.

Comments

Obstetric Ultrasound

ENRIQUE REMARTÍNEZ and CARMEN KRAEMER

Case 10: Extralobar Infradiaphragmatic Pulmonary Sequestration

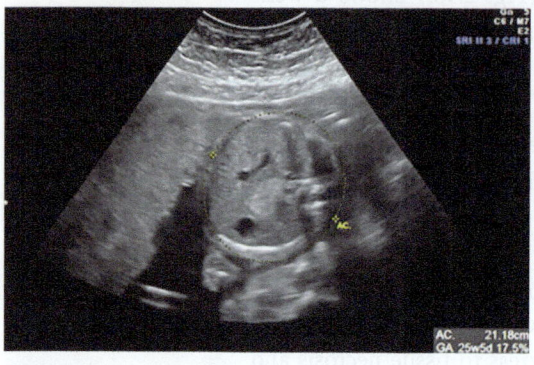

Fig. 2.10.1

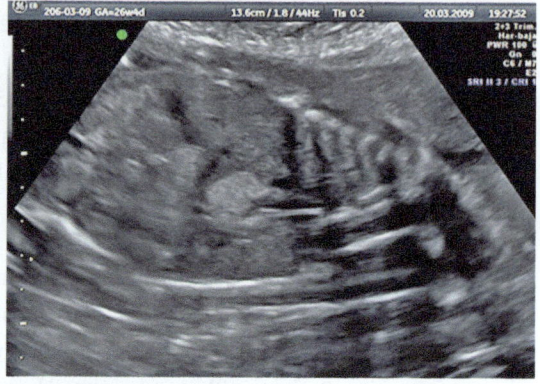

Fig. 2.10.2

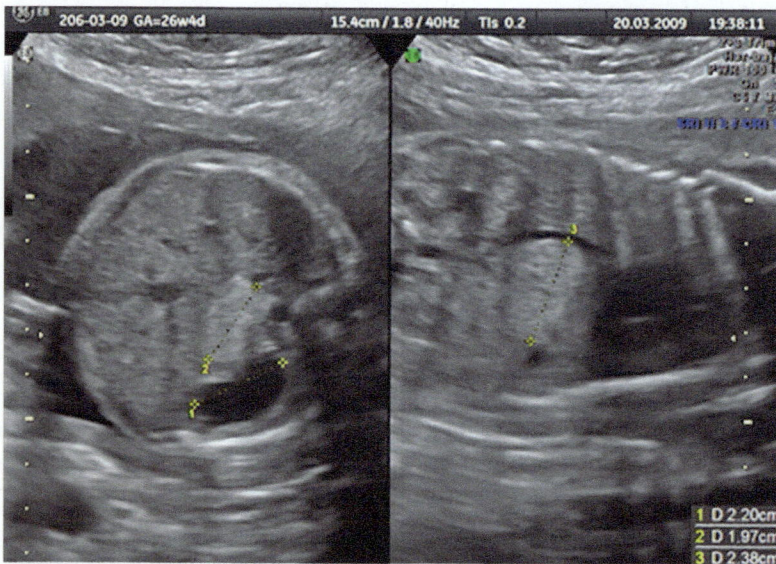

Fig. 2.10.3

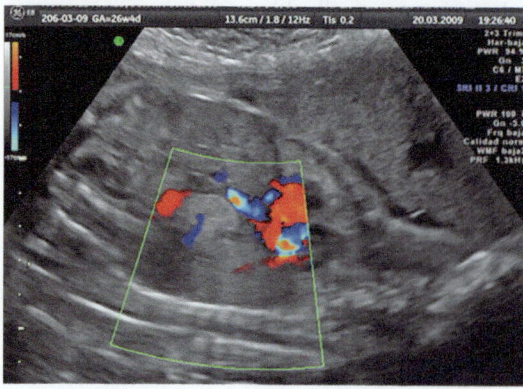

Fig. 2.10.4

Pulmonary sequestration is a relatively rare congenital anomaly first noted in the medical literature in 1861 by Rokitansky and Rektorzik. Subdiaphragmatic sequestration is a rare form of bronchopulmonary foregut malformation occurring in just 2 % of the cases in the largest reported series (1:10,000 live births). Approximately 10–15 % of extralobar sequestrations are found within or below the diaphragm. An extralobar subdiaphragmatic lung sequestration is a mass of nonaerated pulmonary tissue without connection to the normal bronchial tree and is located beneath the diaphragm. It receives its own blood supply from a systemic artery, it is enveloped by its own pleura, and its venous drainage goes to the systemic veins.

It is secondary to an anomalous or supernumerary lung bud that derives its blood supply from the primitive splanchnic vessels that surround the foregut. These vessels migrate distally with the foregut and provide the blood supply to the sequestration. The primary connection with the foregut typically involutes but may persist, allowing communication with the gastrointestinal tract.

Microscopically, extralobar sequestration resembles normal lung except for the diffuse dilatation of parenchymal structures. The bronchioles, alveolar ducts, and alveoli are dilated and tortuous.

The incidence of associated anomalies is >50 %, and these include diaphragmatic defects, gastric and colonic duplications, congenital cystic adenomatoid malformation, vertebral abnormalities, and cardiac defects. There are no associated chromosomal abnormalities.

Several diseases must be considered when an echogenic mass is visualized beneath or within the diaphragm. Neuroblastoma, teratoma, adrenal hemorrhage, or foregut duplication should be considered in the differential diagnosis. Multiple cysts within the mass may be found with associated cystic adenomatoid malformation.

The typical appearance of a subdiaphragmatic sequestration using ultrasound is a nonpulsatile, homogenous, well-circumscribed, hyperechoic mass in the fetal abdomen or retroperitoneum. Ninety percent of extralobar sequestrations are localized to the left side of the fetal abdomen. Cystic areas are commonly found within the lesion. Duplex and color flow Doppler may provide additional information by demonstrating vascular flow from the abdominal aorta and can define the venous drainage pattern.

Comments

Imaging Findings

Figure 2.10.1: Upper abdominal axial US scan at 26 weeks shows hyperechoic mass below the diaphragm, anterior to the spleen and medial to the stomach.

Figure 2.10.2: Abdominal coronal US scan showing hyperechoic mass below left diaphragm near to the aorta.

Figure 2.10.3: Axial and sagittal US scans show a homogeneously echogenic subdiaphragmatic mass, 2.2 cm in size, medial to the stomach, anterior to the spleen, and near to the aorta.

Figure 2.10.4: Left parasagittal color Doppler scan shows an echogenic mass near to the aorta. The proximal feeding vessel is visible.

Case 11: Hypoplastic Left Heart Syndrome

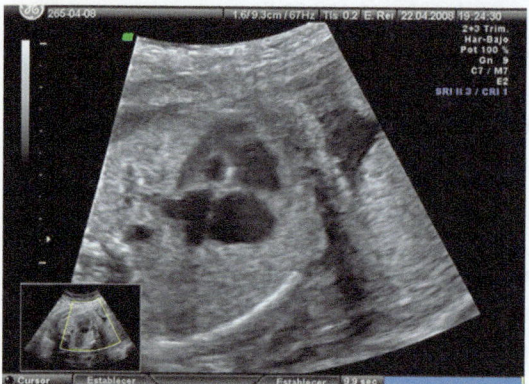

Fig. 2.11.1

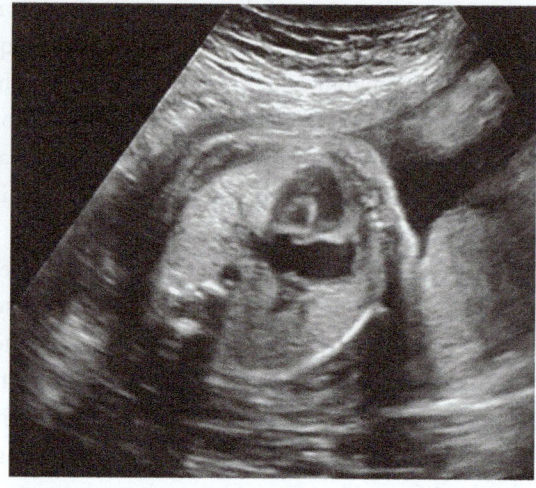

Fig. 2.11.2

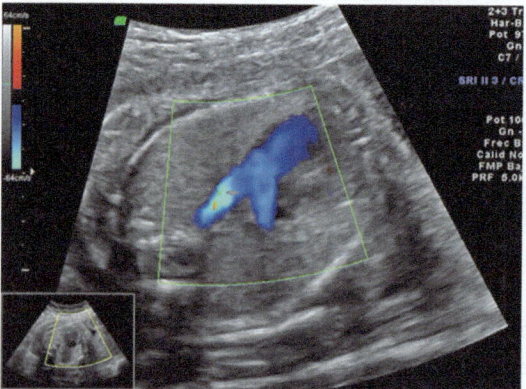

Fig. 2.11.3

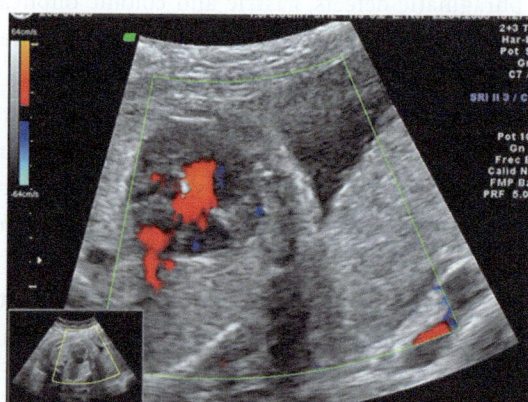

Fig. 2.11.4

Comments

Hypoplastic left heart syndrome is a group of congenital anomalies characterized by underdevelopment of the left ventricle, left atrium, aorta, and aortic and mitral valves. It is the congenital heart anomaly that imposes the most severe form of impedance to aortic blood flow in humans. For years, this condition has been erroneously called aortic atresia. However, aortic atresia is not always synonymous, and about 6 % of patients with aortic atresia will have a normal-sized left ventricle.

Its incidence varies from 1.7 to 6.7 per 10,000 live births according to different studies. Hypoplastic left heart syndrome is the most common cause of death from congenital heart disease in the early neonatal period, accounting for 7–9 % of all structural heart defects.

Ultrasound gray-scale findings include a four-chamber view markedly abnormal with a small and hypokinetic left ventricle, the heart apex is therefore formed by the right ventricle. In most cases, the aortic valve is atretic or hypoplastic, and the mitral valve is patent but dysplastic. The left atrium is small relative to the right atrial size with a paradoxical movement of the leaflet of the patent foramen ovale from the left to right atrium. The aortic outflow is difficult to visualize due to its hypoplastic size (<3 mm). A typical finding is usually visualized at the level of the three-vessel view: a compensatory dilated pulmonary trunk is seen adjacent to the superior vena cava with a nonvisible transverse aortic arch.

Color Doppler ultrasound demonstrates minimal to absent filling of the left ventricle. The five-chamber view confirms absence of forward flow through the atretic aortic valve. At the level of the three-vessel view, color Doppler ultrasound shows a reversal flow through the aortic isthmus and transverse aortic arch.

Differential diagnosis typically includes cardiac malformations that result in a diminutive left ventricle. The single ventricles, hypoplastic right ventricles, and the severe forms of endocardial cushion defect may all appear similar in the four-chamber view. A careful observation of the position of the atria, AV valves, and great vessels often allows the correct diagnosis. Aortic stenosis, aortic coarctation, and interruption of the aortic arch (hypoplasia of the isthmic region), which also imposes severe impedance to aortic blood flow, should also be ruled out.

The recent evolution of palliative surgical procedures (modified Norwood procedure, bidirectional cavo-pulmonary shunt, modified Fontan procedure, aortic valvuloplasty, and heart transplantation) has increased the survival rate of children with left hypoplastic heart syndrome. Staged surgical palliation is preferred over cardiac transplantation as the initial therapeutic approach. The overall survival rate after staged surgery varies, and rates between 25 and 48 % have been reported.

Imaging Findings

Figure 2.11.1: Four-chamber US view of fetal heart shows a diminutive left ventricle, enlarged right ventricle, echogenic bundle in mitral valve (atretic), and enlarged right atrium.

Figure 2.11.2: Panoramic four-chamber US scan shows a small non-apical-forming left ventricle with brightly echogenic left endocardium (fibroelastosis), large oval foramen and right atrium, and dilated pulmonary veins. Thoracic descending aorta is normal.

Figure 2.11.3: Three-vessel view shows compensatory dilated pulmonary trunk adjacent to the superior vena cava with a nonvisible aortic arch.

Figure 2.11.4: Four-chamber color Doppler US demonstrates absence of flow through the mitral valve.

Case 12: Branchio-Oto-Renal Syndrome

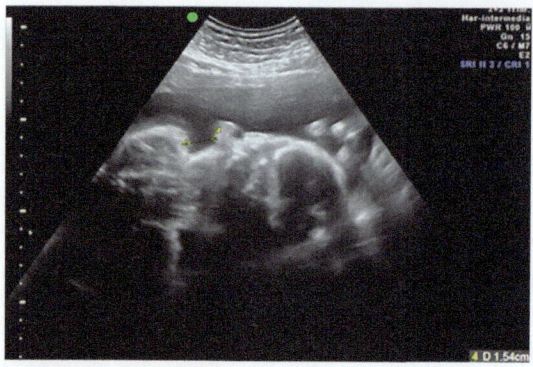

Fig. 2.12.1

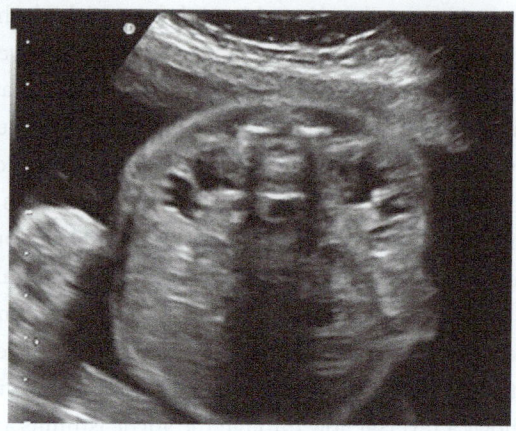

Fig. 2.12.3

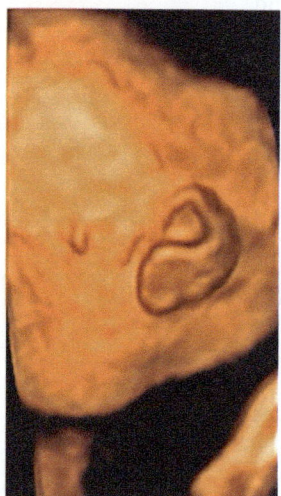

Fig. 2.12.2

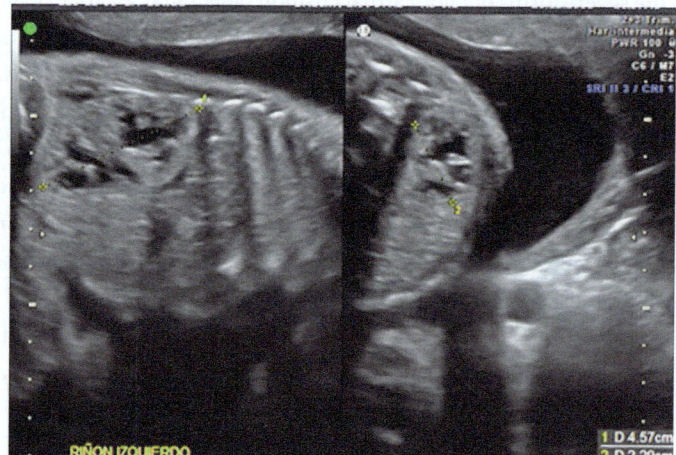

Fig. 2.12.4

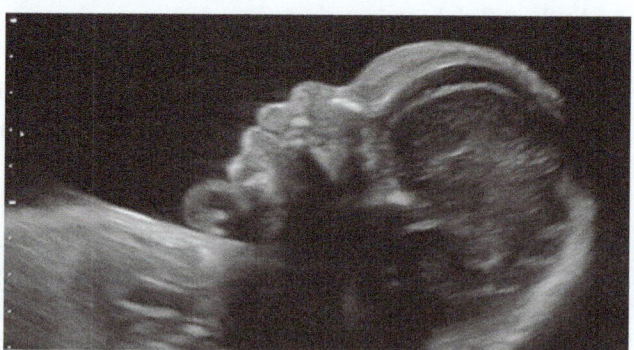

Fig. 2.12.5

Branchio-oto-renal (BOR) syndrome is a dominant genetic disorder that can result in ear pits, hearing loss, branchial (neck) cysts or fistulas, and kidney anomalies. Individuals with BOR usually do not suffer all these symptoms; thus, BOR is said to have variable expression. Although these are the most common symptoms, many others have been reported but are not common.

The most common symptom is hearing loss that is found in more than 90 % of patients and can be highly variable. Ear pits, that are small holes immediately in front of the top of the ear, are found in about 80 % of patients. Some individuals have deformed outer ear(s), middle ear(s), and/or inner ear(s) and 13 % have preauricular tags.

About 60 % of the BOR patients have branchial cysts or fistulas which are small holes located on the front, external lower third of the neck. Some of these open into the throat and may drain fluid. Branchial cysts or fistulas are usually bilateral but may also be unilateral.

Renal anomalies are found in about 67 % of BOR patients. Most of the anomalies do not have clinical significance and involve minor changes in the anatomy of the kidney or urinary tract. They include renal agenesis (29 %), hypoplasia (19 %), dysplasia (14 %), ureteropelvic junction calyceal cyst/diverticulum (10 %), obstruction (10 %), pelviectasis, hydronephrosis, and vesicoureteral reflux (5 % each).

In the absence of a family history, three or more of the following major criteria or two major and two minor criteria must be present to make the clinical diagnosis of BOR syndrome:

1. Major criteria:
   (a) Second branchial arch anomalies
   (b) Preauricular pits
   (c) Auricular deformity
   (d) Renal anomalies
2. Minor criteria:
   (a) External auditory canal anomalies
   (b) Inner ear anomalies
   (c) Preauricular tags
   (d) Other: facial asymmetry and palate abnormalities

Comments

Figure 2.12.1: Coronal US scan of the head at 29 weeks shows abnormal ear.

Imaging Findings

Figure 2.12.2: 3D US scan of the external ear shows deformity, preauricular pits, and tags.

Figure 2.12.3: Transverse US scan of the upper abdomen shows bilateral mild caliectasis.

Figure 2.12.4: Longitudinal and transverse US scan of the left kidney shows mild caliectasis without pelviectasis (megacalycosis).

Figure 2.12.5: Sagittal US scan of the face shows short palate.

Case 13: OEIS Syndrome

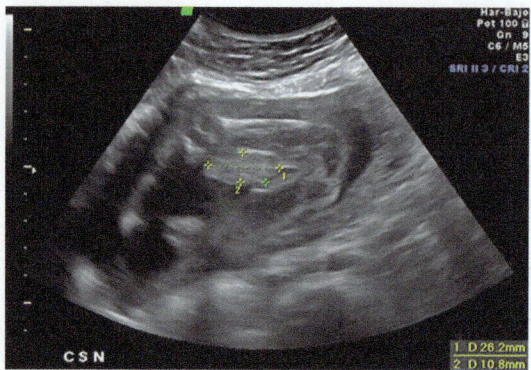

Fig. 2.13.1

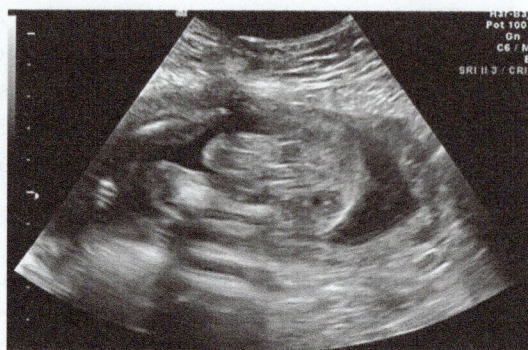

Fig. 2.13.2

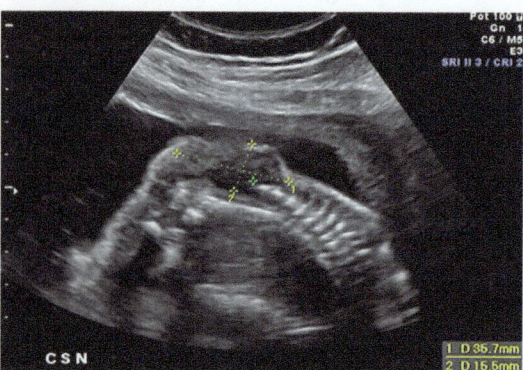

Fig. 2.13.3

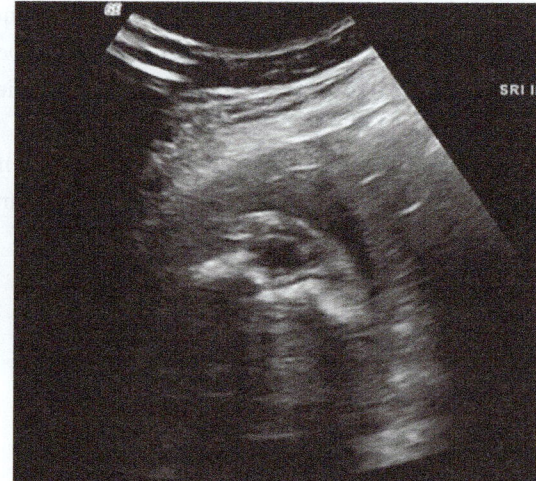

Fig. 2.13.4

The OEIS malformative complex associates an omphalocele, cloacal exstrophy, imperforated anus, and spinal defects. This rare complex is believed to represent the most severe end of a spectrum of birth defects, the exstrophy-epispadias sequence, which, in order of increasing severity, includes phallic separation with epispadias, pubic diastasis, bladder exstrophy and cloacal exstrophy, and OEIS complex.

The incidence of the OEIS complex is very low and has been reported to be 1 in 200,000–400,000 pregnancies. The majority of cases are sporadic, but it has been rarely reported in patients with family members having similar malformations. The etiology of the OEIS complex is still unclear. It is believed to result from a single defect in development of infraumbilical mesoderm, a precursor to infraumbilical mesenchyme, cloacal septum, and caudal spine.

In the OEIS (omphalocele-exstrophy-imperforate anus-spinal defects) complex, exstrophy of the cloaca includes the persistence and exstrophy of a common cloaca that receives the ileum, the ureters, and a rudimentary hindgut and is associated with a wide range of urinary tract anomalies with failure of fusion of the genital tubercles, widely separated pubic bones, congenital vertebral malformations with spinal dysraphism, imperforate anus, cryptorchidism and bifid penis in males, and anomalies of the mullerian duct derivatives in females. Moreover, omphalocele is common, and most patients have a single umbilical artery.

The prenatal diagnosis of OEIS is possible by the detection of:
1. A persistent cloaca; a midline infraumbilical defect with an irregular mass can be detected in the inferior abdominal wall or cystic anterior wall structure (persistent cloacal membrane) or with omphalocele.
2. Nonvisualization of the bladder between the two umbilical arteries.
3. Lumbosacral myelomeningocele. Always found. Common spinal defects include hemivertebrae, sacral anomalies, and either tethered cord and meningocystocele. The spinal defects are not restricted to the lumbosacral region.
4. Omphalocele.
5. Anomalies of the inferior limbs.
6. Wide pubic arch is usually present with symphysis pubis diastasis and congenital hip dislocation.
7. Single umbilical artery.
8. Genital anomalies. The sex determination is often not possible.
9. Anal atresia.

The prognosis is variable and depends on the severity of the structural defects. Survival will depend on the extension of the cloacal exstrophy and the neural tube defect. In mild forms, a good outcome with corrective surgery is possible. Cloacal exstrophy is lethal due to obstruction of the urinary tract and association with renal and pulmonary complications.

Comments

Figure 2.13.1: Transverse US scan of the pelvis at 21 weeks shows a mass between the legs.

Imaging Findings

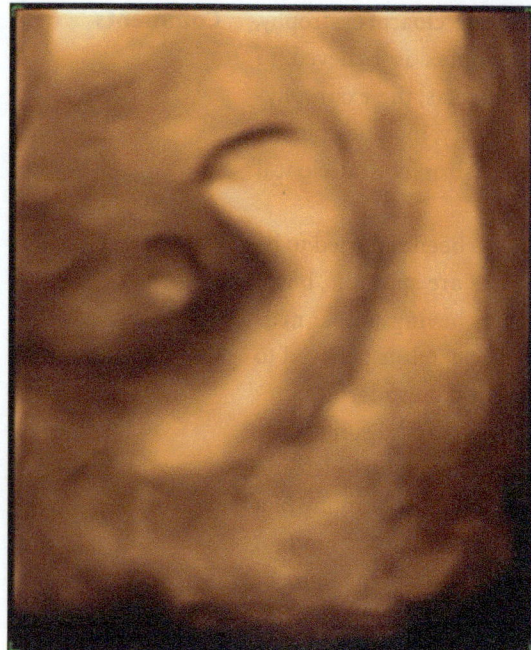

Fig. 2.13.5

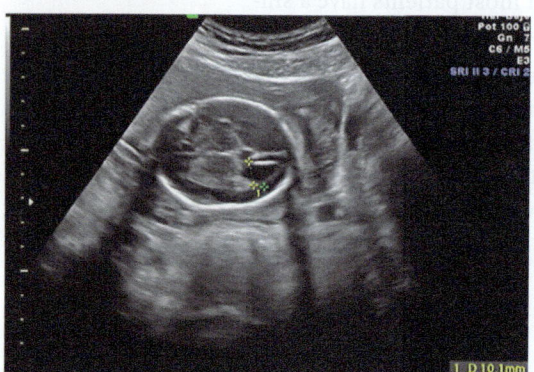

Fig. 2.13.6

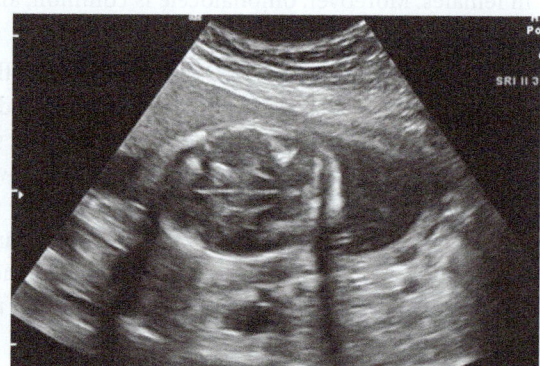

Fig. 2.13.7

Fig. 2.13.8

Figure 2.13.2: Transverse US scan of the low abdomen shows a large anterior wall defect with an echoic mass floating in the amniotic fluid. There is no evidence of bladder.

Figure 2.13.3: Sagittal view shows the spinal defect with myelomeningocele over the lower back of the fetus. The skin seems intact.

Figure 2.13.4: Transverse view shows the lumbosacral spinal defect.

Figure 2.13.5: 3D view of left leg shows the clubfoot.

Figure 2.13.6: Color Doppler US shows a single umbilical artery.

Figure 2.13.7: Transverse US scan of the brain shows mild ventriculomegaly (11 mm).

Figure 2.13.8: Transverse US scan of the posterior fossa shows a banana-shaped cerebellum, no visible cisterna magna, and nuchal skin fold thickness of 7 mm.

Case 14: Exencephaly

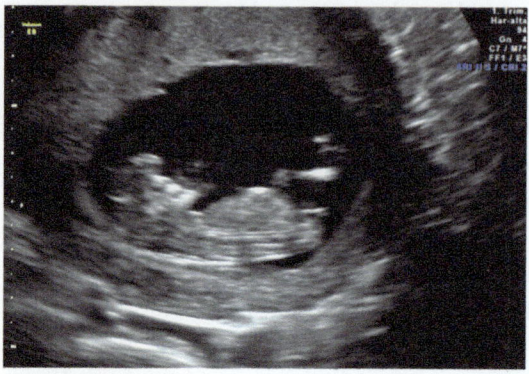

Fig. 2.14.1

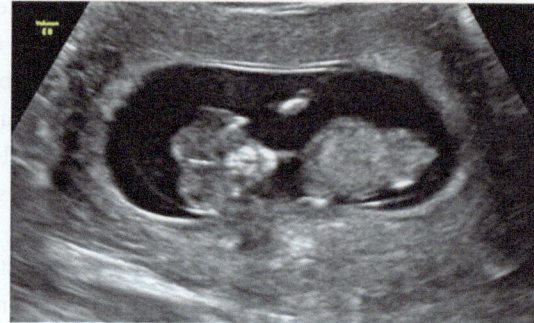

Fig. 2.14.2

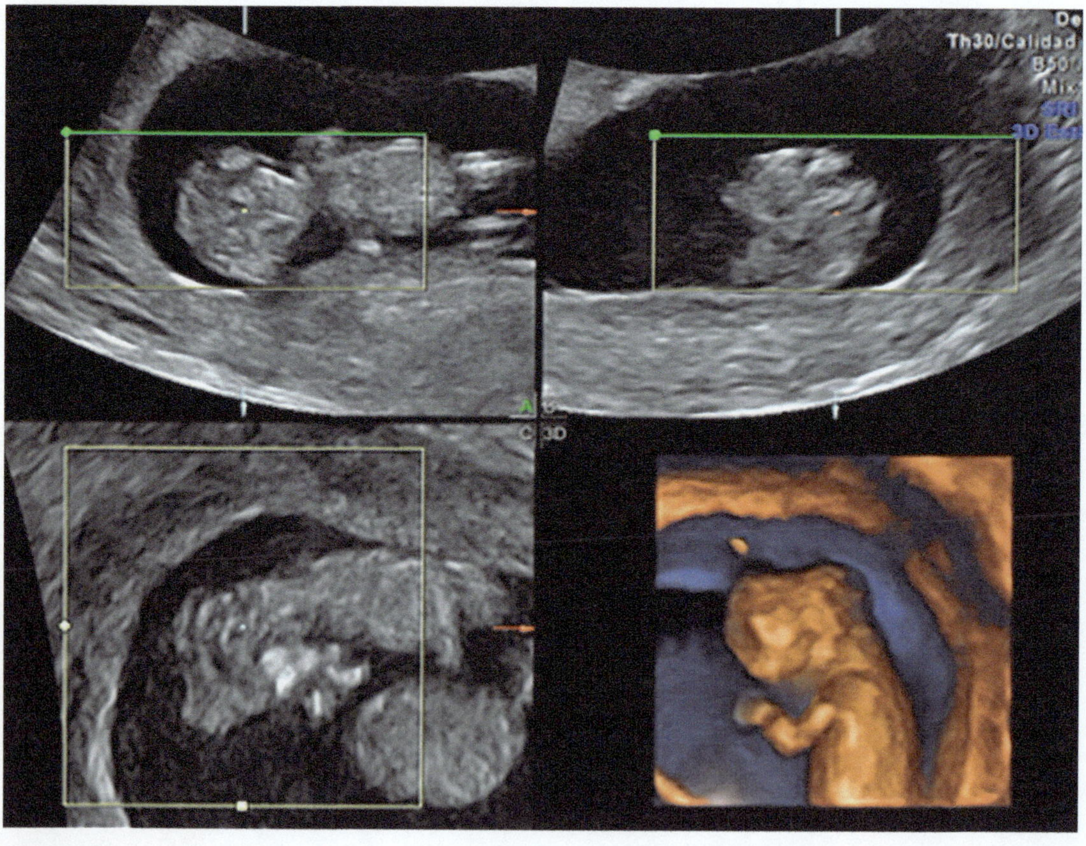

Fig. 2.14.3

Exencephaly, considered part of acrania/exencephaly/anencephaly sequence, is a rare and fatal anomaly characterized by absence of the bones of the cranial vault with a large amount of protruding brain tissue into the amniotic cavity. It is secondary to the failure of the closing of the neural tube during the fourth week of embryonic development, similar to spina bifida but in the proximal fetal pole. This anomaly can be detected early in gestation, when the normal calcification of the cranial bones is not detected. Later in gestation, the most common finding is the presence of a large quantity of disorganized brain tissue. Exencephaly is a rare embryological precursor of anencephaly in which a large amount of brain tissue is present despite the absence of the calvaria. In these cases, the brain consists of a disorganized, anarchic outgrowth of nervous tissue with polymicrogyria and nodular heterotopia. It can be associated with other anomalies such as spinal abnormalities, cleft lip, cleft palate, amniotic bands, omphalocele, and pentalogy of Cantrell.

Sonographic diagnosis of anencephaly is usually possible in early second trimester (10–14 weeks). Conventional 2D ultrasound is accurate in diagnosing anencephaly, and the sensitivity is virtually 100 % after 14 weeks. 3D US has been shown to be equally effective in detecting anencephaly, but 3D is preferred to provide information to the parents.

On US, the cranial vault (bony calvarium) is symmetrically absent. Rudimentary brain tissue (area cerebrovasculosa) is covered by a layer, but not bone. This can be seen protruding from the base of the skull in the early second trimester and gradually degenerates until the appearance of the head is completely flattened behind the facial structures. Facial views reveal a frog-like appearance and prominent bulging eyeballs. Associated polyhydramnios can be detected in the second trimester and is likely due to absent or ineffective fetal swallowing. High degree of fetal activity is often observed. Sonographic pitfalls in the diagnosis of anencephaly usually revolve around difficulties in imaging such as vertex presentation with deep head location. Differentiation of anencephaly from severe microcephaly or large encephaloceles can also be difficult, but in these conditions, the cranial vault is always present. Amniotic band syndrome associated with cranial disruption may also mimic anencephaly, but usually the cranial defect is asymmetric.

The key points for early US diagnosis of exencephaly are:
1. Absent cranium.
2. A large amount of disorganized brain tissue extending from a malformed skull base.
3. Exposed brain had a lobulated or spiked appearance (Mickey Mouse or Bart Simpson head shape).
4. Crown-rump length (CRL) less than expected.
5. Often protuberant eyes.
6. Often contiguous with cervical spine defect or associated with lumbar myelomeningocele.

Comments

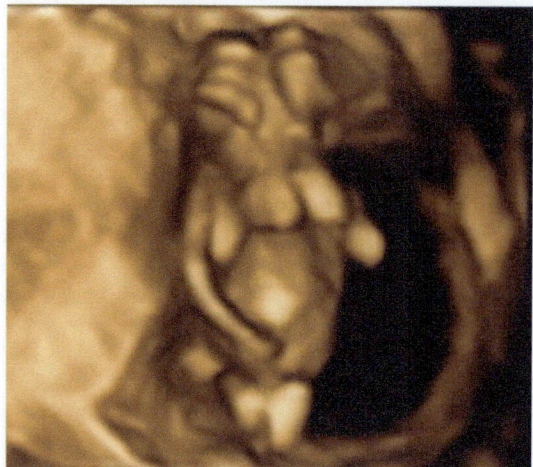

Fig. 2.14.4

Figure 2.14.1: Sagittal transabdominal US scan of a 13-week fetus shows absence of cranial vault and large amount of brain tissue into the amniotic cavity.

Figure 2.14.2: Coronal transabdominal US scan demonstrates heterogeneous and disorganized brain tissue into the amniotic cavity (Mickey Mouse head shape).

Figure 2.14.3: Transabdominal US shows absence of cranial vault and large amount of disorganized brain tissue into the amniotic cavity.

Figure 2.14.4: Transabdominal 3D US scan demonstrates a symmetrically absent bony calvarium and disorganized, heterogeneous, and lobulated brain tissue.

Imaging Findings

Further Reading

Allen RH, Benson CB, Haug LW (2005) Pregnancy outcome of fetuses with a diagnosis of hypoplastic left ventricle on prenatal sonography. J Ultrasound Med 24:1199–1203

Anandakumar C, Nuruddin M, Wong YC, Chia D (2002) Routine screening with fetal echocardiography for prenatal diagnosis of congenital heart disease. Ultrasound Rev Obtet Gynecol 2:50–55

Austin PF, Homsy YL, Gearhart JP, Porter K, Guidi C, Madsen K, Maizels M (1999) The prenatal diagnosis of cloacal exstrophy. J Urol 160:1179–1181

Bardo DM, Frankel DG, Applegate KE, Murphy DJ, Saneto RP (2001) Hypoplastic left heart syndrome. Radiographics 21:705–717

Becker R, Mende B, Stiemer B et al (2000) Sonographic markers of exencephaly at 9 + 3 weeks of gestation. Ultrasound Obstet Gynecol 16:582–584

Calderaro J, Espie M, Duclos J, Giachetti S, Wehrer D, Sandid W, Cahen-Doidy L, Albiter M, Janin A, de Roquancourt A (2009) Breast intracystic papillary carcinoma: an update. Breast J 15:639–644

Caoili EM, Hertzberg BS, Kliewer MA, DeLong D, Bowie JD (2000) Refractory shadowing from pelvic masses on sonography: a useful diagnostic sign for uterine leiomyomas. AJR Am J Roentgenol 174:97–101

Chang EH, Menezes M, Meyer NC, Cucci RA, Vervoort VS, Schwartz CE, Smith RJ (2004) Branchio-oto-renal syndrome: the mutation spectrum in EYA1 and its phenotypic consequences. Hum Mutat 23:582–589

Chang HC, Bhatt S, Dogra VS (2008) Pearls and pitfalls in diagnosis of ovarian torsion. Radiographics 28:1355–1368

Chatzipapas IK, Whitlow BJ, Economides DL (1999) The 'Mickey Mouse' sign and the diagnosis of anencephaly in early pregnancy. Ultrasound Obstet Gynecol 13:196–199

Chung J, Son EJ, Kim J et al (2011) Giant phyllodes tumors of the breast: imaging findings with clinicopathological correlation in 14 cases. Clin Imaging 35:102–107

Drose JA (2010) Fetal echocardiography, 2nd edn. Saunders Elsevier, St. Louis, pp 131–144

Eisenberg P, Cohen HL, Coren C (1992) Color Doppler in pulmonary sequestration diagnosis. J Ultrasound Med 11:175–176

Hall DA, Yoder IC (1994) Ultrasound evaluation of the uterus. In: Callen PW (ed) Ultrasonography in obstetrics and gynecology, 3rd edn. Saunders, Philadelphia, pp 586–614

Hata T et al (2000) Three-dimensional sonographic features of fetal central nervous system anomaly. Acta Obstet Gynecol Scand 79:635–639

Jeong YY, Outwater EK, Kang HK (2000) Imaging evaluation of ovarian masses. Radiographics 20:1445–1470

Keppler-Noreuil KM (2001) OEIS (omphalocele-exstrophy-imperforate anus-spinal defects): a review of 14 cases. Am J Med Genet 99:271–279

Logan WW, Hoffman NJ (1989) Diabetic fibrous breast disease. Radiology 172:667–670

Machado RA, Brizot ML, Carvalho MH et al (2005) Sonographic markers of exencephaly below 10 weeks' gestation. Prenat Diagn 25:31–33

Neetua G, Pathmanathana R, Wengb NK (2010) Diabetic mastopathy: a case report and literature review. Oncol 3:245–251

Outwater EK, Siegelman ES (2001) Ovarian teratomas: tumor types and imaging characteristics. Radiographics 21:475–490

Park SB, Kim JK, Kim KR (2008) Imaging findings of complications and unusual manifestations of ovarian teratomas. Radiographics 28:969–983

Puglisi F, Zuiani C, Bazzocchi M, Valent F, Aprile G, Pertoldi B, Minisini AM, Cedolini C, Londero V, Piga A, Di Loreto C (2003) Role of mammography, ultrasound and large core biopsy in the diagnostic evaluation of papillary breast lesions. Oncology 65:311–315

Romero R, Chervenak FA, Kotzen J, Berkowitz RL, Hobbins JC (1982) Antenatal sonographic findings of extralobar pulmonary sequestration. J Ultrasound Med 1:131–132

Rosen PP (2001) Rosen's breast pathology, 2nd edn. Lippincott Williams & Wilkins, Philadelphia, pp 73–74

Sanerbrei E (1991) Lung sequestration: duplex Doppler diagnosis at 19 weeks gestation. J Ultrasound Med 10:101–105

Schut D, Stovall DW (1993) Leiomyoma of the fallopian tube: a case report. J Reprod Med 38:741–742

Stavros AT (2003) Breast ultrasound, 1st edn. Lippincott Williams & Wilkins, Philadelphia

Tan H, Zhang S, Liu H et al (2011) Imaging findings in phyllodes tumors of the breast. Eur J Radiol. doi:10.1016/j.ejrad.2011.01.085

Verheijen PM, Lisowski LA, Plantinga R et al (2003) Prenatal diagnosis of the fetus with hypoplastic left heart syndrome. Herz 28:250–256

Vijayaraqhavan SB (2004) Sonographic whirlpool sign in ovarian torsion. J Ultrasound Med 23:1643–1649

Weinbaum PJ, Bors-Koefoed R, Green K (1989) Antenatal ultrasonographic findings in a case of intra-abdominal pulmonary sequestration. Obstet Gynecol 73:860–861

Musculoskeletal Ultrasound

3

Angel Bueno, Jose Martel, and Ana Sanz

Introduction

Until the beginning of the millennium, ultrasound had offered, in the musculoskeletal system, a performance well below those of magnetic resonance, thus contributing to a poor penetration and limited use of this technique. However, the gradual improvement in ultrasound technology has had a special impact on the exploration of the musculoskeletal system, making ultrasound to become from a complementary test into an exploration of choice for many lesions, especially in the muscle and the surface. The most important factor has been the emergence of high-resolution linear transducers, sometimes of very small size, which allow exploring superficial structures with a spatial resolution that exceeds that obtained with conventional magnetic resonance and at lower cost.

In addition, ultrasound explorations have, in experienced hands, a lower scan time than magnetic resonance scans and are far more available than magnetic resonance. Also, there are portable ultrasound platforms with excellent image quality that allow point-of-care explorations in the sports world. Furthermore, MRI has a poor performance in identifying calcium and calcifying tendinitis or enthesopathy.

Ultrasound allows also performing dynamic studies, which are useful in several circumstances, for example, in the differential diagnosis of partial or complete tear of a tendon, demonstrating the latter by provocative maneuvers of separation of tendon ends, and also in subluxation or dislocation of muscles, tendons, or nerves which can occur only with specific movements or maneuvers. These dislocations may be reduced in neutral position and therefore cannot be detected with conventional magnetic resonance. And finally, ultrasound allows performing a wide range of image-guided interventional procedures. Ultrasound and MRI are now, therefore, complementary and both necessary techniques in the evaluation of musculoskeletal pathology.

However, it should be kept in mind that musculoskeletal ultrasound is a heavily operator-dependent technique. The quality and reliability of the study depends on the experience of the performer and requires detailed knowledge of anatomy, ultrasound artifacts, and normal and abnormal appearance of different structures. This technique requires a long learning curve, and it is not always easy to find centers or training programs to learn it.

J.L. del Cura et al. (eds.), *Learning Ultrasound Imaging*, Learning Imaging,
DOI 10.1007/978-3-642-30586-3_3, © Springer-Verlag Berlin Heidelberg 2012

Case 1: Gastrocnemius Muscle Tear and Thrombosis of the Gastrocnemius Veins

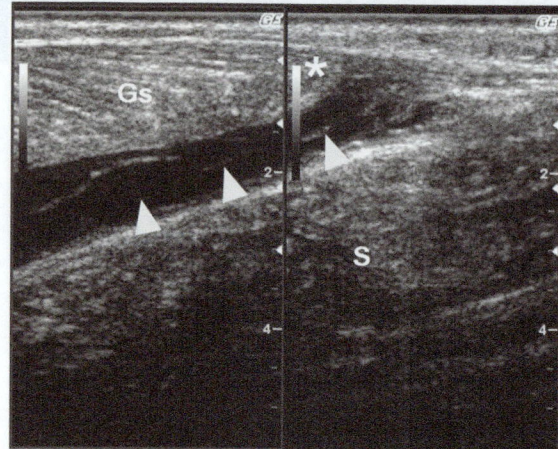

Fig. 3.1.1

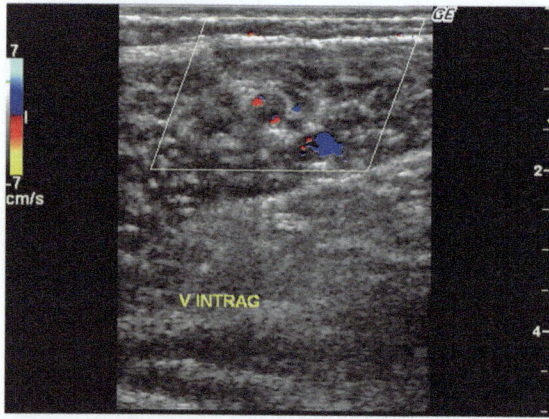

Fig. 3.1.2

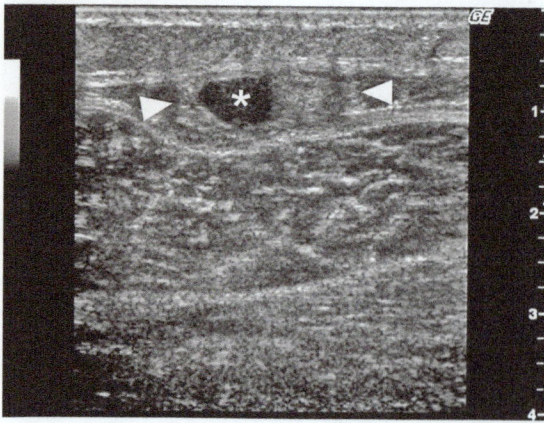

Fig. 3.1.3

Muscular lesions are caused by direct or indirect traumatisms, frequently during sporting activity. Usually, the patient remembers the event that caused the lesion because of having felt sudden pain and functional impotence. In the case of gastrocnemius tear, the patient reports the sensation of being beaten in the leg from behind.

Lesions can be intramuscular or located in the muscular attachments to fascias or tendons. Gastrocnemius tears typically occur in the distal musculotendinous junction of the inner gastrocnemius and are generally due to distension after stretching, indirect traumatism.

As in the rest of muscle tears, gastrocnemius tears can be classified in grades:
- Grade I or stretching is indistinguishable from muscular, persistent contraction and is usually a microscopic lesion. US may show a normal appearance or a discrete alteration in focal echogenicity with mild edema.
- Grade II (partial rupture) is a wider tear, and grade III (complete rupture) is a full-thickness tear with threaded edges and muscular retraction. Both show functional impotence, pain to local palpation, and tumefaction with cutaneous hematoma. Complete rupture can even show discontinuity on palpation. US shows both the muscle disruption and a hematoma that extends along the fascia between the gastrocnemius and the soleus muscles. When exploring with ultrasound, it is important not to press with the probe to avoid the collapse of the hematoma and thus underestimate the lesion grade. Those collections slowly reabsorb within weeks.

A dynamic study can be performed doing muscular contraction to evaluate the grade of separation between the broken stumps (separation of the torn extremes with contraction is the so-called clapper sign that is specific for muscular ruptures, though it can be observed both in partial and complete tears).

Lesion repair used to be the product of a dense fibrous scar formation. On recuperation, the follow-up US study will show a hyperechogenic wall corresponding to granulation tissue that is thicker with time and replenishes the hematic cavity. Muscular tear healing is slow, taking 3–16 weeks, but calf lesions take more time for healing than other localizations.

US can be also useful to diagnose possible secondary complications of gastrocnemius tears, like the thrombosis of the gastrocnemius veins, and to perform percutaneous evacuations of the hematoma to accelerate the healing process.

Comments

Figure 3.1.1 Longitudinal image of the posterior compartment of the leg showing a tear in the distal musculotendinous junction of the medial gastrocnemius with retraction of the muscular mass (clapper sign) (*asterisk*). An anechoic hematoma extends along the fascia between the gastrocnemius (Gs) and the soleus (S) muscles (*arrowheads*).

Figure 3.1.2 Intramuscular vein thrombosis in the same patient. The color Doppler study shows noncompressible veins inside the gastrocnemius muscle with echogenic inner content and no flow.

Figure 3.1.3 Transversal image of gastrocnemius tear evolution demonstrating peripheral fibrosis (*arrowheads*) and central residual hematoma (*asterisk*).

Imaging Findings

Case 2: Achilles Tendon Rupture

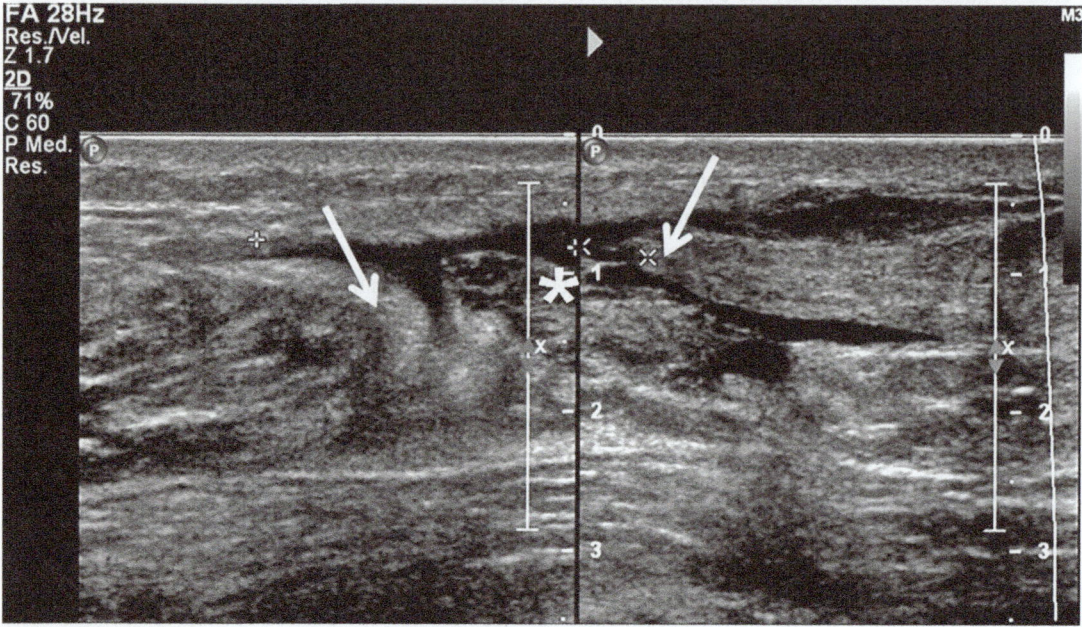

Fig. 3.2.1

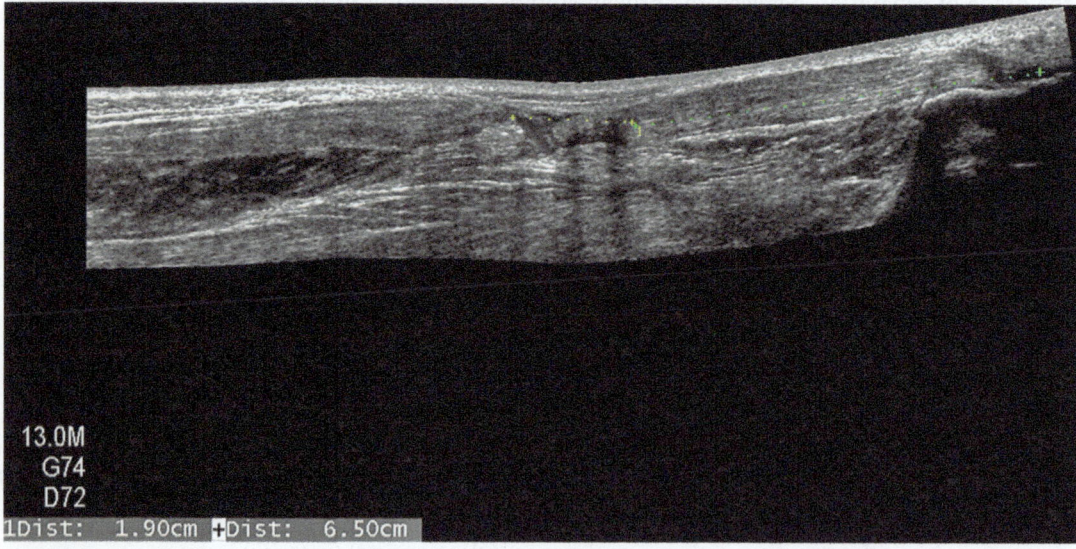

Fig. 3.2.2

Tendon tears can be the result of a direct penetrating traumatism or of an indirect traumatism due to overload, mainly during sporting activity. When ruptures are not associated to previous traumatism, they usually occur in weakened areas of the tendon because of previous tendinopathy. Tendon ruptures frequently occur near the attachment to the bone.

Achilles tendon ruptures are more frequent in male, between 30 and 50 years old. They appear 4–6 cm proximal to the calcaneal insertion, because this is the less vascularized part of the tendon. Degenerative changes with chronic tendinopathy predispose to Achilles tendon rupture, an acute traumatism being the immediate cause of the tear. Ruptures in the muscle-tendon junction and in the calcaneal insertion are less frequent.

The patient experiences an acute pain that is felt by the patient as a kick from behind, with functional impotence to dorsiflexion.

A positive Thompson test consistent on failure of plantar flexion with squeezing of the calf used to be enough to diagnose an Achilles tendon complete rupture. However, under suspicion of Achilleal tear, US is usually indicated to distinguish partial- from full-thickness ruptures (essential for treatment planning), to measure the extension and separation between the torn extremes (tendons which have their fibers oriented longitudinally show a remarkable retraction of the broken stumps), and to describe the localization of the tear (important for therapeutic planning as lacerations in the muscle-tendon junction usually do not require surgical treatment). Moreover, US evaluates plantaris tendon integrity that should not be mistaken with Achilles tendon preserved fibers.

Sonographic evaluation of the patient is performed on decubitus position, with patient's foot hanging over the edge of the bed and exploring from the origin in the junction of gastrocnemius muscles to the calcaneal insertion.

A sonographic diagnosis of Achilleal rupture is done after seeing a full interruption of the tendon thickness. In the acute phase, a hematoma is frequently seen between the torn extremes of the tendon. This hematoma is hyperechoic initially and, together with the ill delimitation of the tendon extremes, can make the diagnosis difficult and lead to the underestimation of the extent of the rupture. For that reason, it is better to perform the US evaluation 24–48 h after the onset of the symptoms, when the hematoma becomes anechoic.

A dynamic study of ankle in dorsiflexion is also useful to detect tears and distinguish complete from partial ruptures.

Comments

Imaging Findings

Figure 3.2.1 Longitudinal scan of the Achilles tendon showing full-thickness tear of Achilles tendon, with distraction of extremes (*arrows*). Fluid and hyperechoic content can also be observed in the tear (*asterisk*).

Figure 3.2.2 Panoramic image of the Achilles tendon showing the tear and two measurements: the distance between both extremes of the torn tendon and the distance to the calcaneal insertion.

Case 3: Myositis Ossificans

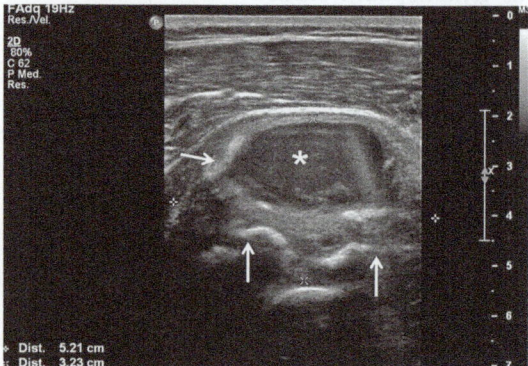

Fig. 3.3.1

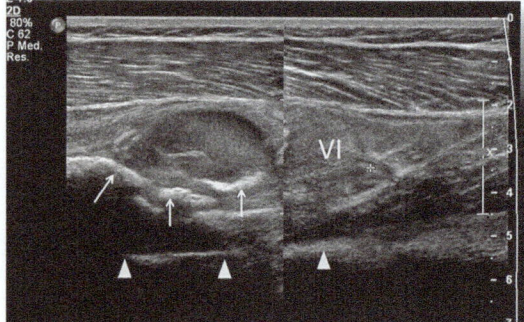

Fig. 3.3.2

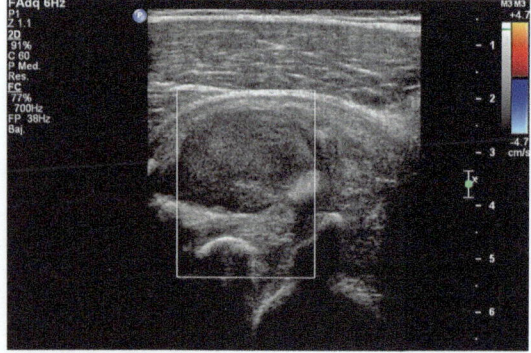

Fig. 3.3.3

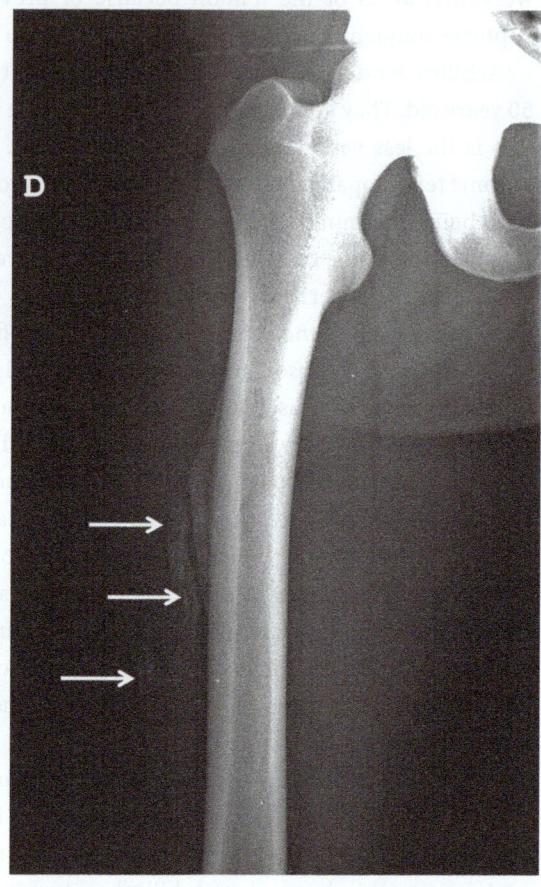

Fig. 3.3.4

Case Presentation   Young sportsman with a painful tumor in the thigh of 1-month evolution time

Comments   Myositis ossificans is a rare and benign complication of muscular lesions that usually appears following a traumatism with hematoma. Frequently, the traumatism is not severe, and the lesion is not linked to a traumatism in up to 40 % of the cases. In most of the cases, it occurs in the extremities, the thighs being the most frequent localization, especially the vastus intermedius muscle.

Patients are usually young adults that after a mild traumatism present a painful and persistent mass disproportionate to the initial lesion. The identification of myositis ossificans is an important issue as its growth causes chronic pain. Documentation of those lesions can avoid diagnostic errors because they can be mistaken with malignant processes.

Histologically, myositis ossificans is made of nonneoplastic metaplastic bone in subcutaneous tissues or musculature, which develops on the original hematoma. The process is long lasting, representing the different phases of myositis ossificans.

At the onset of the process, X-ray films are not useful as no calcifications exist yet. In the first 3 weeks, ultrasound study identifies a heterogeneous soft tissue mass. On Doppler US, it usually shows no evidence of vascularization, although occasionally it can be seen. In this phase, myositis ossificans is difficult to distinguish from an organized hematoma or from a soft tissue neoplasm. However, the combination of the US findings – well-defined lesion, poorly or not vascularized – and the history can orientate the diagnosis. In this phase, MRI may also show edema and a heterogeneous pattern that can be misinterpreted as a sarcoma. A biopsy taken from the center of the lesion may lead to diagnose a malignant tumor due to the presence of immature and mitotic cells.

At weeks 3–4, the first calcifications appear. Those calcifications can be identified earlier on US than using conventional X-ray. They usually present a characteristic peripheral distribution.

At months 5–6, ossification appears and mature bone can be observed. The main differential diagnosis in this phase is with periosteal or parosteal sarcoma. On US, ossifications present acoustic shadowing. Sometimes, shadowing is strong and avoids the visualization of the intact periosteum of the underlying bone, thus making it difficult to rule out an aggressive condition. Changing the angle of the probe is useful in order to visualize the adjacent normal periosteum. It is also important to check that no abnormal soft tissue mass appears outside the calcification, as this can help to distinguish myositis ossificans from parosteal sarcoma.

Imaging Findings

Figure 3.3.1 Axial sonogram of the vastus intermedius muscle demonstrating an oval heterogeneous intramuscular mass with central hypoechogenic content (*) and coarse calcifications in the periphery (*arrows*).

Figure 3.3.2 Longitudinal view of vastus intermedius muscle (*VI*). Lesion with peripheral calcifications (*arrows*) in the muscle. The femur (*arrowheads*) can be seen at the bottom of the image.

Figure 3.3.3 Color Doppler ultrasound. The lesion shows no vascularization.

Figure 3.3.4 A radiograph of the femur demonstrates soft tissue calcifications adjacent to the cortical of the diaphysis (*arrows*).

Case 4: Morel-Lavallée Lesion

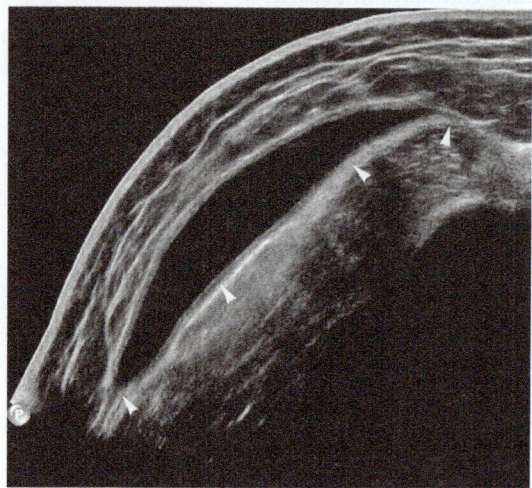

Fig. 3.4.1

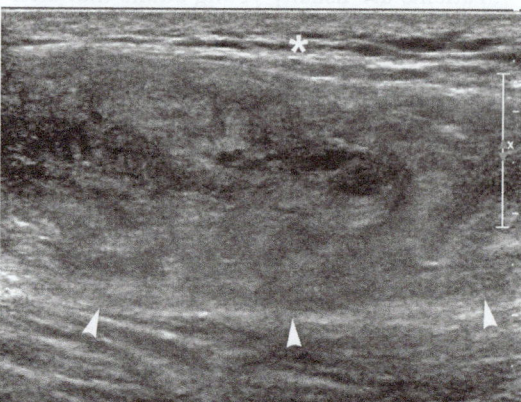

Fig. 3.4.2

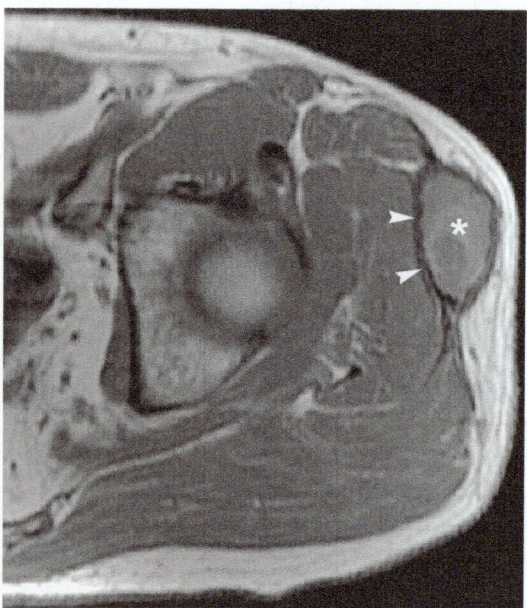

Fig. 3.4.3

Morel-Lavallée lesion is a posttraumatic seroma which most commonly develops along the trochanteric region and the proximal thigh between the deep layer of the subcutaneous tissue and the fascia. This lesion is defined as a blunt soft tissue injury caused by direct/tangential impact trauma that separates the hypodermis from the underlying fascia, causing a shearing injury. The sheared hemolymphatic supply of the involved tissues fills the perifascial plane with blood, lymph, and necrotic fat, creating a fluid-filled cavity.

US depicts Morel-Lavallée lesion as a fluid collection located just superficial to the echogenic fascia. Depending on the time of evolution and predominant contents of the lesion, the fluid collection can appear as hyperechoic (blood-predominant) or anechoic (lymph-predominant).

The differential diagnosis of Morel-Lavallée lesions includes abscesses, hematomas, fat necrosis, and neoplasms. In long-standing lesions, a reactive pseudocapsule may develop around the collection, and the organization of blood and debris can give it a heterogeneous appearance that may make it to be mistaken with a soft tissue tumor. In chronic lesions, the diagnosis can be difficult due to the slow growth of the mass, the local pain, and the absence of clear relationship with a previous trauma. Biopsy could be necessary in selected cases.

Morel-Lavallée lesions have a tendency to recur and can therefore become chronic sources of pain and infection. US-guided aspiration of fluid followed by local compression helps to prevent local recurrence.

Comments

Extended field-of-view US image obtained over the vastus lateralis in a patient with a mass in the thigh after a bike traumatism (Fig. 3.4.1) reveals a well-defined anechoic collection within the subcutaneous tissue in close relationship with the fascia (*arrowheads*). These are the typical findings of acute Morel-Lavallée lesions.

After 4 months, a new US exam is performed. Ultrasonography (Fig. 3.4.2) shows a well-defined hyperechoic lesion with slightly internal anechoic cystic-like lesions. The mass is separating the subcutaneous fatty tissue (*asterisk*) from the underlying fascia (*void arrowheads*). No Doppler signal was demonstrated. On MRI, axial T1-weighted image of hip (Fig. 3.4.3) shows long-standing Morel-Lavallée lesion (*asterisk*) in deep subcutaneous plane adjacent to fascia lata. The lesion is mildly hyperintense and appears surrounded by a thick hypointense capsule (*arrowheads*) suggesting a subacute hematoma.

Imaging Findings

Case 5: Primary Hydatid Cyst of the Skeletal Muscle

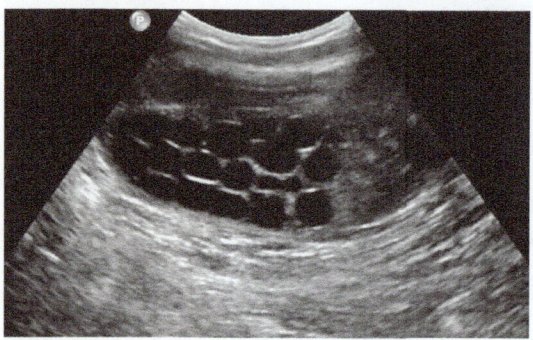

Fig. 3.5.1

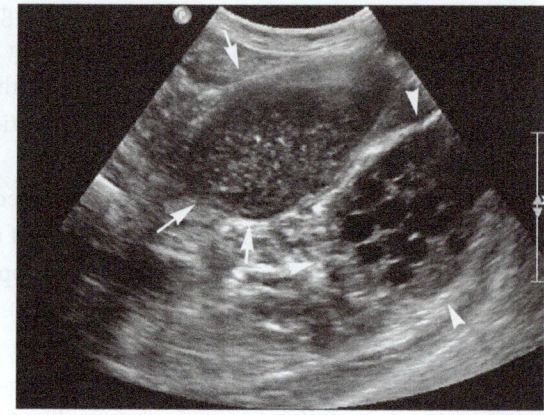

Fig. 3.5.2

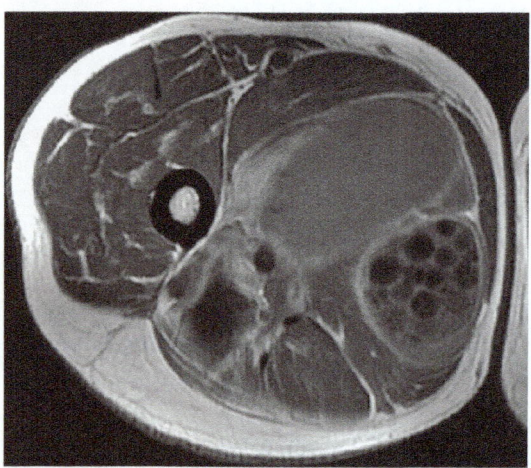

Fig. 3.5.3

Hydatid disease is a parasitic disease that is endemic in many parts of the world. Hydatid disease can occur almost anywhere in the body and demonstrates a variety of imaging features that vary according to growth stage, associated complications, and involved organs. There are two types of *Echinococcus* infections. *E. granulosus* is the more common type, whereas *E. multilocularis* is less common but more invasive, mimicking a malignancy. The liver is the most frequent site of involvement.

Primary muscular hydatid disease is rare, with only some cases described in the literature. The low frequency of muscular involvement is explained by the fact that continual muscular contractions and the production of lactic acid prevent scolex implantation. It is often asymptomatic and progresses slowly, thus delaying the diagnosis.

Ultrasound is most often the key examination for orienting the diagnosis of any tumor of the soft tissues. Hydatid disease in the soft tissues may have variable appearances:

- Type I is a simple cyst with no internal architecture.
- Type II is a unilocular cyst with daughter vesicles or detached membranes.
- Type III is characterized by calcification
- Type IV comprises hydatid cyst complications including rupture and infection.

MRI can be useful to provide a full picture of the locoregional extension of the lesion and its relations with the nerve and vascular pedicles. After injection of gadolinium, the cysts can present moderate peripheral enhancement because of the pericystic vascularization.

Treatment of muscular echinococcosis is surgical. The first-choice technique is pericystectomy.

Figure 3.5.1 On ultrasound imaging, a cyst with multiple daughter cysts is detected in the right thigh.

Figure 3.5.2 Transversal ultrasound image through the right thigh from a medial approach. Two different lesions are detected: a simple hypoechoic cyst (*white arrows*) and a cyst formation with daughter cysts (*arrowheads*).

Figure 3.5.3 Axial MRI T1-weighted image after gadolinium injection shows both cysts localized in the adductor compartment. Daughter cysts have a hypointense signal and showed relatively peripheral enhancement.

Comments

Imaging Findings

Case 6: Massive Rotator Cuff Tear

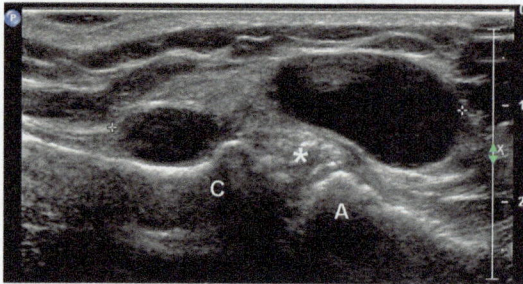

Fig. 3.6.1

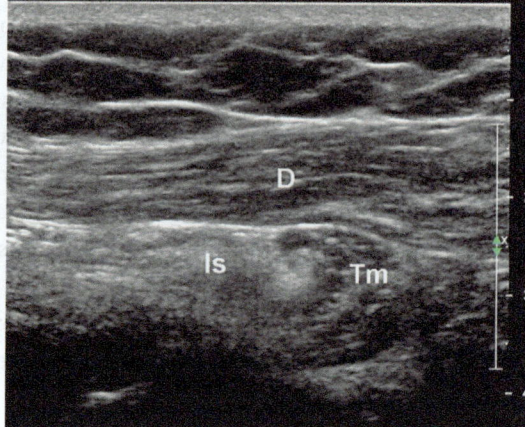

Fig. 3.6.3

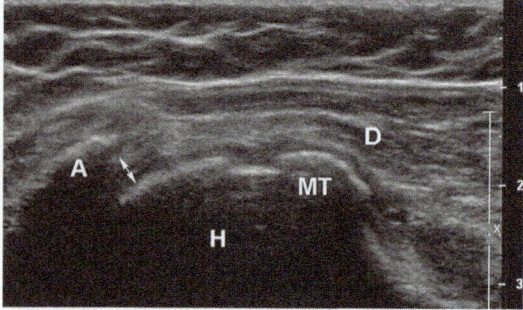

Fig. 3.6.2

Comments

The shoulder is the joint with more range of motion of our anatomy. The rotator cuff includes, from front to back, the subscapular, supraspinatus, infraspinatus, and torus minor tendons. The most frequent rotator cuff tear involves the supraspinatus tendon. Rotator cuff tears can be classified as full- or partial-thickness tears, depending on if there is communication between both surfaces of the tendon (articular and bursal surfaces) or not. If the full-thickness tears cannot involve the whole wide of the tendon (on its short axis), then they are incomplete tears. Incomplete full-thickness tears have several grades and shapes of fiber retraction (C, U, and L shapes). When the tear involves the whole wide of the tendon, it is called complete tear, and it usually has several grades of whole tendon retraction. Massive rupture is when the tear involves more than the whole wide of one tendon. The most frequent, massive rotator cuff ruptures involve the supraspinatus and infraspinatus tendons, which are the superior component of rotator cuff, located between the acromioclavicular arc and the humeral head. This subacromial space gets narrow when the massive rupture is chronic, with marked retraction of the tendons (bald humeral head sign), and upward displacement of the humeral head happens. Evident signs of long-standing massive rupture are fatty atrophic changes in the supraspinatus and infraspinatus muscles. The humeral head motion would be only covered by the deltoid muscle (anterior-laterally) and by the acromioclavicular joint and acromion (superior-posteriorly). The chronic microtrauma on the acromioclavicular joint produces degenerative changes, such as disk joint degeneration, capsule joint hypertrophic changes, osteophytosis, and synovial cysts, due to tearing of the acromioclavicular joint capsule. These cysts can only grow superiorly because there is no space under acromioclavicular joint. They can reach big size as a column of fluid extending from the glenohumeral joint, through the massive rotator cuff rupture, into the acromioclavicular joint. The acromioclavicular joint cyst and the massive rotator cuff tear are easily seen on ultrasound exploration. Dynamic ultrasound, pressing with the probe on the cyst, could demonstrate debris of the synovial fluid moving across the acromioclavicular joint. It is called "geyser sign" because of its similarity. The communication between the acromioclavicular joint cyst and the glenohumeral joint is better demonstrated on magnetic resonance and arthrography images. Acromioclavicular joint cysts may be associated with calcium pyrophosphate dihydrate deposition disease.

The clinical differential diagnoses include any tumor in the superior aspect of the shoulder. The lump may have soft- or firm-elastic consistency to the touch. Ultrasound quickly demonstrates its cystic nature. However, sometimes there are internal septa, synovial thickening, and debris leading to a more echogenic appearance. It is important to realize the relation between the pseudotumor and the chronic massive rotator cuff tear on ultrasound in order not to interpret it as a true tumor. US-guided aspiration and arthrography can be useful. On the other hand, it is important to be aware of the high recurrence rate after simple excision of the cyst, if the tear and joint pathology are not simultaneously treated.

Imaging Findings

Figure 3.6.1 Longitudinal ultrasound image through the acromioclavicular joint. There is a cystic lesion next to the acromioclavicular joint (*C*: clavicle, *A*: acromion). The joint disk and the hypertrophic articular capsule are seen as hyperechoic bulging tissue at the superior aspect of the joint (*).

Figure 3.6.2 Ultrasound image through the long axis of the superior rotator cuff. The cortex of the major tuberosity of the humerus (*MT*) is irregular. The superior aspect of the rotator cuff (supraspinatus and infraspinatus tendons) is missing due to tendon retraction after chronic massive rupture. The deltoid muscle (*D*) rests directly on the humeral head. Acromiohumeral space is narrowed (*double arrow*). *A*: acromion, *H*: humeral head.

Figure 3.6.3 Ultrasound image through the short axis of the infraspinatus (*Is*) and torus minor (*Tm*) muscles. The massive and chronic tear of supraspinatus and infraspinatus tendons causes atrophic changes in the muscles. This posterior approach ultrasound image to the short axis of these muscles, under scapula spine, shows the infraspinatus muscle smaller and hyperechoic relative to the torus minor muscle, due to fat atrophic changes.

Case 7: Hand Angiomyoma

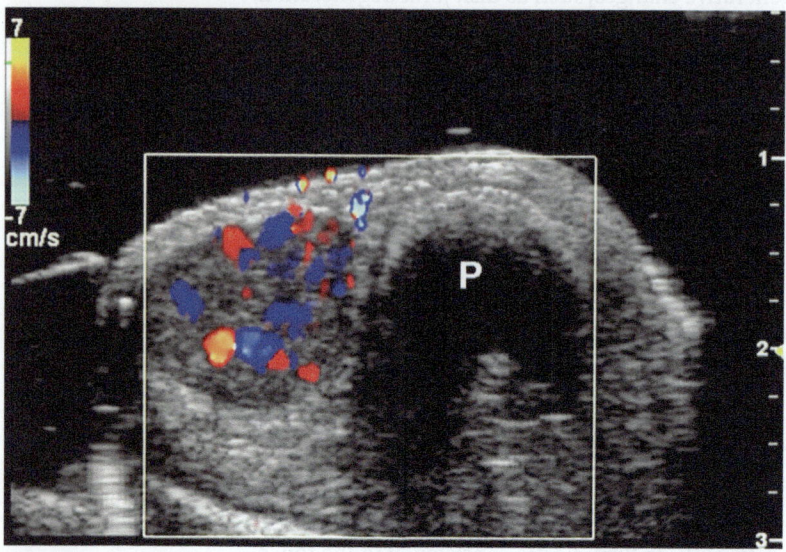

Fig. 3.7.1

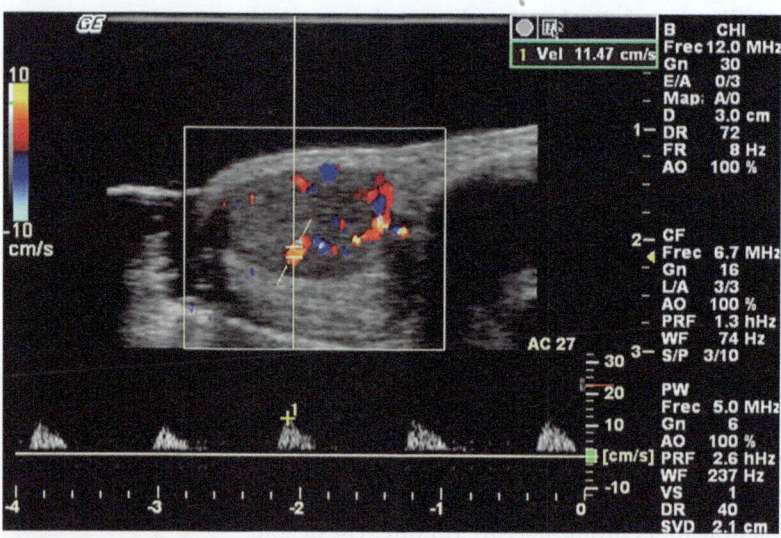

Fig. 3.7.2

Angiomyoma is a rare benign soft tissue tumor which arises from the muscularis media of small vessels, so it belongs to the group of smooth muscle benign tumors. The most frequent variety of angiomyoma is the solid subtype, like the tumor shown above. Angiomyoma is a small, elastic, and slowly growing tumor (frequently several years duration) with a predilection for subcutaneous fat limb location. The fact that it is an uncommon tumor and that its radiological appearance has seldom been described makes it very difficult to make a preoperative diagnosis. Gray-scale and Doppler US characteristic features allow distinguishing easily angiomyoma from more frequent soft tissue tumors in this location, such as ganglion/synovial cysts, inclusion epidermoid cysts, tendinous sheath tumors, or lipomas. It might be more difficult to distinguish it from some subcutaneous hemangiomas or vascular malformations which may also show arterial flow, but hemangiomas usually have a more heterogeneous structure, with fat tissue and frequent phleboliths. Another possible differential diagnosis is nerve sheath tumor, which may present dependence of the fibrillar nerve structure and less conspicuous flow, with a peripheral distribution. Also, nerve sheath tumors may show a target pattern, with a more echogenic center. Another very characteristic feature of angiomyoma is the presence of an afferent arterial vessel, which may be frequently demonstrated after a careful sonographic examination. Resistive indexes may be variable, even in vessels in the same tumor. Rarely, angiomyoma presents calcifications. From a clinical standpoint, angiomyoma may be asymptomatic, although not uncommonly, they may be painful.

Figure 3.7.1 Color Doppler ultrasound image, obtained from a dorsal approach, of a soft tissue mass in the third finger of the hand. There is an oval soft tissue mass with smooth borders within the dorsal and radial aspects of the subcutaneous fat. Skin and cortical bone are not involved, and the lesion does not show dependence of the tendinous sheath. Small vessels with arterial flow in different directions are seen within an echogenic homogeneous background. *P*: Phalanx.

Figure 3.7.2 Pulsed Doppler US of an intralesional vessel showing a high-resistance waveform.

Case 8: Giant Cell Tumor of the Tendon Sheath

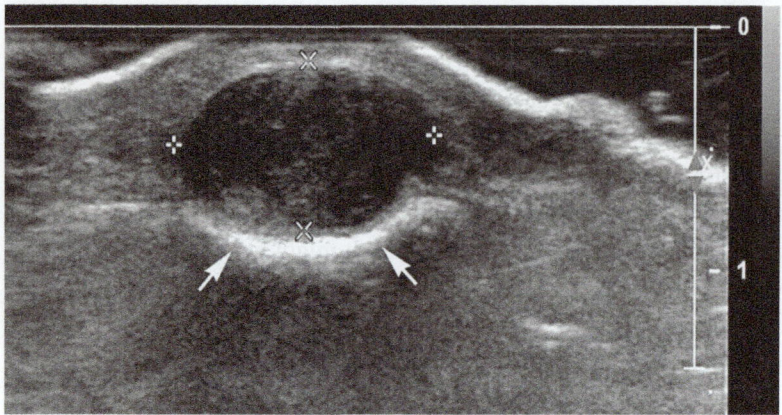

Fig. 3.8.1

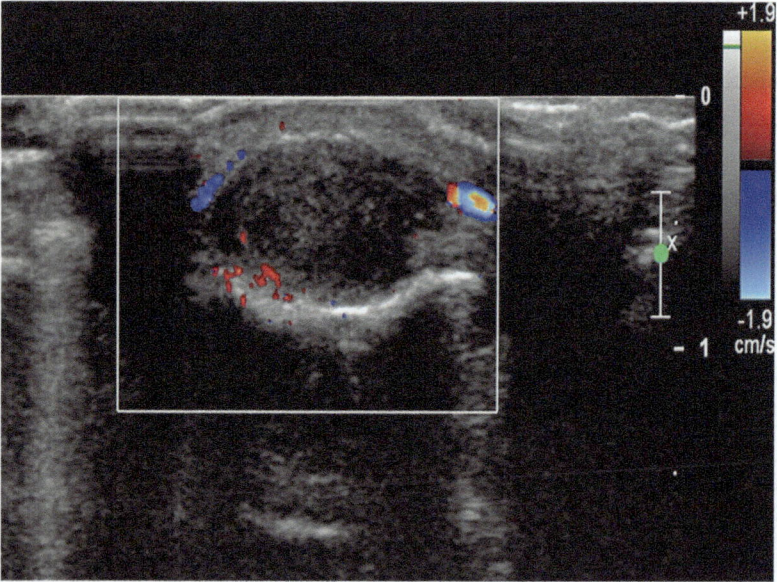

Fig. 3.8.2

The localized form of giant cell tumor of tendon sheath or nodular tenosynovitis is a process histologically similar to pigmented villonodular synovitis and represents its extra-articular analogue. It belongs to the group of benign fibrohistiocytic soft tissue tumors. It is one of the most common soft tissue masses of the hand, second in frequency after ganglion (it is approximately seven times more common than pigmented villonodular synovitis). The lesion most commonly affects the volar aspect of the digits, although lesions may be lateral or circumferential. It is most commonly located in the first three fingers. The second more frequent localization is in the foot (5–15 % of lesions), most often in the first two toes. Patients present with a slowly growing mass that may be painful, mainly with activity. It is freely mobile under the skin, but typically it has hard consistency and is attached to deeper structures (the tendon sheath from which it arises). Local recurrence is much less frequent than in the diffuse form, but it may be seen in about 7–44 % of cases. The lesion is typically a small (smaller than 2–4 cm), well-encapsulated multinodular mass. They are hypoechoic, slightly heterogeneous, lobulated, and well-defined lesions. Calcifications are rare. They usually are hypovascular on color Doppler, although in some cases they may appear hypervascular and softer on clinical palpation. Usually they grow eccentric from the tendon sheath, although occasionally they may be intrinsic. Sometimes, they cause erosion or remodeling of the cortex of the adjacent phalanx. They usually do not provoke trigger finger. As they grow, they displace but do not infiltrate the adjacent structures, such as the neurovascular bundle of the finger.

Differential diagnosis includes tendon sheath fibroma, nearly indistinguishable using imaging but much less frequent. However, presurgical differentiation between both tumors is not important. The hypervascular variety is difficult to distinguish from hypertrophic tenosynovitis, or even from a rare acral sarcoma with tendon sheath infiltration.

Figure 3.8.1 Longitudinal ultrasound image of right third finger from a dorsal and radial approach. There is a well-defined hypoechoic soft tissue mass which causes bone remodeling in the middle phalanx (*arrows*).

Figure 3.8.2 Color Doppler ultrasound image shows that the tumor is hypovascular and displaces but does not infiltrate the neurovascular bundle.

Case 9: Subungual Glomus Tumor

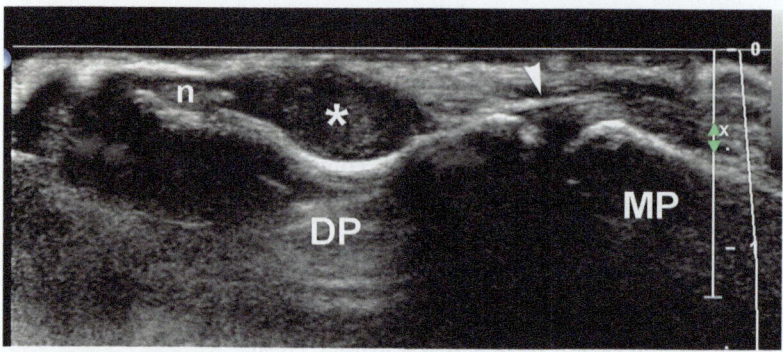

Fig. 3.9.1

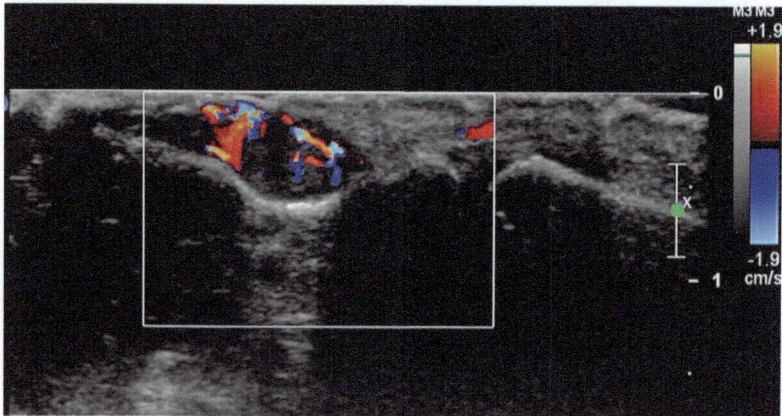

Fig. 3.9.2

Glomus tumor is a small, benign tumor which arises from the neuromyoarterial plexus. It belongs to the pericytic (perivascular) tumors in the WHO 2002 classification of the soft tissue tumors (group 5). Pathologic variants include glomangioma, with large cavernous spaces (20 % of the cases); glomangiomyoma, with smooth muscle component (less than 10 % of the cases); and malignant glomus tumor (less than 1 %).

It is commonly localized in the nail bed of a finger, although it may also be located subcutaneously in the wrist, forearm, and foot. Unusual locations include the thigh, patella, stomach, colon, nerve, face, trachea, and mediastinum. Subungual lesions present a striking female predilection in ages 20–40.

The classic clinical triad includes pain, point tenderness, and cold sensitivity (30 % of patients). Patients have typically a small red-blue nodule with paroxysms of pain with changes of temperature or pressure. There are some trophic changes in the nail and keratosis, erythema, etc.

Ultrasound imaging features consist of a small focal hypoechoic nodule located in the nail bed, with erosion or remodeling of the cortex of the adjacent phalanx (22–82 % of cases), which is hypervascular on echo-Doppler exploration. The lesion usually is located parasagittal inside the nail bed and sometimes even on the marginal aspect of the nail bed growing to the palmar aspect from the dorsal aspect of the finger tip. Multiple lesions are present in about 10 % of patients.

The differential diagnosis includes several tumors. Subungual epidermoid inclusion cyst produces bone erosion in the same location but does not show Doppler flow or paroxystic pain. Subungual hemangioma has Doppler flow but does not have bone erosion or paroxystic pain. Phalanx enchondroma and bone giant cell tumor usually do not have soft tumor component or paroxystic pain.

Comments

Figure 3.9.1 Longitudinal ultrasound image through the fingertip of the left thumb from a dorsal approach. There is a well-defined, round, homogeneous, and hypoechoic soft tissue mass within the nail bed (*asterisk*), causing bone remodeling of the dorsal aspect of the distal phalanx (*DP*). *MP*: middle phalanx, *n*: nail, *arrowhead*: insertion of the terminal extensor tendon.

Figure 3.9.2 Color Doppler ultrasound at the nail bed. The tumor appears hypervascular.

Imaging Findings

Further Reading

Baek HJ, Lee SJ, Cho KH et al (2010) Subungual tumors: clinicopathologic correlation with US and MR imaging findings. Radiographics 30:1621–1636

Bianchi S, Martinoli C (2007) Ultrasound of the musculoskeletal system. Springer, Berlin/Heidelberg

Bureau NJ, Cardinal E, Cchem R (1998) Ultrasound of soft tissue masses. Semin Musculoskelet Radiol 2:283–298

Choudhary AK, Methratta S (2010) Morel-Lavallée lesion of the thigh: characteristic findings on US. Pediatr Radiol 40(Suppl 1):S49

Craigh EV (1984) The geyser sign and torn rotator cuff: clinical significance and pathomechanics. Clin Orthop Relat Res 191:213–215

Fessell DP, Van Holsbeeck MT (1999) Foot and ankle sonography. Radiol Clin North Am 37:831–857

Fornage BD et al (1983) Ultrasonography in the evaluation of muscular trauma. J Ultrasound Med 2:549–554

Gibbons CL, Khwaja HA, Cole AS, Cooke PH, Athanasou NA (2002) Giant-cell tumour of the tendon sheath in the foot and ankle. J Bone Joint Surg Br 84:1000–1003

Hachisuga T, Hashimoto H, Enjoji M (1984) Angioleiomyoma: a clinicopathologic reappraisal of 562 cases. Cancer 54:126–130

Horcajadas AB, López Lafuente J, de La Cruz Burgos R et al (2003) Ultrasound and MR findings in tumor and tumor-like lesions of the fingers. Eur Radiol 13: 672–685

Kransdorf MJ, Murphey MD (2006) Vascular and lymphatic tumors. In: Soft tissue tumors, 2nd edn. Lippincott Williams & Wilkins, Philadelphia, pp 150–188

Marchadier A, Cohen M, Legre R (2006) Subungual glomus tumors of the fingers: ultrasound diagnosis. Chir Main 25:16–21

Mellado JM, Pérez del Palomar L, Diaz L et al (2004) Long standing Morel-Lavallée lesions of the trochanteric region and proximal thigh: MRI features in five patients. Am J Roentgenol 182:1289–1294

Neal C, Jacobson JA, Brandon C, Kalume-Brigido M, Morag Y, Girish G (2008) Sonography of Morel-Lavallee lesions. J Ultrasound Med 27:1077–1081

Omezzine SJ, Abid F, Mnif H, Hafsa C, Thabet I et al (2010) Primary hydatid disease of the thigh. A rare location. Orthop Traumatol Surg Res 96:90–93

Pedrosa I, Saiz A, Arrazola J, Ferreiros J, Pedrosa CS (2000) HD: radiologic and pathologic features and complications. Radiographics 20:795–817

Peh WC, Wong Y, Shek TW, Ip WY (2001) Giant cell tumour of the tendon sheath of the hand: a pictorial essay. Australas Radiol 45:274–280

Polat P, Kantarci M, Alper F, Suma S, Koruyucu MB, Okur A (2003) Hydatid disease from head to toe. Radiographics 23:475–494

Scheller AD, Kasser JR, Quigley TB (1980) Tendon injuries about the ankle. Orthop Clin North Am 11:811

Shirkoda A, Armin AR, Bis KG, Makris J, Irwin RB, Shetty AN (1995) MR imaging of myositis ossificans: variable patterns at different stages. J Magn Reson Imaging 5:287–292

Thermann H, Hoffmann R, Zwipp H (1992) The use of ultrasound in the foot and ankle. Foot Ankle Int 13:386–390

Tshering Vogel DW, Steinbach LS, Hertel R et al (2005) Acromioclavicular joint cyst: nine cases of a pseudotumor of the shoulder. Skeletal Radiol 34:260–265

Wang Y, Tang J, Luo Y (2007) The value of sonography in diagnosing giant cell tumor of the tendon sheath. J Ultrasound Med 26:1333–1340

Yoo HJ, Choi JA, Chung JH et al (2009) Angioleiomyoma in soft tissue of extremities: MRI findings. Am J Roentgenol 192:W291–W294

Small Parts

4

PEDRO SEGUÍ, ELENA ELIZAGARAY, CARLOS NICOLAU, XIMENA WORTSMAN, ROSA ZABALA, JOSE LUÍS DEL CURA, and MONTSERRAT DOMINGO

Introduction

The main problem with ultrasound as a diagnostic technique is the loss of acoustic signal and resolution as the distance to the structure studied increases. So, ultrasound achieves its highest performance in the study of superficial structures (when they contain no bone or air). In these structures, the so-called small parts, the ultrasound is the diagnostic procedure of choice.

Ultrasound is the most used and also the highest-resolution imaging technique in neck pathology. In thyroid disease, the most frequent pathology in the neck, ultrasound is currently the primary imaging test, and most of the management of these conditions is based on sonographic findings. The accessibility of ultrasound has contributed to the increased prevalence of thyroid diseases: while the prevalence of palpable thyroid nodule is 4–8 %, detection by imaging is 67 %. The management of thyroid nodule is, therefore, one of the commonest ultrasound applications in daily practice.

Soft parts of the face are easily accessible to ultrasound exploration. For example, salivary gland pathology is diagnosed with excellent accuracy, and ultrasound is a quick and available image technique to study these glands. The orbits, almost entirely composed of fluid, transmit ultrasound very well, thus being excellently explored by ultrasound. Ultrasound is particularly useful when the eyeball is not accessible to direct visual examination through the iris.

Ultrasound is also the main technique for the study of testicular conditions, both acute and chronic. It is especially valuable in acute disease, being the key test in the decision to operate or not a patient with acute scrotum. And in recent years, due to the emergence of high-resolution probes that allow an accurate study of very superficial planes, the skin has emerged as a field of study for ultrasound, opening a vast field of new possibilities for the development of this technique.

J.L. del Cura et al. (eds.), *Learning Ultrasound Imaging*, Learning Imaging,
DOI 10.1007/978-3-642-30586-3_4, © Springer-Verlag Berlin Heidelberg 2012

Neck

Rosa Zabala, Pedro Seguí, and Jose Luís del Cura

Case 1: Hodgkin's Disease

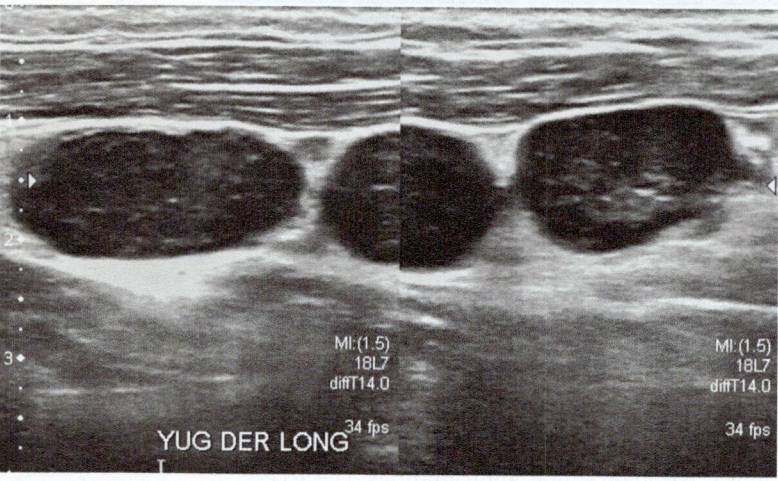

Fig. 4.1.1

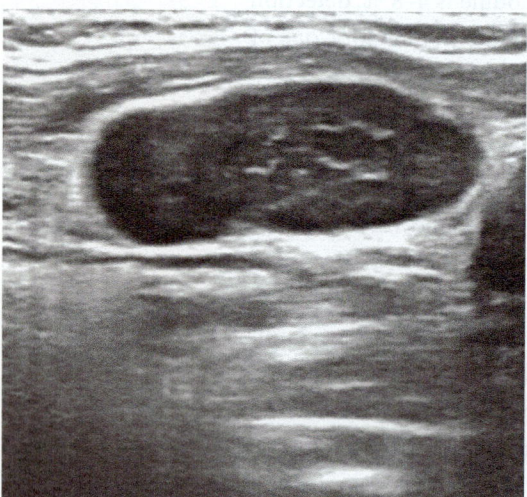

Fig. 4.1.2

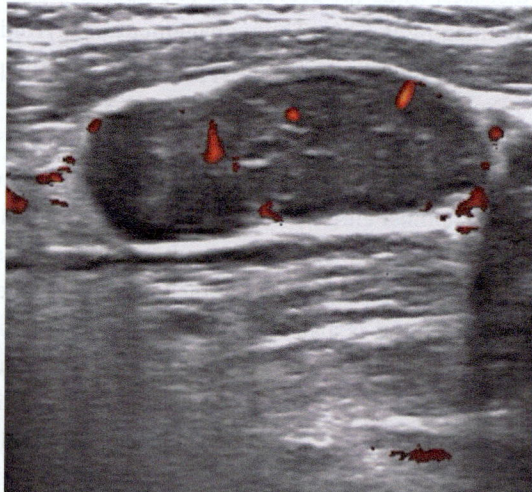

Fig. 4.1.3

A 33-year-old male patient presented with a 2-month history of bilateral neck masses, without fever or weight loss. A cervical US scan was performed.

Longitudinal gray-scale sonogram of the right cervical jugular chain (Fig. 4.1.1) showed multiple rounded or oval, enlarged lymph nodes. Nodes appear homogeneously hypoechoic and without echogenic hilus. Figure 4.1.2 shows a detailed US image of a jugular lymph node that shows intranodal reticulation and absent hilus. On power Doppler sonogram (Fig. 4.1.3), the node has a chaotic vascularity.

An adenopathy was surgically excised and diagnosed at histological examination as Hodgkin's disease, nodular sclerosing type. Staging CT and PET (Fig. 4.1.4) showed pathologic cervical (*arrows*) and mediastinal adenopathies, without abdominal involvement. Patient received chemotherapy treatment.

Case Presentation and Imaging Findings

Hodgkin's disease is a B-cell lymphoma. In 80–90 % of patients, the first manifestation of Hodgkin's disease is lymphadenopathy, most frequently located in the neck. High-resolution sonography can be used as the first-line modality for evaluating cervical soft tissue masses.

Sonography is a useful imaging tool in the assessment of peripheral lymph nodes. Gray-scale sonography is widely used in the evaluation of the number, size, site, shape, borders, soft tissue edema, and internal architectures of lymph nodes. Spectral Doppler sonography with measurement of vascular resistance, color Doppler, and power Doppler may be helpful. High-resolution ultrasound is currently used in the diagnostic evaluation of lymph node involvement in patients with head and neck carcinomas (cervical lymph nodes), breast cancer (axillary nodes), melanoma (regional peripheral nodes), and many other malignancies. Normal and reactive nodes are usually oval and have an echogenic hilus. The upper limit in minimal axial diameter of normal and reactive nodes varies with the location (5–8 mm for cervical nodes). Malignant lymph nodes (metastatic and lymphomatous) are usually round and without echogenic hilus; central necrosis (echogenic-coagulative or anechoic-cystic) is sometimes present. Eccentric cortical hypertrophy is a useful sign to indicate focal tumor infiltration in a node.

In both Hodgkin's and non-Hodgkin's lymphoma, usually, lymph nodes are round or oval, hypoechoic, without echogenic hilum, and show intranodal reticulation.

Fine-needle biopsy and core biopsy are usually diagnostic for Hodgkin's disease but may not yield enough material to enable the histological classification. Thus, excisional lymph node biopsy is sometimes required to fully appreciate the architecture of the lymph node.

Staging in Hodgkin's disease consists of determining the location and extent of disease, defining prognostic factors and manifestations that can be evaluated and will determine the choice of treatment. In essence, the staging

Comments

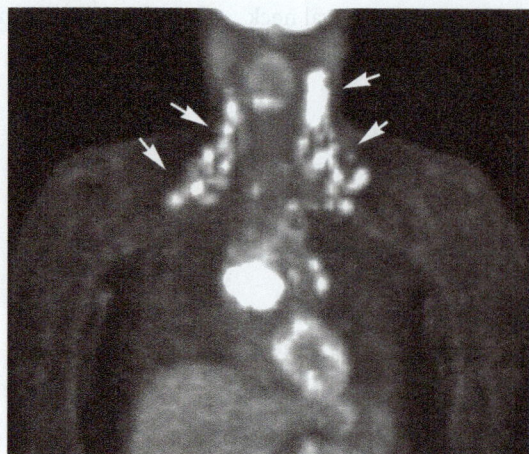

Fig. 4.1.4

is based on the number of sites of lymph node involvement, whether lymph nodes are involved on both sides of the diaphragm, whether there is visceral involvement, and whether B symptoms (fever, weight loss, drenching night sweats) are present.

Thoracic CT scanning is useful as it has a considerable potential to influence the initial treatment. Staging below the diaphragm is hampered by false-negative results of CT scanning due to inability to detect Hodgkin's disease in normal-sized nodes and the difficulties in detecting Hodgkin's disease in the spleen by CT scanning or ultrasound. Although bone marrow involvement is relatively uncommon, a bone marrow biopsy is usually recommended. Magnetic resonance appears to be sensitive for the evaluation of bone and/or bone marrow involvement. However, this modality has the disadvantage that only a limited area of the body can be investigated. Positron emission tomography is a very useful noninvasive modality for the diagnosis of lymphoma and complete assessment of the extent of disease.

Case 2: Papillary Thyroid Carcinoma

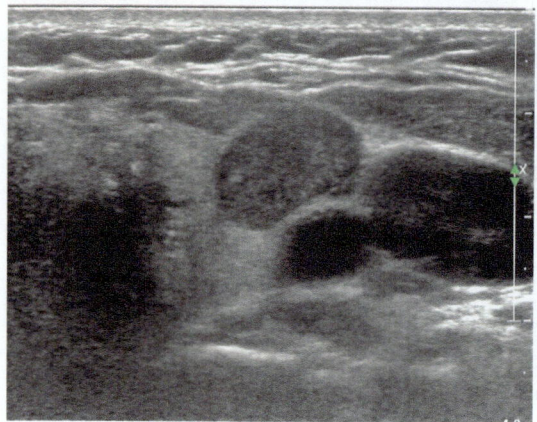

Fig. 4.2.1

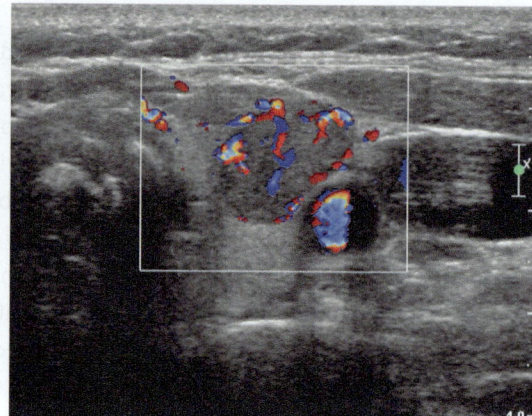

Fig. 4.2.2

A thyroid nodule was incidentally discovered in a 42-year-old female during a cervical Doppler ultrasound exam performed after some episodes of dizziness. Ultrasound (Figs. 4.2.1 and 4.2.2) showed a solid nodule in the middle left thyroid lobe. The nodule appeared well delimited and hypoechoic to the parenchyma (Fig. 4.2.1) and showed central vascularization on color Doppler (Fig. 4.2.2). An ultrasound-guided biopsy performed on the nodule yields the diagnosis of papillary thyroid carcinoma, which was confirmed on surgery.

Case Presentation and Imaging Findings

Thyroid carcinoma is the most frequent endocrinological cancer. The improvement and more frequent use of the diagnostic techniques in recent years have induced an exponential increase in the diagnosis of thyroid pathology, including thyroid cancer. In fact, thyroid nodules can be found in 60 % of the population on ultrasound. Of them, between 0.6 and 12 % are malignant.

Comments

Papillary carcinoma is the most frequent of the malignant thyroid tumors (75–80 %). It is more frequent in women and around 45 years. Exposure to radiation, especially in the area of the neck, increases the risk of papillary carcinoma. Its prognosis is excellent, with survival over 95 % at 10 years. Age over 45 years and the presence of adenopathies or distant metastases are linked to a worse prognosis.

Ultrasound has a central role in the management of thyroid pathology because it is the most effective technique for the evaluation of the thyroid. Ultrasound should be the first image technique indicated when thyroid disease is suspected.

When exploring a thyroid nodule with ultrasound, there are several signs that are linked to a higher probability of cancer and should be carefully searched:

- A predominantly solid nature. A cystic or a spongiform pattern is usually benign.
- Anteroposterior diameter larger than the latero-lateral diameter.
- Spiculated or lobulated margins.
- Hypoechogenicity with respect to the parenchyma of the thyroid.
- Intranodular calcification. It can be observed as microcalcifications (more suspicious) or as thick calcifications.
- Central vascularization on color Doppler.

The detection of any of these signs implies the need to perform a biopsy of the nodule. The biopsy of the nodules should be better performed using ultrasound guidance because it has demonstrated higher accuracy than biopsy by palpation.

When performing an ultrasound exam of the thyroid, it is also important to explore the lymph node chains of the neck, especially when a papillary carcinoma has been previously diagnosed. The presence of metastatic lymph nodes is linked to a worse prognosis and requires the specific surgical excision of the involved lymph node chains.

Case 3: Medullary Thyroid Carcinoma

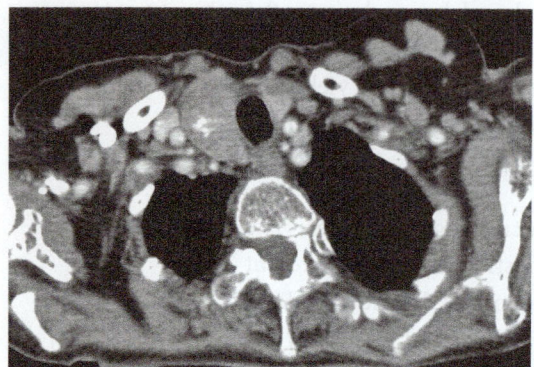

Fig. 4.3.1

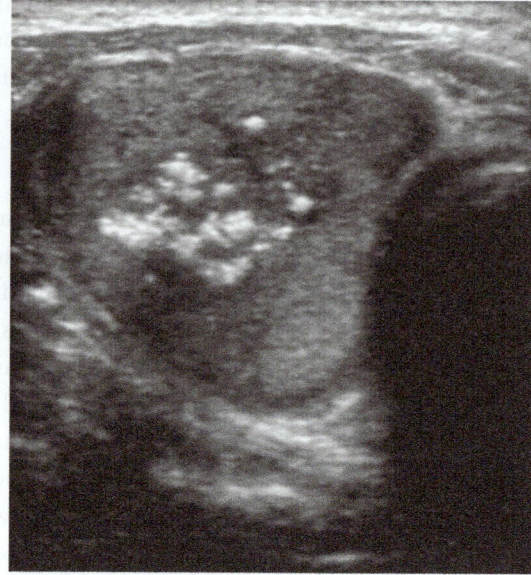

Fig. 4.3.2

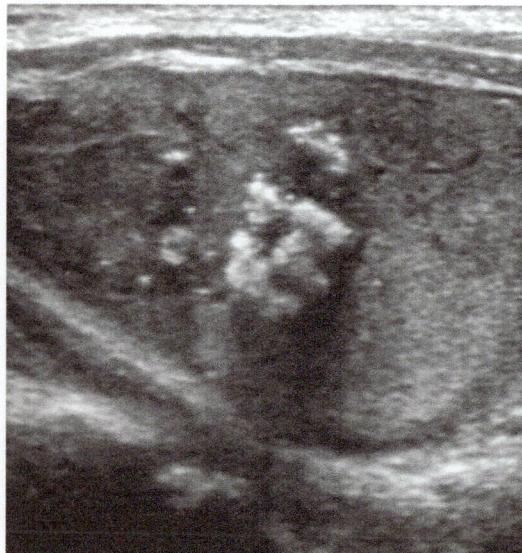

Fig. 4.3.3

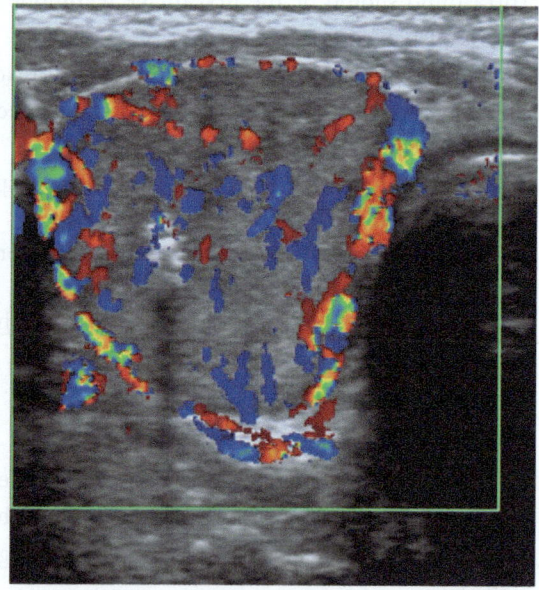

Fig. 4.3.4

A CT was performed to a 77-year-old female who was studied for anemia, weight loss, and tumor marker increase. In Fig. 4.3.1, an axial contrast-enhanced CT scan shows an enlarged right thyroid lobe with gross calcifications. No pathologic lymph node was detected. The patient, upon interrogation, reported having palpated this nodule for more than 10 years but had not consulted about it.

An ultrasound was performed. Transverse and longitudinal US images through the right thyroid gland (Figs. 4.3.2 and 4.3.3) showed a solid, hypoechoic, well-defined nodule with micro- and macro-calcifications. Color Doppler US image (Fig. 4.3.4) showed that the nodule was hypervascular. Ultrasound findings were suspicious of malignancy.

Ultrasound-guided fine-needle aspiration was performed with result suggestive of malignancy. The histological analysis of the thyroidectomy specimen yielded the result of medullary thyroid carcinoma. Immunohistochemistry showed strong positivity for calcitonin and negativity for thyroglobulin.

Case Presentation and Imaging Findings

Medullary thyroid carcinoma is a neuroendocrine neoplasm derived from C-cells. It represents 5–10 % of the malignant thyroid tumors. Eighty percent are sporadic, and the rest are of the familial type, associated or not to the multiple endocrine neoplasia (MEN) type 2 syndrome. Nearly all the patients present high levels of serum calcitonin. Sporadic cases usually appear in middle age as a solitary nodule or mass. Familial cases are usually detected in young patients and are, more frequently, bilateral or multicentric. Around half of the cases of medullary carcinoma present cervical adenopathies at the time of their initial diagnosis. Prognosis depends to a great extent on the initial stage with a 10-year survival of near 100 % in patients with disease limited to the thyroid. This survival goes down to 80 % when cervical adenopathies are present and to 50 % with distant metastasis (more frequent in lung, liver, and bone).

As said above, nonfamilial medullary carcinoma typically appears as a palpable thyroid nodule or cervical adenopathy, and the initial imaging method usually used is ultrasound. Ultrasound characteristics that suggest malignancy are similar for medullary and for papillary carcinomas: micro- or macro-calcifications, hypoechogenicity, irregular or spiculated margin, anteroposterior diameter bigger than transverse, and predominantly solid appearance. In general, it is not possible to differentiate the papillary and the medullary carcinoma with ultrasound. Medullary thyroid carcinoma usually appears as a solid, hypoechogenic, and circumscribed nodule. It presents micro- or macro-calcifications in 60 % of the cases. Cystic areas are more frequent than in the papillary thyroid carcinoma (up to a third of the cases).

Fine-needle aspiration presents up to 25 % of false negatives for the medullary thyroid carcinoma. Thus, a negative result in presence of ultrasound characteristics suggestive of malignancy should lead to the repetition of the biopsy or to the surgical excision of the nodule.

Comments

Face

PEDRO SEGUÍ, JOSE LUÍS DEL CURA, and ROSA ZABALA

Case 4: Pleomorphic Adenoma of Parotid Gland

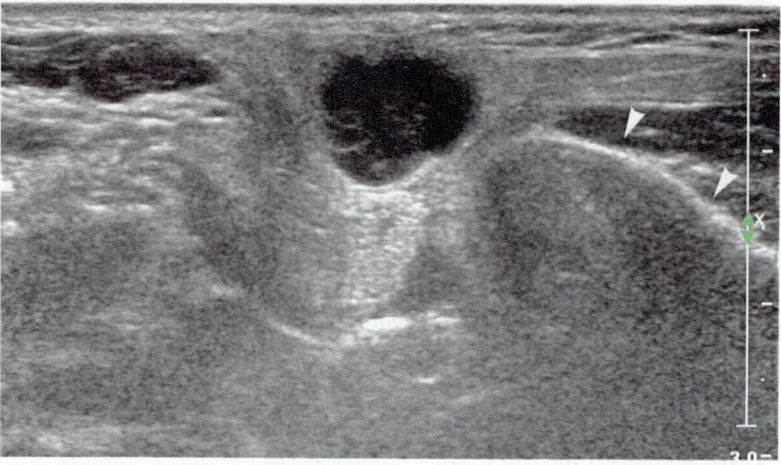

Fig. 4.4.1

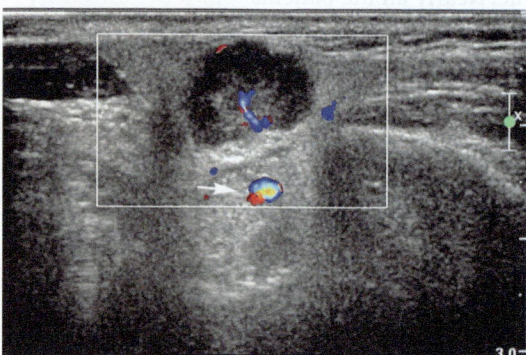

Fig. 4.4.2

A 42-year-old female presented a palpable lump on the right side of her face, below the ear. Sonography (Fig. 4.4.1) showed a hypoechoic nodule of 1 cm in diameter located in the superficial lobe of the parotid gland. The *arrowheads* indicate the anterior border of the jaw. The nodule is spherical and well delimited with lobulated borders. Color Doppler ultrasound shows only a thick central vessel (Fig. 4.4.2). Also, color Doppler ultrasound demonstrates the retromandibular vein (*arrow*), which can be used as a reference to differentiate the superficial and the deep lobes of the parotid gland.

Case Presentation and Imaging Findings

Pleomorphic adenoma is the most frequent tumor of the salivary glands. In the parotid gland, 80 % of the tumors are benign. Of them, 80 % are pleomorphic adenomas. It is also the most frequent tumor in the submandibular glands. It usually appears in patients over 50 years of age, and it is more frequent in women.

Comments

It normally appears as a solitary slow-growing, firm to palpation, and not painful tumor. As a small part of them become malignant, they should be surgically removed. Malignant degeneration should be suspected when observing sudden growth, skin retraction, pain, or paralysis of the facial nerve.

Ultrasound is the first-choice imaging technique, given the superficial location of the salivary glands. They appear as hypoechoic tumors, usually homogeneous and well delimited, with a round, ovoid, or polylobulated morphology. They can present calcifications in their interior. It is common to find isolated central vessels in the Doppler study.

Differentiation between pleomorphic adenoma and other salivary tumors using only imaging techniques is difficult. It is frequent that benign and malignant salivary tumors present with very similar findings in the ultrasound as well as in other imaging techniques. Therefore, ultrasound-guided biopsy is indicated for any nodule in the salivary glands when a rapid and reliable diagnosis is desired.

Case 5: Warthin's Tumor

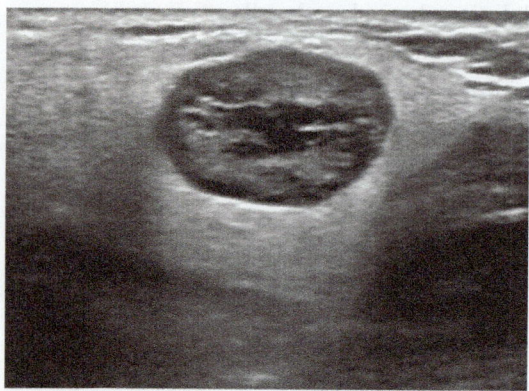

Fig. 4.5.1

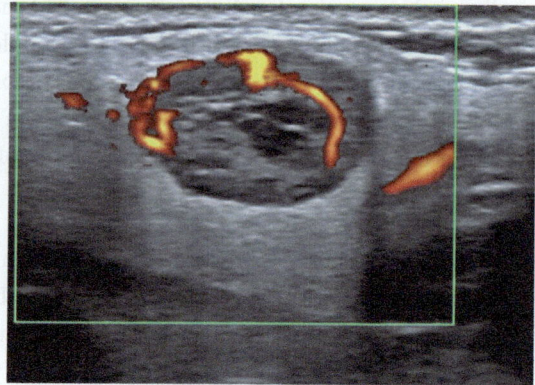

Fig. 4.5.2

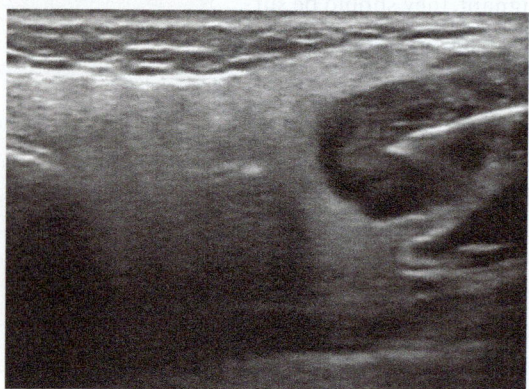

Fig. 4.5.3

A 51-year-old male consulted after noting a painless, left preauricular palpable nodule. An ultrasound was performed.

Longitudinal sonogram of the left parotid gland (Fig. 4.5.1) shows a hypoechoic lesion with a well-circumscribed margin, distal acoustic enhancement, and internal cystic changes. Power Doppler sonogram (Fig. 4.5.2) shows moderate intralesional vascularization.

An ultrasound-guided fine-needle aspiration was scheduled (Fig. 4.5.3). Transverse sonogram shows the needle tip inside the lesion during the procedure. The cytological sample corresponded to a Warthin's tumor. The histological analysis of the surgical piece confirmed the diagnosis.

Case Presentation and Imaging Findings

Warthin's tumor is the second most frequent benign tumor of the salivary glands. It is exclusive of the parotid gland. Nearly half of the cases are multifocal or bilateral, being the most common tumor with this presentation, sometimes in metachronic form. It is more frequent in men and after 50 years old. Treatment is surgical and it rarely recurs. Malignant transformation to carcinoma of squamous cells or lymphoma has been described but is very rare. Histologically, it is characterized by a layer of epithelial cells with oncocytic characteristics and an underlying polyclonal lymphoid component that forms germinal centers. The formation of inner cystic areas is very frequent.

On ultrasound, it appears as focal, oval or rounded, well-defined, hypoechogenic lesions, often with anechoic macrocystic or multiple microcystic areas inside. On color Doppler, it frequently appears hypervascular. It usually shows high uptake on Tc-99 scintigraphy and is hypermetabolic in the PET. Although the presence of cystic areas (and especially of microcystic areas) is highly characteristic and Warthin's tumor is the most frequent lesion with this presentation, this is not a pathognomonic sign, since benign lesions such as pleomorphic adenoma and malignant lesions such as the mucoepidermoid carcinoma and acinar cell carcinoma can also present cystic areas. Occasionally, Warthin's tumor can also appear as a simple cyst, being the differential diagnosis in these cases with the lymphoepithelial cysts and the infrequent cystic carcinomas.

Histological confirmation before surgery can be achieved with fine-needle aspiration. This technique has a high accuracy in Warthin's tumors, with the exception of completely cystic tumors. Several cases of tumor infarction after performing fine-needle aspiration have been reported.

Comments

Case 6: Lymphoma of the Parotid Gland

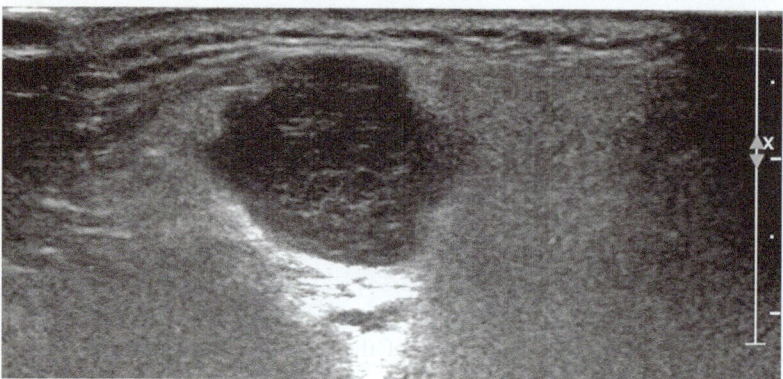

Fig. 4.6.1

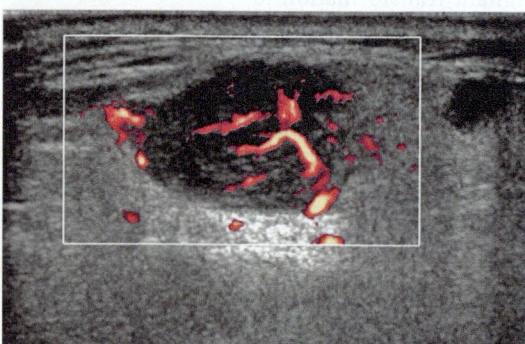

Fig. 4.6.2

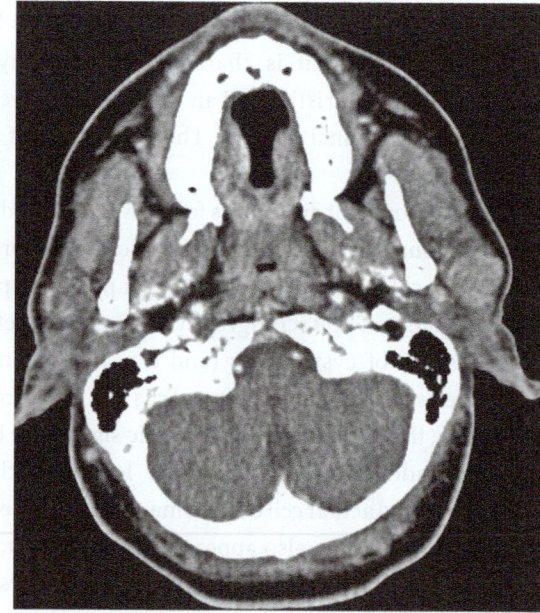

Fig. 4.6.3

A 71-year-old female, with no significant history, consults her doctor about the appearance of a lump on her face, before her left ear. She relates that the lump appeared some months ago and that it has been growing slowly. An ultrasound exam was performed showing (Fig. 4.6.1) that the lump was caused by a 15-mm-diameter, hypoechoic, lobulated tumor with well-defined borders, in the left parotid gland. Power Doppler examination (Fig. 4.6.2) showed the presence of central vessels. On CT, the nodule presented similar morphological characteristics and enhanced with contrast more than the parotid gland parenchyma (Fig. 4.6.3).

An ultrasound-guided biopsy of the mass was performed. The diagnosis was large B-cell lymphoma.

Parotid lymphomas make up 0.3 % of all the malignant tumors of the body, 5 % of the extranodal lymphomas and 2.5 % of the salivary gland tumors. Of them, 85 % are non-Hodgkin's lymphomas. The most frequent histological type is the low-grade MALT lymphoma, which can evolve in a variable interval of time (up to 29 years has been described) into a high-grade B-cell non-Hodgkin's lymphoma, as in the case presented here.

It is most frequently diagnosed in elderly persons (60–80 years old). The relation between the appearance of salivary gland lymphoma and some benign processes such as chronic sialadenitis or benign lymphoepithelial lesions has been described. The relation between parotid gland lymphoma and Sjögren syndrome is especially strong, increasing by a factor of 40 the risk of developing this tumor.

It usually appears as a palpable, firm facial mass. Ultrasound is an excellent technique to identify it as a tumor and to define its extension. It usually appears as a hypoechoic mass, usually polylobulated and well delimited, indistinguishable from other parotid gland tumors. Also, on MRI and CT, lymphoma appears as a solid nodule, indistinguishable from other tumors.

Given that the radiological diagnosis is difficult, an excellent alternative for obtaining the diagnosis is the percutaneous biopsy. This can be easily performed guided by ultrasound, given the accessibility of the parotid gland. Once the diagnosis is confirmed, it is important to carry out an appropriate staging.

The treatment includes surgical excision of the lesion, as well as chemotherapy and radiotherapy. The patients with low-grade lymphoma of the parotid gland have an excellent prognosis due to the low aggressiveness of the disease as well as the usual excellent response to the treatment.

Case 7: Mucoepidermoid Carcinoma of the Submaxillary Gland

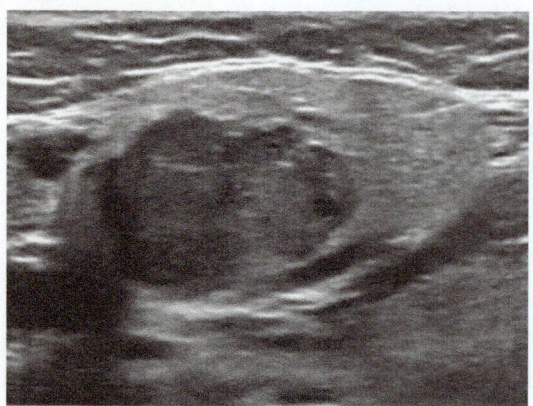

Fig. 4.7.1

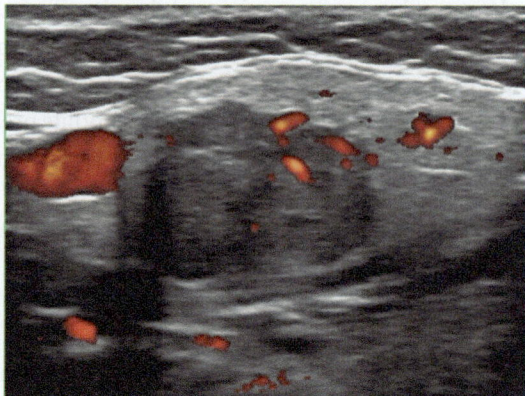

Fig. 4.7.2

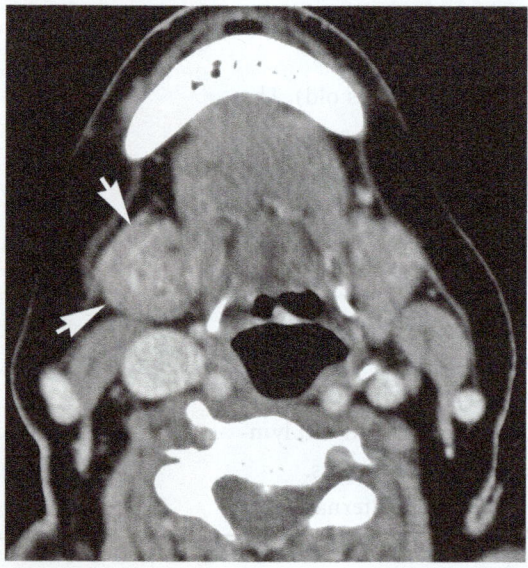

Fig. 4.7.3

A 69-year-old female has noticed for the last 2 years a painless nodule in the region of the right submandibular gland. Apparently, it has not grown.

An ultrasound was performed. Longitudinal sonogram (Fig. 4.7.1) shows a hypoechoic, microlobulated, solid lesion in the submandibular gland. The power Doppler (Fig. 4.7.2) shows some blood vessels in the lesion.

A contrast-enhanced CT was performed (Fig. 4.7.3), showing a nodule in the right submandibular gland (*arrow*) with no specific features. Ultrasound-guided fine-needle aspiration was performed with the result of "epithelial tumor of uncertain biological behavior." The histological diagnosis of the surgical resection specimen was low-grade mucoepidermoid carcinoma.

Case Presentation and Imaging Findings

Neoplasms are much less frequent in the submaxillary glands than in the parotid, representing only 10 % of all the salivary gland neoplasms. In contrast with the parotid gland in which 80 % of the neoplasms are benign, about 50 % of the lesions of the submaxillary glands are malignant. The most frequent malignant salivary gland neoplasms are mucoepidermoid carcinoma and adenoid cystic carcinoma. They usually appear in middle age, although they can also present in children, being in fact the most frequent pediatric salivary gland carcinoma. The most common form of clinical presentation is a slow-growing painless mass. Treatment includes wide local resection. The prognosis depends mainly on the differentiation grade of the tumor, which can be quite variable, with a 5-year survival above 90 % for low-grade tumors and around 50 % for high-grade tumors.

Imaging characteristics of mucoepidermoid carcinoma depend to a great extent on its grade. High-grade or advanced tumors present irregular shape, poorly defined or irregular borders, and hypoechogenic or heterogeneous pattern, varying from completely solid to predominantly cystic. On the other hand, low-grade tumors are smaller in size and indistinguishable from the benign tumors, with smooth, well-defined borders and a more homogeneous solid appearance. Doppler is not useful in reliably differentiating benign from malignant tumors, although some authors state that high resistance index is linked to a higher probability of malignancy.

Fine-needle aspiration is the procedure of choice for the initial characterization of the focal lesions of salivary glands, being necessary for planning the surgery. A negative or non-diagnostic result of the fine-needle aspiration does not guarantee that the lesion is benign since only 60 % of the malignant salivary gland tumors are correctly classified with fine-needle aspiration. Especial caution should be taken with the "non-diagnostic" or "undetermined epithelial tumor" cytological diagnosis because they include many low-grade malignant tumors. Many of these incorrectly classified malignant tumors present large cystic changes. Because of this, some authors use the core-needle biopsy to improve the results, especially in the parotid, with excellent accuracy.

Comments

Orbit

Elena Elizagaray

Case 8: Retinal Detachment

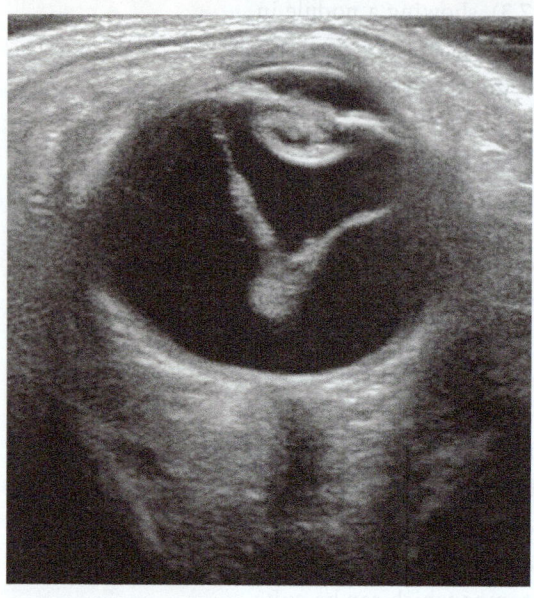

Fig. 4.8.1

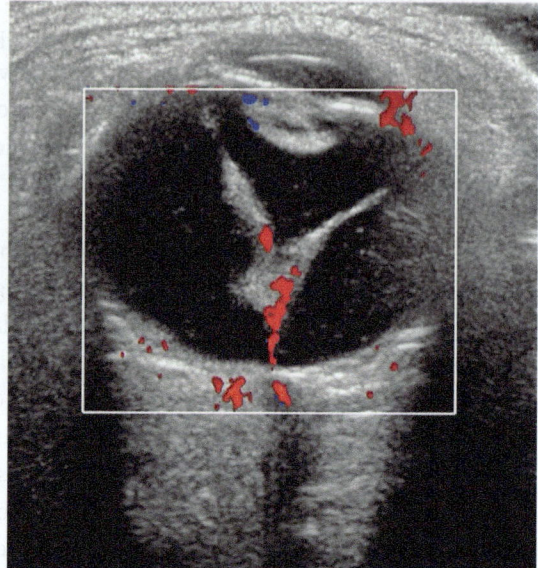

Fig. 4.8.2

The retina is normally attached to the rest of the elements of the posterior ocular globe and is not visible as a distinct structure. When a detachment happens, fluid fills the virtual space beneath the retinal epithelium and accumulates, pushing the retina away from the outer layers of the globe. Acute retinal detachment is a sight-threatening condition requiring urgent diagnosis and treatment.

The most common type of retinal detachment is termed "rhegmatogenous" (from the Greek *rhegma*, meaning "tear"), which refers to a break or tear in the retinal epithelium. Most cases are due to age-related vitreous detachment, which can create tiny holes that allow fluid to pass into and accumulate in the subretinal space. In younger patients, direct trauma is the most common cause.

Less common types of retinal detachment include "tractional," in which the vitreous contracts and pulls the neural retina off the underlying pigmented layer but does not cause a break in the epithelium, and "exudative," in which serous fluid accumulates beneath the retina because of inflammatory conditions.

Retinal detachment is seen on ultrasound as a prominent, continuous, echogenic membrane that appears to have been lifted off the posterior surface of the eye. Depending on the timing and severity of the detachment, the retinal separation may be visible only as a small peripheral convexity or, in case of an extensive detachment, as the so-called funnel appearance because the retina is firmly attached to the optic disc, and even after a complete detachment, it will appear tethered to this point. Complete detachment appears as an echogenic membrane attaching at the ora serrata anteriorly and at the optic nerve posteriorly.

When performing eye ultrasound in case of suspicion of retinal detachment, it is very important to evaluate the entire globe in order to avoid missing small detachments. This may require asking the patient to gaze upward and downward, left and right to achieve adequate visualization. Because the anterior-most attachment of the retinal epithelium is just lateral to the ciliary bodies, care must be taken to interrogate its entire surface. The entire globe must be examined in sagittal and axial planes.

Differential diagnosis includes other ocular pathologies that may appear similar on sonography as choroid detachment, posterior vitreous detachment, and vitreous hemorrhage. Choroid detachment has a convex shape, is unattached to optic disc, and can extend anterior to the ora serrata. Posterior vitreous detachment may also appear as a hyperechoic linear image that has been lifted off the posterior globe; however, it typically appears thinner and less echogenic than retinal detachment, has no color Doppler signal, and is unattached to the periphery of the globe. Vitreous hemorrhage typically appears as medium-low-level echoes within the vitreous body that are unattached to optic disc. Vitreous hemorrhage is mobile on dynamic scanning and has no Doppler signal.

Comments

Eye sonogram (Fig. 4.8.1) showing a thick hyperechogenic V-shaped membrane, attached to the ora serrata anteriorly and to the optic nerve posteriorly. Color Doppler imaging (Fig. 4.8.2) shows vessels in the membrane.

A complete retinal detachment was diagnosed.

Imaging Findings

Case 9: Vitreous Hemorrhage

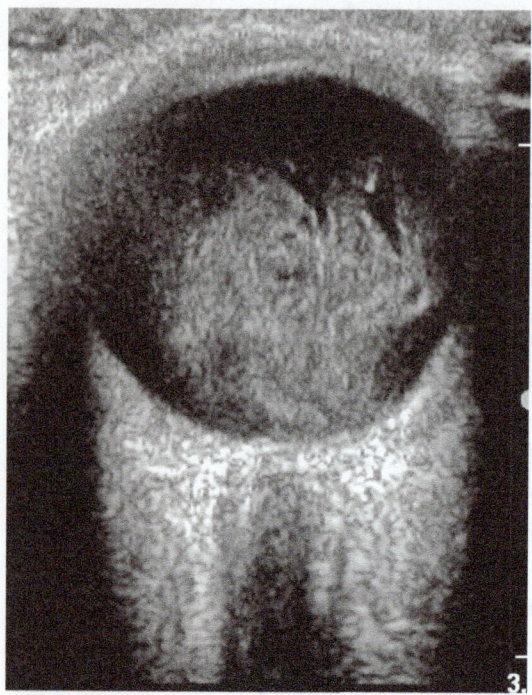

Fig. 4.9.1

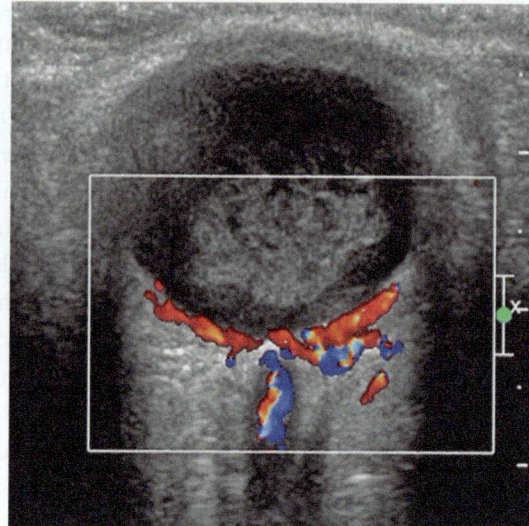

Fig. 4.9.2

Vitreous hemorrhage can occur in different situations such as after a trauma or a retinal tear, a retinal vein occlusion, or a complication of diabetes mellitus (abnormal blood vessels in proliferative diabetic retinopathy are prone to bleed). Vitreous hemorrhage can be caused by disruption of normal or diseased retinal vessels and extension of hemorrhage to the vitreous from other sources.

Blood may be trapped between the posterior hyaloid (vitreous layer separating the vitreous from the retina) and the retina, also called subhyaloid hemorrhage, or it may enter the vitreous cavity. Vitreous hemorrhage is often found on ultrasound because vitreous hemorrhage is one of the main reasons to examine the eye to rule out other pathologies obscured by the vitreous hemorrhage.

Sonographic pattern of a vitreous hemorrhage depends on time and severity. Fresh hemorrhage can appear as small dots or linear areas (within the vitreous chamber) that can affect partially or totally the vitreous chamber. Vitreous hemorrhage may also appear as low echogenic mobile vitreous opacities, which tend to settle down, appearing as dependent echoes. In older hemorrhages, blood organizes and forms membranes that sway as the eye moves from side to side.

During the ocular US examination, the gain setting should be adjusted to achieve acceptable imaging, using the highest gain setting to visualize weak signals. It is important to ask the patient to move the eyes while performing the examination to see the hemorrhage sway. Vitreous is not attached to the optic nerve. Color Doppler does not show any signal within the vitreous hemorrhage.

Eye ultrasound image (Fig. 4.9.1) shows the vitreous body filled with echoes. No color signal can be observed inside the lesion on color Doppler ultrasound (Fig. 4.9.2). A massive vitreous hemorrhage was diagnosed.

Comments

Imaging Findings

Case 10: Choroidal Detachment

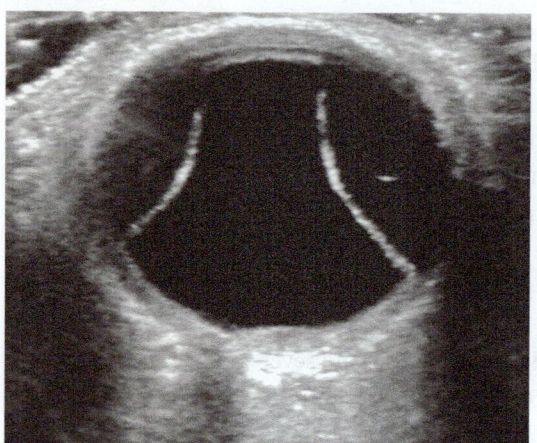

Fig. 4.10.1

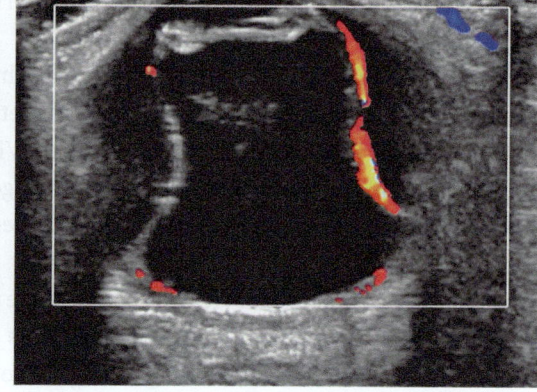

Fig. 4.10.2

Choroidal detachment refers to a collection of fluid in the suprachoroidal space in the eye, a virtual space between the choroid and the sclera. When fluid accumulates between both structures, this space becomes real, and the choroid is separated from its normal position. The fluid accumulated can be either serum or blood. Serous choroidal detachment may be caused by an increased transmural pressure, most frequently because of globe hypotony (low intraocular pressure) or by inflammation, which causes exudation of serum resulting from increase in vascular permeability. A hemorrhagic choroidal detachment occurs when blood accumulates within the suprachoroidal space from rupture of a choroidal vessel following contusion, penetrating ocular trauma, or as a complication of ocular surgery. Sudden globe decompression during ocular surgery also predisposes to choroidal detachment.

Sonography shows choroidal detachment as thick, smooth, dome-shaped, echogenic membranes. When large, the choroidal detachment can be seen as a biconvex membrane that almost touches at the center of the vitreous body. During dynamic scanning, this appearance does not change with eye movement. Choroidal membranes may extend anterior to ora serrata, but not to the optic nerve. Color Doppler shows vascularization within the membranes.

Figure 4.10.1: Choroidal detachment after cataract surgery: echogenic biconvex membrane (unattached to the optic nerve head) involving the nasal and temporal quadrants of the globe.

Figure 4.10.2: Color Doppler ultrasound of the same patient shows vessels in the choroidal membrane.

Case 11: Optic Disc Drusen

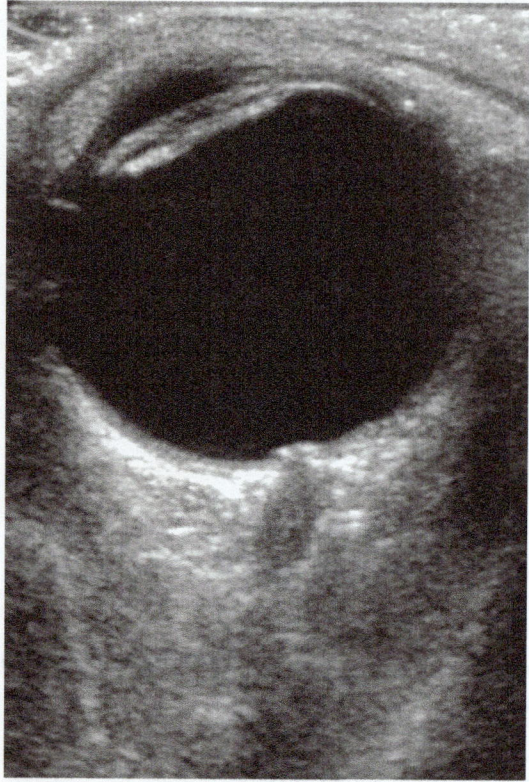

Fig. 4.11.1

Optic disc drusen are frequent incidental ophthalmologic findings during routine exams. They appear in 3.4–24 per 1,000 population and are bilateral in approximately 75 %. Optic disc drusen are a form of calcific degeneration in some of the axons of the optic nerve head. Disturbance in the axonal metabolism in the presence of a small scleral canal is considered responsible for its development.

The drusen usually increase in size with age due to continuing calcium apposition. Visual acuity is often not affected, but the visual fields of these patients can be abnormal and deteriorate over time. Patients do not usually notice these defects, despite their progression over the years, due to its insidious course. Currently, there is no cure or direct treatment for the progressive vision loss or the complications that may develop from optic nerve drusen.

Bilateral optic disc drusen can mimic papilledema, raising the question of intracranial hypertension and sometimes prompting unnecessary or invasive procedures. Since children as well as adults are affected, it is important to consider optic nerve head drusen in the differential diagnosis of papilledema or optic nerve swelling at any age. The diagnosis can be established using clinical findings combined with ultrasound. Ocular ultrasound demonstrates an echogenic focus of variable size within or on the surface of the optic nerve head. It can be unilateral or bilateral. Posterior acoustic shadowing may be present in larger lesions. Ultrasound is useful to diagnose and also to follow up the progression of this condition.

Comments

Figure 4.11.1: Small echogenic focus on the surface of the optic nerve head, without posterior acoustic shadowing.

Imaging Findings

Case 12: Choroidal Melanoma

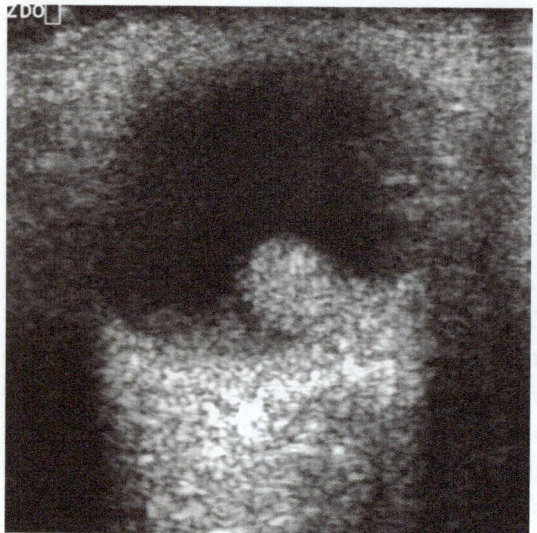

Fig. 4.12.1

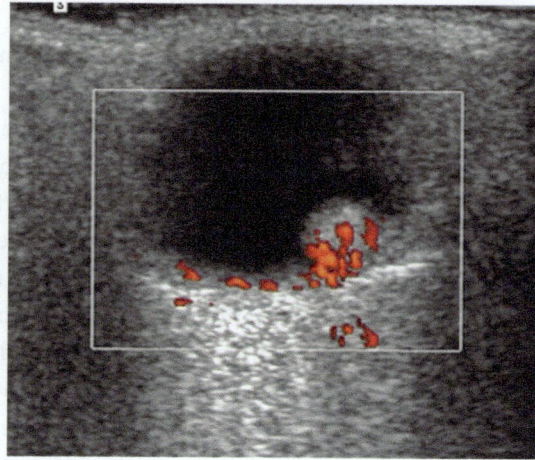

Fig. 4.12.2

Comments

Malignant melanoma of the uvea is the most common primary malignant intraocular tumor in adults. It is nevertheless an infrequently found tumor. The ocular tissue where these tumors arise, the uvea, is a vascular tissue, with fenestrated capillaries and stroma containing melanocytes, that forms part of the wall of the eye. The uvea is subdivided into the iris, the ciliary body, and the choroid. The choroid underlies the retina. Uveal melanomas may develop, in order of decreasing frequency, in the choroid, ciliary body, and iris.

Uveal melanomas can be classified as anterior uveal melanomas, in which the tumor arises in the iris, and posterior uveal melanomas, in which the tumor arises in either the choroid or the ciliary body. Commonly, melanomas are seen posteriorly, but intraocular melanomas can involve more than one uveal structure. These are nearly always unilateral.

Choroidal melanomas may remain asymptomatic for long periods of time. In general, the farther the tumor's location is from the optic nerve and fovea, the larger the tumor can become before the patient notices a visual defect.

Exudation of fluid into the subretinal space can lead to a retinal detachment. Rarely, choroidal melanomas can impinge into underlying posterior ciliary nerves, causing severe ocular pain. At diagnosis, melanomas can be quite large and fill a significant portion of the vitreous chamber or may be very small.

Melanoma has a great propensity to metastasize. If the tumor does not show extraocular extension, it can only spread hematogenously, because there are no lymphatic vessels in the eye. It most often metastasizes to the liver. Other involved organs include lung, bone, skin, and central nervous system. Local spread occurs through the overlying Bruch membrane, with access to the subretinal space, or toward the orbit, through the sclera, most often along ciliary vessels and nerves. Choroidal melanoma almost never extends through the optic nerve; when it does, it is usually in juxtapapillary tumors or in diffuse choroidal melanomas.

Sonography is used to help establish the diagnosis, to evaluate possible extraocular extension, to estimate tumor size and localization, and to plan therapeutic intervention. On ultrasound, melanomas are usually homogeneous, echogenic solid masses, which may show a wide range of shapes. Small choroidal melanomas typically appear as a nodular, dome-shaped, and well-circumscribed mass. As they grow, they may adopt more irregular configurations, adopting bilobular, multilobular, or mushroom shapes. Duplex Doppler and color flow examination of these tumors show evidence of perfusion. Ultrasound is also useful in monitoring the tumor response to treatment.

In about 5 % of the cases, the involvement can be diffuse, with lateral growth throughout the choroid with minimal elevation. These diffuse, flat melanomas are quite difficult to diagnose. Rarely, choroidal melanomas may appear multicentric or in both eyes.

Retinal detachment is a common associated sonographic finding. This may be a small focal detachment immediately adjacent to the tumor or an extensive detachment involving the entire retina.

Imaging Findings

Figure 4.12.1: Eye sonogram: a well-defined, homogeneous soft tissue mass is seen coming out from the choroid.

Figure 4.12.2: The color Doppler study shows moderate flow in the tumor. A medium-size choroidal melanoma was confirmed at surgery.

Testis

Montserrat Domingo and Carlos Nicolau

Case 13: Testicular Microlithiasis

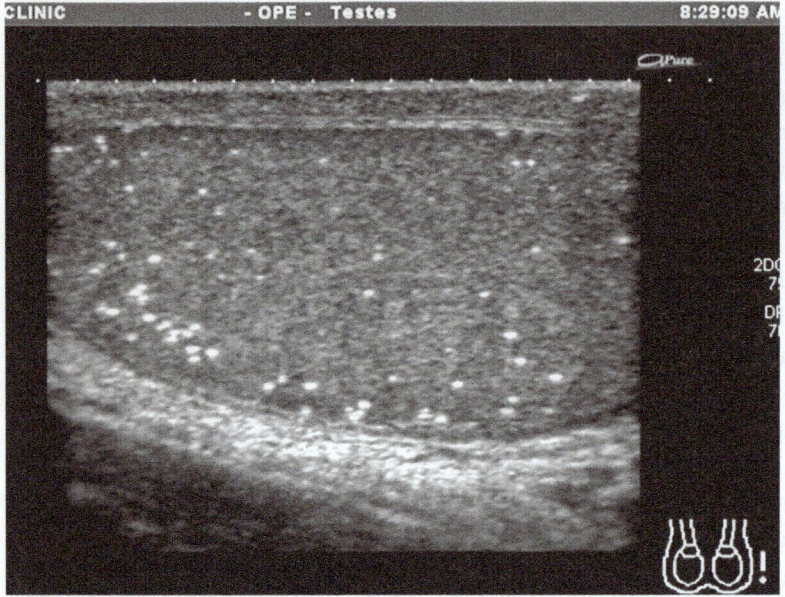

Fig. 4.13.1

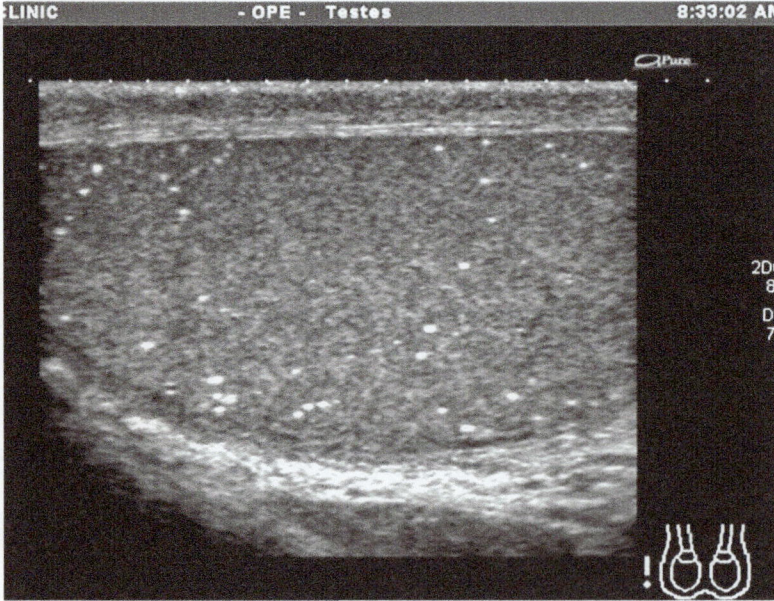

Fig. 4.13.2

A 31-year-old male with infertility and intermittent nonspecific scrotal pain was referred for scrotal ultrasound examination.

Longitudinal US scan of the left (Fig. 4.13.1) and right testicles (Fig. 4.13.2). Composed images of both testicles (Fig. 4.13.3). Multiple bilateral small scattered echogenic foci of 1–2 mm in size without posterior acoustic shadowing in testicular parenchyma, compatible with microlithiasis, are shown. No other testicular anomalies were detected.

Testicular microlithiasis is uncommon, with unknown true prevalence (0.6–9 %). This condition is seen at all ages but is more common in childhood and more prevalent in black men. The presence of microlithiasis has an uncertain significance that has been associated with various genetic anomalies, cryptorchidism, and infertility but also with testicular tumors. It has been considered as a potential marker of elevated testicular cancer risk with an increased prevalence of intratubular germ cell neoplasia or germ cell tumors (GCT) (histological types in decreasing order of frequency: seminoma, teratoma, and mixed GCT). There are reports of an incidence of GCT between 6 and 46 % and an association with contralateral testicular cancer following orchiectomy for testicular cancer. But, currently, there is no evidence that microlithiasis is either a premalignant condition or a causative agent in testicular neoplasia. This fact is supported by two reasons: first, most patients (>90 %) with microlithiasis do not show tumor at presentation and no interval development of GCT; second, prevalence among different racial groups and the geographic distribution of microlithiasis are different from those of testicular tumor. Therefore, it is likely that both microlithiasis and testicular cancer are caused by a common condition such as tubular degeneration.

Testicular microlithiasis is usually diagnosed as an incidental finding on US evaluation of the testis performed for nonspecific reasons. On US, testicular microlithiasis appears as multiple small echogenic foci of calcifications of 1–3 mm in size, without posterior acoustic shadowing. They are usually bilateral, with a symmetric, uniform, and diffuse distribution and appear randomly scattered throughout the testicular parenchyma, but they can be unilateral, asymmetric, and/or focal. There are no widely accepted criteria about how many echogenic foci should be detected to make the diagnosis of testicular microlithiasis, but some authors classify them as classic if there are five or more microliths in one US image and limited microlithiasis if there are less than five. No Doppler specific findings have been reported in testicles with microlithiasis. Histologically, they are characterized by calcification of degenerate intratubular cells. Testicular microlithiasis is located within the seminiferous tubules.

When microcalcifications are focal, they should be differentiated from a solitary focus of echogenicity (present in scar tissue, fibrosis, or burned-out

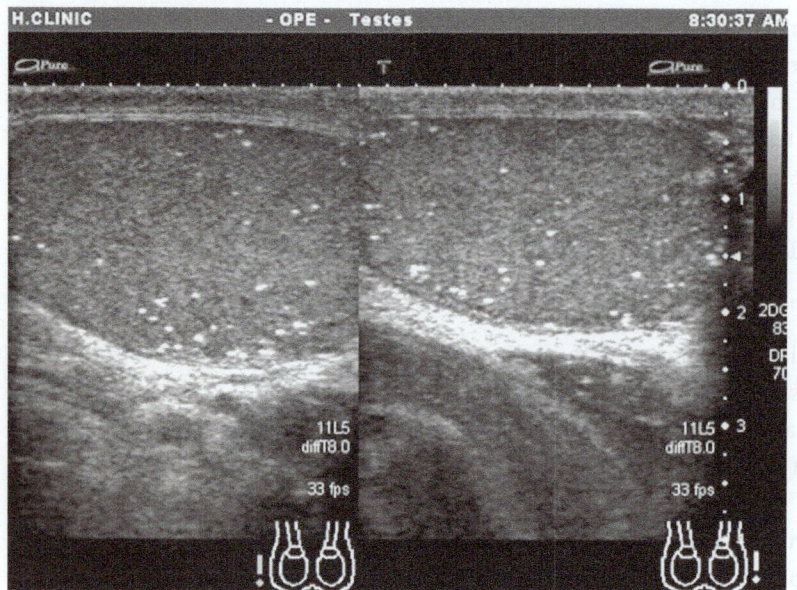

Fig. 4.13.3

tumors) and from multiple focal echogenicities (that can be seen in benign processes such as orchitis, scar, granulomas, sarcoidosis, chronic infarction, and after chemotherapy or radiation therapy). In these cases, calcifications are irregular, larger, and ill defined compared to microlithiasis appearance.

As the malignant potential of microlithiasis is controversial, there is no consensus about the management of testicular microlithiasis. There is no wide agreement about the necessity, interval, duration, and diagnostic modality of monitoring. The most extended practice in asymptomatic patients is the physical self-examination and annual US examination. The use of biochemical tumor markers, abdominal and pelvic CT, or testicular biopsy is not recommended.

Case 14: Testicular Non-seminomatous Germ Cell Tumor

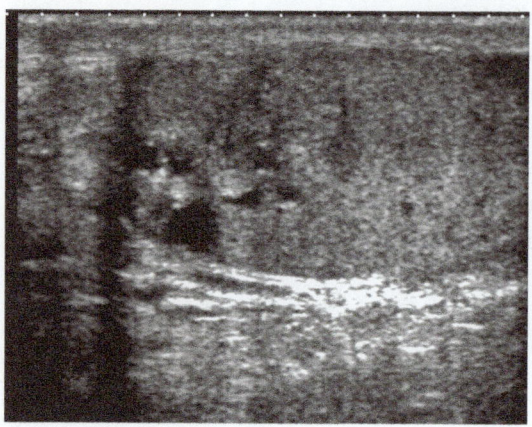

Fig. 4.14.1

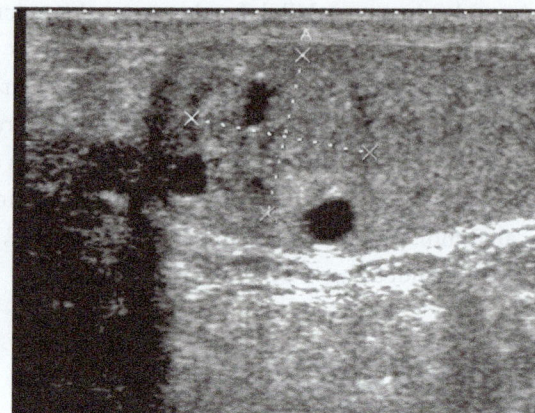

Fig. 4.14.2

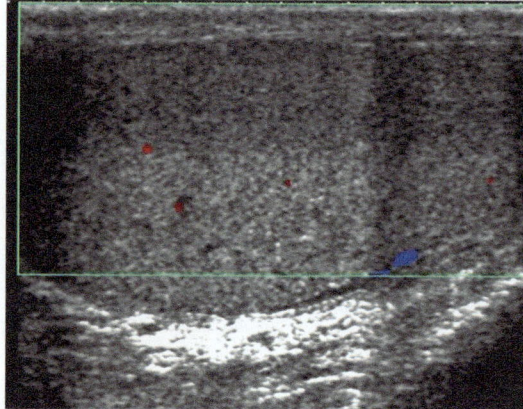

Fig. 4.14.3

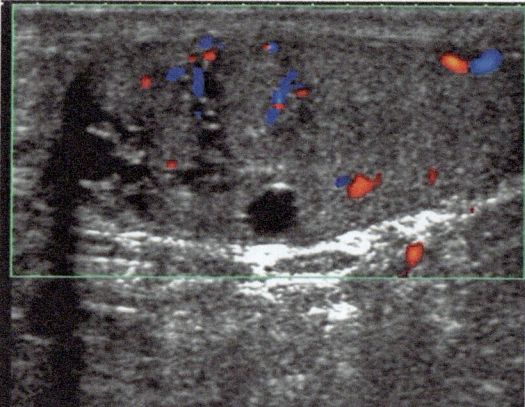

Fig. 4.14.4

Case Presentation and Imaging Findings

A 23-year-old man was referred to the ultrasound department due to small nodularity on the right testicular surface.

Gray-scale US shows a heterogeneous mass in the upper pole of the right testicle with hyperechoic and hypoechoic areas including some intratumoral small cysts (Figs. 4.14.1 and 4.14.2). Small cysts were also detected at the periphery of the tumor. Left testicular parenchyma was homogeneous with no focal lesions (Fig. 4.14.3). Color Doppler US shows vascularization of the testicular mass being compatible with testicular carcinoma (Fig. 4.14.4). The final diagnosis obtained after orchiectomy was non-seminomatous germ cell tumor.

Testicular carcinoma accounts for 1 % of all neoplasms in men, but it is the most common malignancy in the 15–34-year-old age group. Germ cell tumors are the most common subtype and account for 95 % of the cases. They are divided into seminomas (35–50 %) and non-seminomatous germ cell tumors (50–65 %). Seminoma is seen in older population and is associated with the best prognosis. Non-germ cell tumors accounts for only 4 % of all tumors, and they derive from the sex cord (Sertoli cells) and interstitial stroma (Leydig cells). Non-primary tumors (lymphoma, leukemia, and metastases) are rare (1 % of all tumors).

The most common presentation is a painless scrotal mass. Ten percent of the cases present with scrotal pain that has been related to the presence of intratumoral necrosis or hemorrhage. In about 10 % of patients with metastatic disease, metastases are the first symptom of the disease.

US is the preferred imaging modality to evaluate scrotal masses. US examination is used to determine its origin (testicular or extratesticular) and to recognize benign intratesticular conditions that can mimic a testicular neoplasm. Testicular neoplasms can be solitary or multiple and up to 10 % are bilateral. Seminomas are typically well-defined, homogeneous, and hypoechoic lesions. Non-seminomatous germ cell tumors are usually more heterogeneous and ill-defined lesions that may contain calcium and cystic areas. However, some seminomas can present as large heterogeneous lesions that even replace the testicular parenchyma. Most testicular tumors show increased intravascular signals on color Doppler, with irregular distribution and architecture. However, testicular tumors are frequently hypovascular because the detection of blood flow using color Doppler depends on the tumor size. Thus, it is especially difficult to demonstrate blood flow when incidental small tumors (<1 cm) are detected. Doppler US features of the different subtypes of testicular tumors are nonspecific, but it has been described that Leydig cell tumors may have a peripheral circumferential blood flow on color Doppler. On US, other testicular tumors such as teratomas may present as a well-defined and heterogeneous mass containing cystic areas (anechoic or complex) and echogenic foci with/without shadowing, representing cartilage, calcification, and fibrous components of the teratoma.

The differential diagnosis of testicular tumors should include changes secondary to infarction, hematomas, focal orchitis, granulomatous diseases, and lymphomas. Previous history and clinical findings are essential to achieve a correct diagnosis, and color Doppler is also very helpful especially in the differential diagnosis with hematomas and ischemic lesions showing absence of color signal. The differential diagnosis with inflammatory disease can be difficult because of an increased vascularization in both entities using color Doppler. Even if inflammatory disease is highly suspected, a short follow-up after treatment is recommended to rule out a tumor and confirm the resolution of the inflammatory disease.

Comments

Case 15: Testicular Trauma

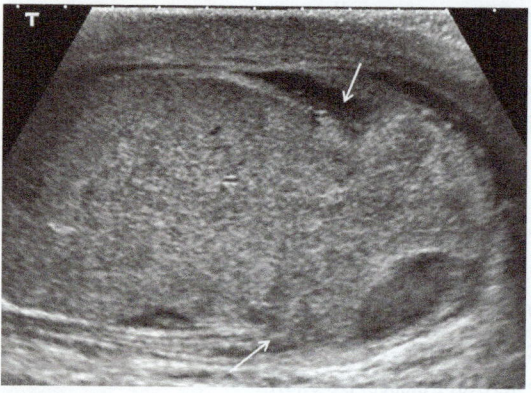

Fig. 4.15.1

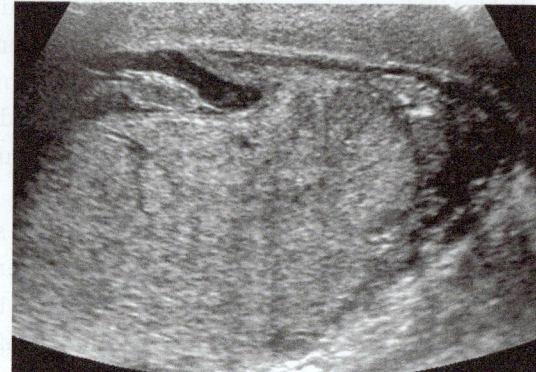

Fig. 4.15.2

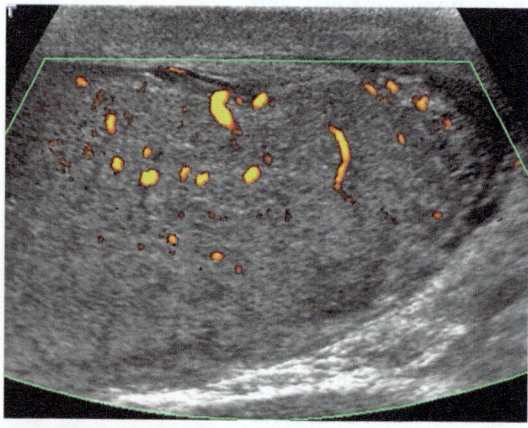

Fig. 4.15.3

Case Presentation and Imaging Findings

A 28-year-old man with scrotal pain and swelling secondary to direct trauma from a motorbike accident.

Gray-scale longitudinal US scan (Figs. 4.15.1 and 4.15.2) shows the characteristic features of a testicular rupture: disruption of the tunica albuginea (*arrows*) with loss of oval morphology at inferior pole, extrusion of testicular parenchyma through the albuginea rupture, and heterogeneity of the affected testicular parenchyma. Color Doppler US

(Fig. 4.15.3) showed conserve-d but diminished vascularity of the testicular affected area.

Testicular trauma is the third most common cause of acute scrotal pain. It results from athletic injury (>50 %), motor vehicle accident (9–17 %), direct blow, or straddle injury. There are three main mechanisms: blunt injuries, penetrating injuries, and iatrogenic injuries (inguinal herniorrhaphy or orchiectomy).

Testicular trauma may result in testicular contusion, hematoma, fracture, or rupture.

Testicular rupture is a surgical emergency with more than 80 % of cases being saved if surgery is performed within 72 h after injury. On ultrasound (US), the diagnostic criterion is the detection of discontinuity of the tunica albuginea. Other US findings include the presence of heterogeneous echotexture of the testicle, irregularity of the testicular margins, decrease or absence of vascularization on color Doppler of the affected testicular area, hematocele, and thickening of the wall of the scrotum.

Testicular fracture is a discontinuity in the testicular parenchyma. Its detection using US is rare because of the associated heterogeneity of the testicular parenchyma that hampers the identification of the fracture line. On US, the fracture is identified as a linear hypoechoic band crossing the testicular parenchyma. If there is no associated disruption of the tunica albuginea, urgent surgery is not required.

Intratesticular hematoma is very common. Its US appearance depends on the age. Acute hematomas are usually hyperechoic or heterogeneous compared to the surrounding parenchyma; chronic hematomas may have hypoechoic areas or even cystic component. Color Doppler US is essential in the diagnosis and follow-up of avascular testicular hematomas. They should be followed until resolved to rule out testicular cancers since 10–15 % of testicular tumors first manifest after a scrotal trauma.

Other extratesticular findings are common in scrotal trauma such as hematocele, scrotal wall hematomas, and traumatic lesions of the epididymis. Hematocele, the most common finding after blunt injury, is a blood collection within the leaves of tunica vaginalis. Its US appearance also depends on the evolution: an acute hematocele tends to be echogenic, and a chronic hematocele is usually predominantly anechoic with low-level echoes, fluid-fluid level, or septations. Epididymis can be also injuried after testicular trauma, presenting different appearences traumatic epididymitis, which is the most common (heterogeneous enlarged epididymis with increased vascularity); hematoma; and fracture or rupture, which is rare (ill-defined epididymis with a heterogeneous echotexture and absence of blood flow).

Case 16: Epididymo-orchitis

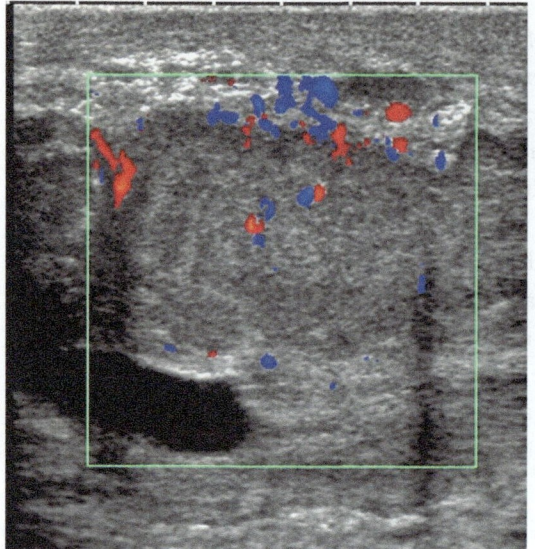

Fig. 4.16.1

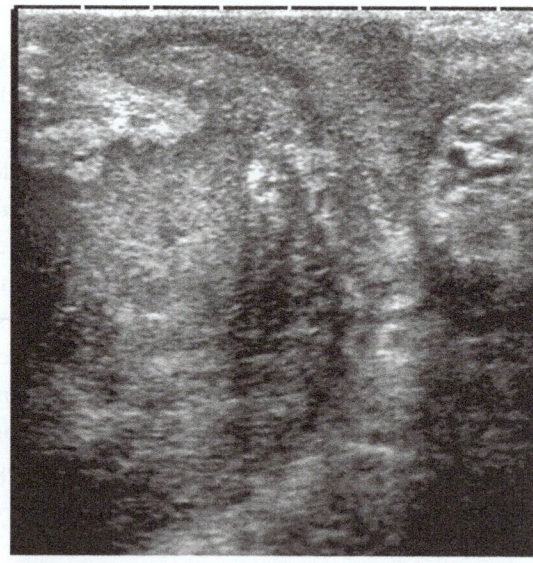

Fig. 4.16.2

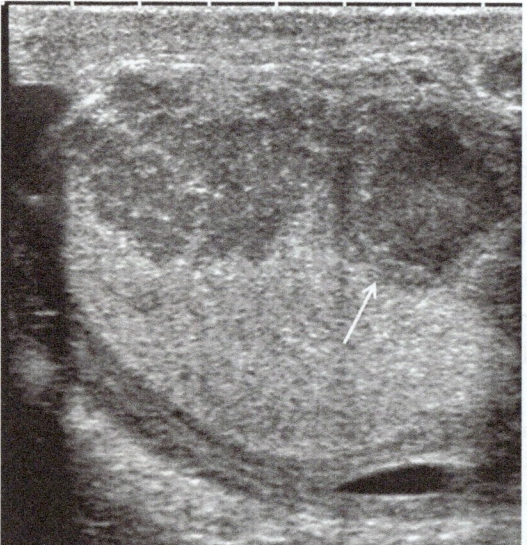

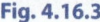

Fig. 4.16.3

Fig. 4.16.4

A 34-year-old man was referred to the ultrasound (US) department complaining of scrotal swelling accompanied by fever, local pain, and suppurative process in scrotal skin.

Longitudinal and transversal color Doppler US image (Figs. 4.16.1 and 4.16.2) demonstrates an enlarged hypoechoic left epididymis with increased vascularization. Transverse B mode US image (Fig. 4.16.3) depicts an extension of inflammation to the left testicle with abscess formation (anechoic center with peripheral capsule) (*arrow*). Longitudinal gray-scale (Fig. 4.16.4) and color Doppler US images (Fig. 4.16.5) show a cutaneous fistula from the epididymis with thickening and increased vascularity of the scrotal wall.

Case Presentation and Imaging Findings

Epididymitis with or without orchitis is a common cause of acute scrotal pain in adolescents and adults. The epididymis is the organ primarily affected, and the testicle is involved diffusely or focally in 20–40 % of cases due to direct spread of infection. Its etiology varies depending on the age: in adolescents, it is caused by sexually transmitted organisms (*Chlamydia trachomatis* and *Neisseria gonorrhoeae*) and in prepubertal boys and in men over 35 years, it is secondary to *Escherichia coli* and *Proteus mirabilis*. Epididymitis is usually unilateral but can be bilateral.

Gray-scale US features of acute epididymitis include the presence of enlargement and thickening of the epididymis. These findings are usually diffuse, affecting all the epididymis. However, inflammation can occur in only an epididymal part (head, body, or tail). In addition, decreased echogenicity or heterogeneity of the epididymis is common and is usually associated with indirect signs of inflammation (reactive hydrocele or pyocele with scrotal wall thickening). The most accurate criterion of epididymal inflammation is the detection of hyperemia of the epididymis detected on color Doppler US, with an increased flow secondary to an increased number and concentration of vessels. If Doppler US spectra are obtained, a high flow, with a decreased resistive index, is often detected.

When there is extension to the testicle, a diffuse involvement with heterogeneous echostructure secondary to edema or focal involvement with hypoechoic parenchymatous lesions can be detected. Color Doppler also shows increased vascularity except in cases of abscess formation that is demonstrated by the presence of hypoechoic lesions without color Doppler signal. These features are characteristic but nonspecific of inflammation because testicular heterogeneous echostructure and increased vascularization can also be seen in neoplastic diseases including leukemia and lymphoma. However, in these entities, the involvement is usually bilateral, while in infection it is usually unilateral. Thus, US follow-up is required to verify the resolution or decrease of the US findings to rule out neoplastic diseases.

Comments

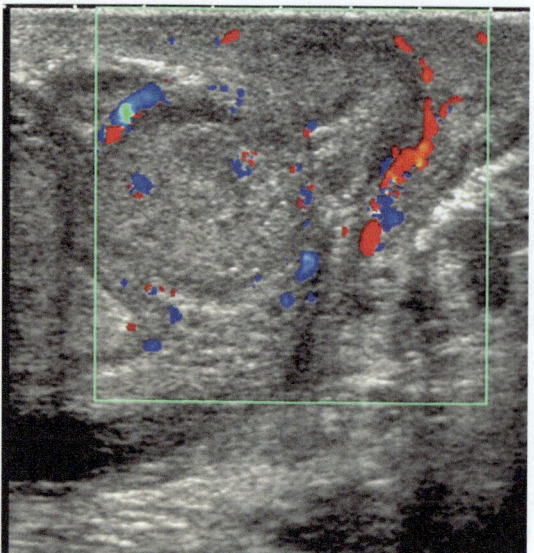

Fig. 4.16.5

Chronic epididymitis is characterized by persistent pain. Its features on gray-scale US include enlarged or shrunken hyperechoic epididymis with or without calcifications. Testicles may be also involved. Granulomatous epididymitis is a type of chronic epididymitis that can be caused by tuberculosis, brucellosis, sarcoidosis, leprosy, and syphilis and has different US appearances (hypoechoic, mixed echogenicity, or hyperechoic epididymis).

Skin

Ximena Wortsman

Case 17: Hemangioma

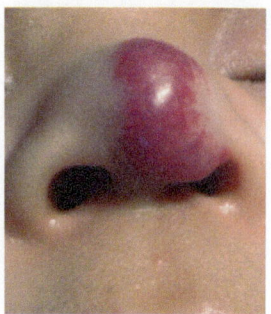

Fig. 4.17.1

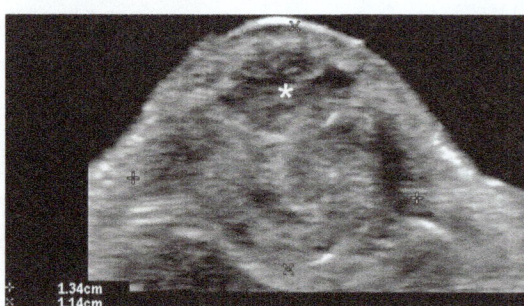

Fig. 4.17.2

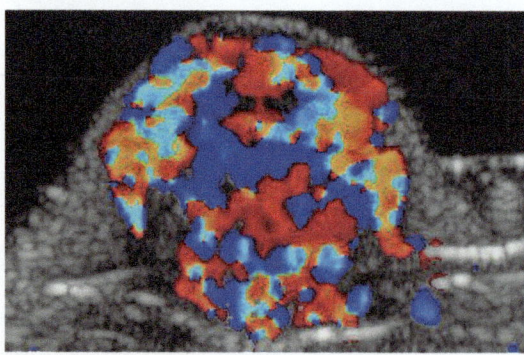

Fig. 4.17.3

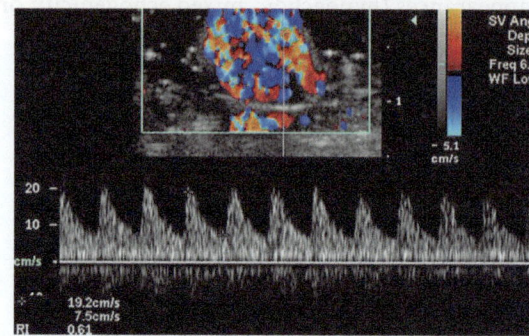

Fig. 4.17.4

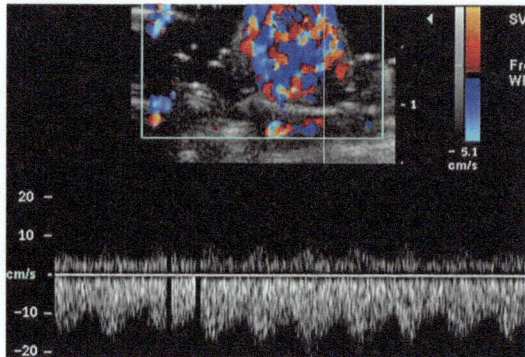

Fig. 4.17.5

A 3-month-old female child presents with fast growing erythematous lesion at the tip of the nose (Fig. 4.17.1).

Hemangiomas are the most common soft tissue tumors in infancy and usually present a fast growth during the first 2 years of life followed by a regression or involuting period of variable duration. These benign tumors are composed of an abnormal proliferation of vessels. Moreover the skin layers, they can easily involve deeper structures such as cartilage, muscle, or glands as well as generate an extrinsic compression or mass effect.

On sonography, hemangiomas appear as ill-defined heterogeneous solid masses that can vary in their echogenicity according to the phase of activity. Hence, during the proliferative phase, hemangiomas tend to appear as hypoechoic, and in the involuting phase, they show hyperechogenicity. In between, during the partial regression or involution period, a mix of echogenicities within the lesional area could be found. During the early phases, high vascularity is detected within the lesions which tend to progressively decrease in the late phases. Arterial and venous vessels, and often arteriovenous shunts, are usually found in hemangiomas. In the final involuting or regression phase, variable degrees of lipodystrophy may be found at the site of the hemangioma which may include hypertrophy and/or atrophy of the fatty component of the subcutaneous tissue. Sonography may support the follow-up of these vascular tumors by providing anatomical information to perform early decisions in their management. Hemangiomas are different from vascular malformations because the latter are errors in morphogenesis and not real tumors. Vascular malformations usually lack solid component and are classified according to the type of vessel: arterial, venous, lymphatic, capillary, or mixed. In contrast to hemangiomas, vascular malformations tend to maintain their morphology over time.

Figure 4.17.2: Gray-scale ultrasound (transverse view) at the tip of the nose shows 1.3-cm (wide) × 1.1-cm (deep) heterogeneous lesion, with some hypoechoic (proliferative) areas (*). Notice that the lesion involves both nasal cartilages.

Figure 4.17.3: Color Doppler image (transverse view) demonstrates a highly vascular lesion.

Figure 4.17.4: Color Doppler spectral curve analysis shows arterial blood flow in part of the lesion.

Figure 4.17.5: Color Doppler spectral curve analysis also demonstrates arterialized venous flow in other part of the lesion. Final diagnosis was hemangioma.

Case 18: Pilomatrixoma

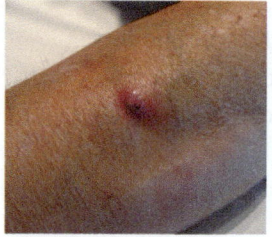

Fig. 4.18.1

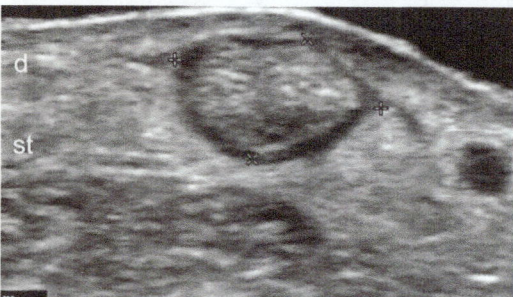

Fig. 4.18.2

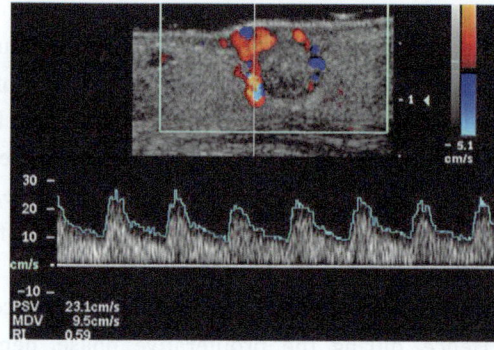

Fig. 4.18.5

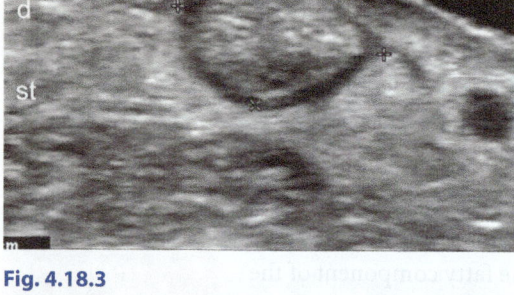

Fig. 4.18.3

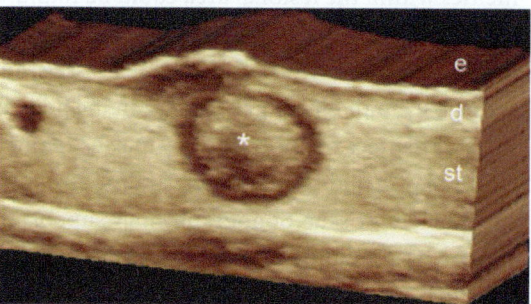

Fig. 4.18.6

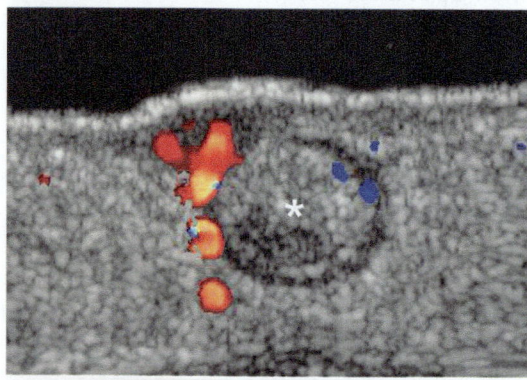

Fig. 4.18.4

A 68-year-old female patient presenting with erythematous lesion in the dorsum of the left forearm (Fig. 4.18.1).

Pilomatrixoma or calcifying epithelioma of Malherbe is a common skin tumor that arises from the hair follicle matrix. Clinically, these benign tumors show as slow-enlarging, erythematous, or bluish nodules commonly affecting the head, neck, and extremities. This cutaneous tumor is more common in children and young adults but can appear at any age. Pilomatrixomas have been reported to present a high rate of clinical misdiagnosis in up to 56 % of the cases, commonly mimicking other entities such as epidermal cysts, foreign body reactions, lymph nodes, and hemangiomas.

On sonography, the classical appearance is a target-shaped nodular lesion with hypoechoic rim and hyperechoic center usually located between dermis and subcutaneous tissue. Hyperechoic spots may be found within the center sometimes producing posterior acoustic shadowing, a typical artifact proper of calcified structures. Variable degrees of vascularity can be found in the periphery and/or central parts of the tumor usually with slow-velocity arterial and venous vessels. Occasionally, pilomatrixomas may show variants such as a vascular presentation that shows prominent blood flow within these tumors and may be clinically mistaken for a hemangioma. Other rare sonographic variant of pilomatrixomas is the cystic form that shows on sonography as an eccentric hypoechoic nodule separated by anechoic fluid from the hypoechoic rim. Septum and echoes may be noticed within the fluid-filled part of the cystic variant of pilomatrixoma. In late phases, a completely hyperechoic (calcified) nodule may be found in the skin layers which conforms another pattern of presentation in the evolution of pilomatrixomas.

Figure 4.18.2: Pilomatrixoma on dermoscopy (Courtesy of Dr. Tirza Saavedra, Department of Dermatology, Hospital Clinico U. Chile, Faculty of Medicine University of Chile). Notice the white areas in the center of the lesion.

Figure 4.18.3: Gray-scale ultrasound (transverse axis) shows a target-shaped nodule (between markers) with a hypoechoic rim and a hyperechoic center that involves dermis (*d*) and the upper subcutaneous tissue (*st*). Increased echogenicity of the subcutaneous tissue and a focal area of decreased echogenicity in the upper dermis that surrounds the lesion are also noticed, suggestive of edema.

Figure 4.18.4: Color Doppler ultrasound (transverse view) demonstrates increased blood flow in the periphery of the lesion (*).

Figure 4.18.5: Color Doppler spectral curve analysis shows arterial blood flow within the vessels.

Figure 4.18.6: 3D reconstruction (5–8 seconds sweep) demonstrates the upward displacement of the epidermis and dermis produced by the lesion (*). *e* epidermis, *d* dermis, *st* subcutaneous tissue.

Case 19: Basal Cell Carcinoma

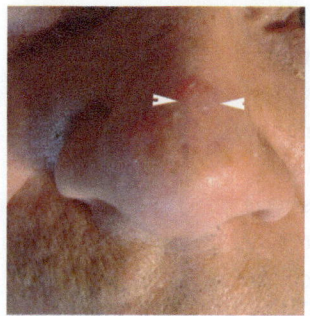

Fig. 4.19.1

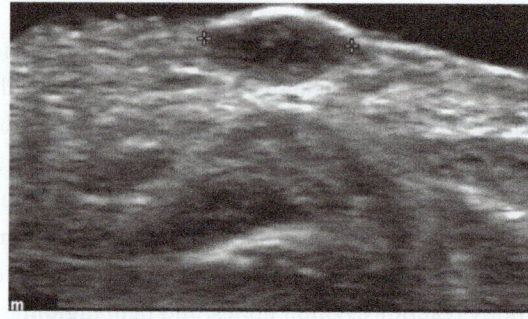

Fig. 4.19.4

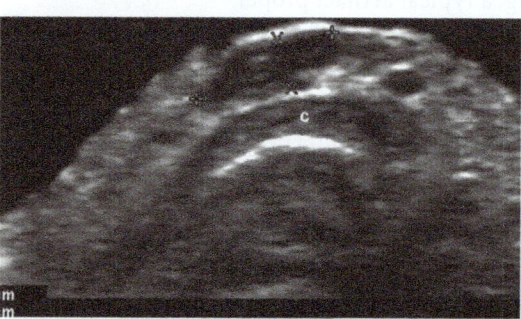

Fig. 4.19.2

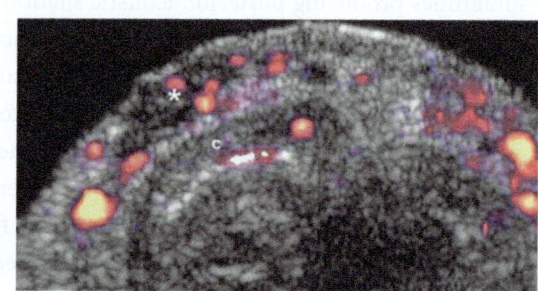

Fig. 4.19.5

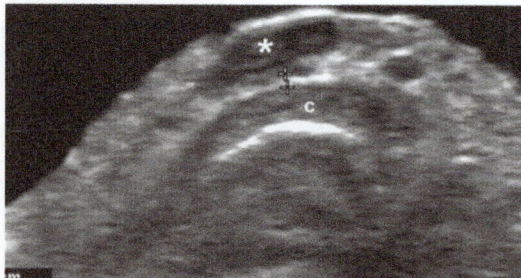

Fig. 4.19.3

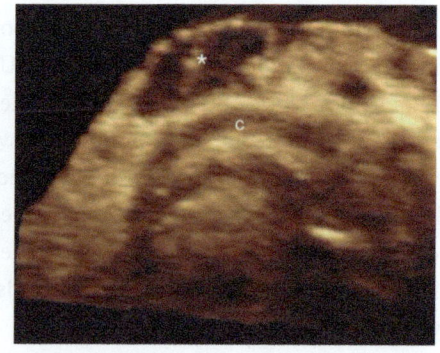

Fig. 4.19.6

Male, 69 years old presenting with an 8-month history of erythematous lesion (*arrowheads*) at the tip of the nose (Fig. 4.19.1).

Basal cell carcinoma is the most common cancer among human beings and composes 75–90 % of all skin cancers. It is a slow-growing cutaneous tumor that occasionally may be aggressive and presents high rates of recurrence. Together with squamous cell carcinoma conforms what is called the non-melanoma skin cancer. Basal cell carcinoma usually appears in exposed-to-sun areas of the skin such as the face, especially in the nose, eyes, lips, and ears, where the cutaneous layers are thin, and presents a high tendency for deep tissues involvement. Thus, the sonographic imaging of the primary tumor may support the planning of the surgery by providing a clear image of the unknown dimension for the clinical naked eye: depth. Also, this noninvasive technique can be of utmost importance for ruling out the involvement of deeper layers such as cartilage or muscle in highly exposed locations. Moreover, the sonographic presurgical anatomical information may support a better cosmetic prognosis which can be critical in difficult-to-treat cases or in patients presenting with multiple or recurrent tumors.

On sonography, basal cell carcinomas appear as hypoechoic lesions with slightly irregular borders and increased blood flow at the bottom of the lesions. Commonly, these tumors affect epidermis and dermis and occasionally may present inner hyperechoic spots and involve deeper layers. Two artifacts have been described on sonography in basal cell carcinomas: the first one is the blurring of the tumor borders in presence of severe sebaceous hyperplasia, and the second is composed by angled hypoechoic borders at the bottom of the lesion which is generated by a giant cell inflammatory reaction. Sonography has been reported to be useful to detect subclinical satellite lesions (≤ 2 cm from the primary tumor). Measurements of the lesions are usually performed in at least two perpendicular axes. Depth measurement is made at the deepest point of the lesion and usually in agreement with the pathologists. To date, depth by sonography has showed an excellent correlation with histology in literature reports.

Figure 4.19.2: Gray-scale ultrasound, transverse view, shows 6.1-mm (wide) × 2.1-mm (deep) hypoechoic oval-shaped lesion affecting the dermis. Nasal cartilage (*c*). Figure 4.19.3: Gray-scale ultrasound, transverse view, shows 0.6-mm distance between the lesion and the right nasal cartilage which is unremarkable (*c*). Lesion is marked (*). Figure 4.19.4 Gray-scale ultrasound, longitudinal view, shows 5.9-mm (long) hypoechoic lesion between markers. Figure 4.19.5 Power Doppler, transverse view, demonstrates slightly increased blood flow within the lesion (*). Figure 4.19.6 3D reconstruction (5–8 seconds sweep, transverse view) highlights the lesion (*). A basal cell carcinoma was the final diagnosis.

Case 20: Plantar Wart

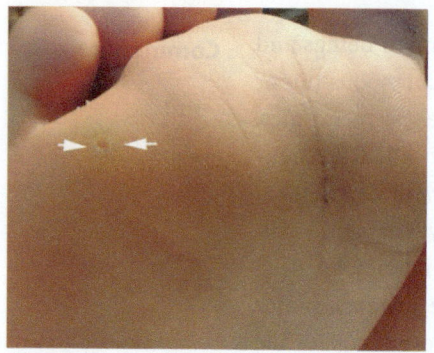

Fig. 4.20.1

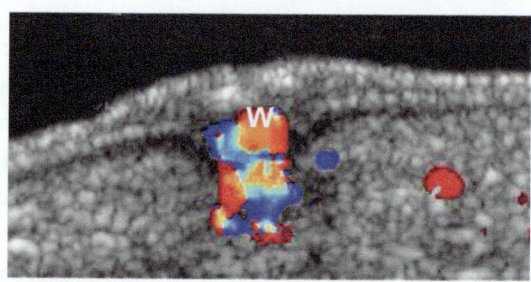

Fig. 4.20.4

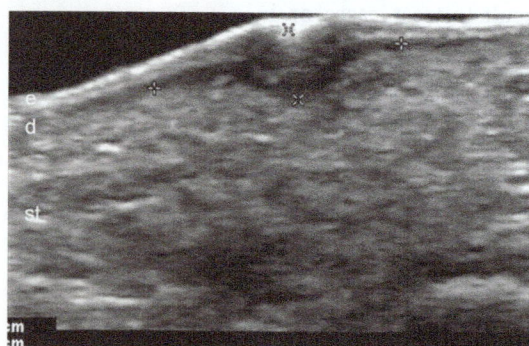

Fig. 4.20.2

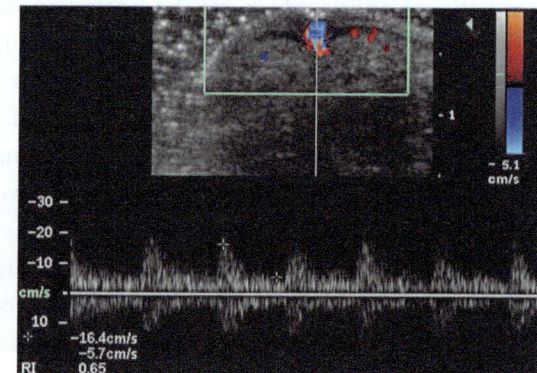

Fig. 4.20.5

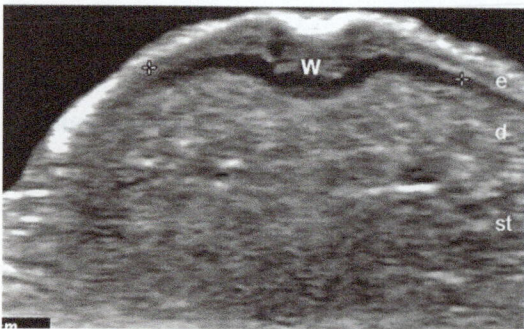

Fig. 4.20.3

Case Presentation

A 12-year-old female presenting with hyperkeratotic painful cutaneous lesion (*arrows*) in the sole of the right foot between the distal parts of the 4th and 5th metatarsal bones (Fig. 4.20.1). A plantar wart was diagnosed.

Comments

Plantar warts are common benign skin lesions produced by the infection of the human papilloma virus. These lesions affect 7–10 % of the US population and up to 22 % of the children in some parts of Australia. Moreover, recurrences are frequently reported. Plantar warts can be very painful and therefore may easily affect the quality of life of individuals. Thus, these viral infiltrations affect the epidermis and dermis, using an endophytic pattern probably generated by the invagination of the viral components secondary to the pressure when walking or standing. Also, plantar warts can be more frequent during immunosuppressive conditions which can add complexity to these already difficult cases. Often, plantar warts may be clinically mistaken by Morton's neuromas or foreign bodies because of the painful symptoms.

On sonography, plantar warts show as fusiform hypoechoic lesions involving epidermis and dermis. Variable degrees of vascularity may be noticed within the lesions usually with slow-velocity arterial vessels in the dermal layer. Furthermore, increased sublesional blood flow has been described in up to 79 % of the cases. Plantar warts can present single or multiple locations and affect one or both feet. Additionally, plantar bursitis has been reported in up to 56 % of the cases in the vicinity of the warts as the result of a strong inflammatory reaction. Also, increased echogenicity of the subcutaneous tissue beneath the lesion can be detected secondary to edema. Sonography can allow support the diagnosis and the noninvasive monitoring of the treatment as well as to provide anatomical data for planning surgery when needed.

Imaging Findings

Figure 4.20.2: Gray-scale ultrasound (transverse view) demonstrates 10.2-mm (wide) × 2.9-mm (deep) hypoechoic fusiform lesion (between markers) affecting epidermis (*e*) and dermis (*d*). Notice the bilaminar appearance of the normal plantar epidermis in the vicinity (*st*) subcutaneous tissue.

Figure 4.20.3: Gray-scale ultrasound (longitudinal view) demonstrates 12.4-mm (long) hypoechoic fusiform lesion (*W*). *e* epidermis, *d* dermis, *st* subcutaneous tissue.

Figure 4.20.4: Color Doppler (transverse view) shows increased blood flow in the dermal component of the lesion (*W*).

Figure 4.20.5: Color Doppler spectral curve analysis demonstrates arterial blood flow within the lesion.

Further Reading

Ahuja AT, Ying M, Ho SY (2008) Ultrasound of malignant cervical lymph nodes. Cancer Imaging 8:48–56

Arbabi EM, Fearnley TE, Carrim ZI (2010) Drusen and the misleading optic disc. Pract Neurol 10:27–30

Bedi DG, Gombos DS, Ng CS, Singh S (2006) Sonography of the eye. AJR Am J Roentgenol 187:1061–1072

Bhatt S, Dogra V (2008) Role of US in testicular and scrotal trauma. Radiographics 28:1617–1629

Bialek EJ, Jakubowski W, Zajkowski P, Szopinski KT, Osmolski A (2006) US of the major salivary glands: anatomy and spatial relationships, pathologic conditions, and pitfalls. Radiographics 26:745–763

Blaivas M, Theodoro D, Sierzenski PR (2002) A study of bedside ocular ultrasonography in the emergency department. Acad Emerg Med 9:791–799

Bobadilla F, Wortsman X, Muñoz C, Segovia L, Espinoza M, Jemec GBE (2008) Pre-surgical high resolution ultrasound of facial basal cell carcinoma: correlation with histology. Cancer Imaging 22:163–172

Chan JM, Shin LK, Jeffrey RB (2007) Ultrasonography of abnormal neck lymph nodes. Ultrasound Q 23:47–54

Cho HW, Kim J, Choi J (2011) Sonographically guided fine-needle aspiration biopsy of major salivary gland masses: a review of 245 cases. Am J Roentgenol 196:1160–1163

Choi N, Moon WJ, Lee JH (2011) Ultrasonographic findings of medullary thyroid cancer: differences according to tumor size and correlation with fine needle aspiration results. Acta Radiol 52:312–316

Choo HJ, Lee SJ, Lee YH, Lee JH, Oh M, Kim MH, Lee EJ, Song JW, Kim SJ, Kim DW (2010) Pilomatricomas: the diagnostic value of ultrasound. Skeletal Radiol 39:243–250

Dogra V, Gottlieb R, Oka M, Rubens D (2003) Sonography of the scrotum. Radiology 227:18–36

Esen G (2006) Ultrasound of superficial lymph nodes. Eur J Radiol 58:345–359

Hilborn MD, Munk PL, Lin DTL, Vellet AD, Poon PY (1993) Sonography of ocular choroidal melanomas. AJR Am J Roentgenol 161:1253–1257

Howlett DC (2003) High resolution ultrasound assessment of the parotid gland. Br J Radiol 76:271–277

Kahn A, Kahn AL, Corinaldi CA, Benitez FL, Fox PJC (2005) Retinal detachment diagnosed by bedside ultrasound in the emergency department. Cal J Emerg Med 6:47–51

Kim B, Winter T, Ryu J (2003) Testicular microlithiasis: clinical significance and review of the literature. Eur Radiol 13:2567–2576

Kim J, Kim EK, Park CS (2004) Characteristic sonographic findings of Warthin's tumor in the parotid gland. J Clin Ultrasound 32:78–81

Kwong JS, Munk PL, Lin DTL, Vellet AD, Levin M, Buckley AR (1992) Real-time sonography in ocular trauma. AJR Am J Roentgenol 158:179–182

Lam DL, Gerscovich EO, Kuo MC, McGahan JP (2007) Testicular microlithiasis: our experience of 10 years. J Ultrasound Med 26:867–873

Lee S, Shin JH, Ko EY (2010) Medullary thyroid carcinoma: comparison with papillary thyroid carcinoma and application of current sonographic criteria. Am J Roentgenol 194:1090–1094

Lindegaard J, Isager P, Prause PJ, Heegaard S (2006) Optic nerve invasion of uveal melanoma: clinical characteristics and metastatic pattern. Invest Ophthalmol Vis Sci 47:3268–3275

McNicholas MMJ, Brophy DP, Power WJ, Griffin JF (1994a) Ocular sonography. AJR Am J Roentgenol 163:921–926

McNicholas MMJ, Power WJ, Griffin JF (1994b) Sonography in optic disk drusen: imaging findings and role in diagnosis when funduscopic findings are normal. AJR Am J Roentgenol 162:161–163

Moon WJ, Jung SL, Lee JH, Na DG, Baek JH, Lee YH, Kim J, Kim HS, Byun JS, Lee DH (2008) Benign and malignant thyroid nodules: US differentiation-multicenter retrospective study. Radiology 247:762–770

Paltiel HJ, Burrows PE, Kozakewich HP, Zurakowski D, Mulliken JB (2000) Soft-tissue vascular anomalies: utility of US for diagnosis. Radiology 214:747–754

Pearl MS, Hill MC (2007) Ultrasound of the scrotum. Semin Ultrasound CT MR 8:225–248

Peer S (2009) The place of sonography in the diagnostic work-up of haemangiomas and vascular malformations. Handchir Mikrochir Plast Chir 41:70–77

Peyster RG, Augsburger JJ, Shields JA, Satchell TV, Markoe AM, Clarke K, Haskin ME (1985) Choroidal melanoma: comparison of CT, fundoscopy, and US. Radiology 156:675–680

Purohit A, Gonzales C (2007) Vitreous hemorrhage: a discussion of etiologies, controversies and current and future therapeutics. Expert Rev Ophthalmol 2:249–254

Ramirez H, Blatt ES, Hibri NS (1983) Computed tomographic identification of calcified optic drusen. Radiology 148:137–139

Smith V, Walton S (2011) Treatment of facial basal cell carcinoma: a review. J Skin Cancer 2011:371–380

Solivetti FM, Elia F, Drusco A, Panetta C, Amantea A, Di Carlo A (2010) Epithelioma of Malherbe: new ultrasound patterns. J Exp Clin Cancer Res 6:29–42

Srinivasan S, Van der Hoek J, Green F, Ratta H (2001) Tractional ciliary body detachment, choroidal effusion, and hypotony caused by severe anterior lens capsule contraction following cataract surgery. Br J Ophthalmol 85:1260

Wittenberg A, Tobias T, Rzeszotarski M, Minotti A (2006) Sonography of the acute scrotum: the four T's of testicular imaging. Curr Probl Diagn Radiol 35:12–21

Woodward P, Sohaey R, O'Donoghue M, Green D (2002) From the archives of the AFIP: tumors and tumorlike lesions of the testis: radiologic-pathologic correlation. Radiographics 22:189–216

Wortsman X, Wortsman J (2010) Clinical usefulness of variable frequency ultrasound in localized lesions of the skin. J Am Acad Dermatol 62:247–256

Wortsman X, Sazunic I, Jemec GBE (2009) Sonography of plantar warts. J Ultrasound Med 28:787–793

Wortsman X, Wortsman J, Arellano J, Oroz J, Giugliano C, Benavides MI, Bordon C (2010a) Pilomatrixomas presenting as vascular tumors on color Doppler ultrasound. J Pediatr Surg 45:2094–2098

Wortsman X, Jemec GBE, Sazunic I (2010b) Anatomical detection of inflammatory changes associated to plantar warts. Dermatology 220:213–217

Wortsman X, Gutierrez M, Saavedra T, Honeyman J (2011) The role of ultrasound in rheumatic skin and nail lesions: a multi-specialist approach. Clin Rheumatol 30:739–748

Wortsman X (2012) Common applications of dermatologic sonography. J Ultrasound Med 31:97–111

Rosa Zabala and Jose Luís del Cura

Introduction

The chest is one of the areas of the body in which the utility of ultrasound appears less likely. Lungs are filled with air, and air is a well-known obstacle to the transmission of ultrasound beam. The rib cage consists of bones that do not transmit ultrasound. Thus, ultrasound has been traditionally considered of little use in thoracic pathology and usually ignored as a diagnostic tool in the chest, especially in the lung. However, this is no longer true.

Ultrasound has gained a progressive acceptation as a highly useful tool in the evaluation of pleural diseases, and in fact, it has become the most sensitive technique in the detection of pleural fluid. Small amounts of pleural fluid can be easily detected without using harmful radiations. Also, as a consequence of its increased use, new applications of ultrasound have been developed in imaging of the lung and mediastinum. Although normal lung is not visible on ultrasound, diseases like pneumonia or tumors are visible, allowing them to be explored with sonography.

Also, ultrasound allows exploring soft tissue lesions involving chest wall with higher resolution than with other image techniques. The thorax includes also some superficial regions like axillas or supraclavicular fossas, with lymph node groups that are key in the dissemination of regional cancers. Both can be readily explored using ultrasound. Some areas of the mediastinum are also easily accessible using an appropriate approach. So, ultrasound is currently one of the imaging techniques to be considered when dealing with thoracic disease and especially to manage pleural fluid.

J.L. del Cura et al. (eds.), *Learning Ultrasound Imaging*, Learning Imaging,
DOI 10.1007/978-3-642-30586-3_5, © Springer-Verlag Berlin Heidelberg 2012

Case 1: Pneumonia

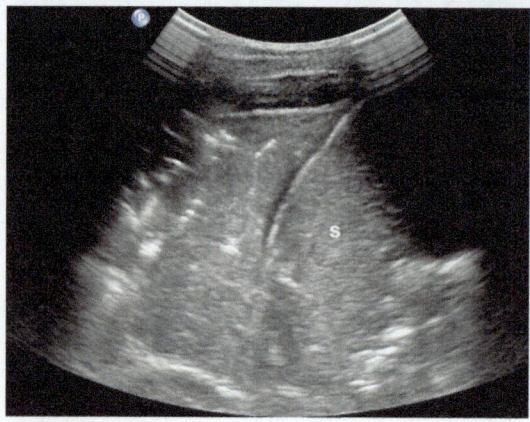

Fig. 5.1.1

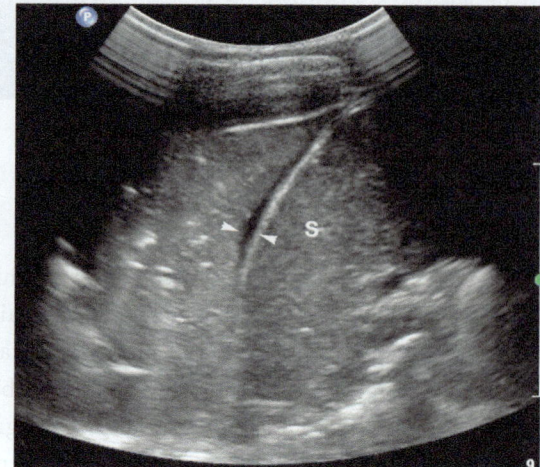

Fig. 5.1.2

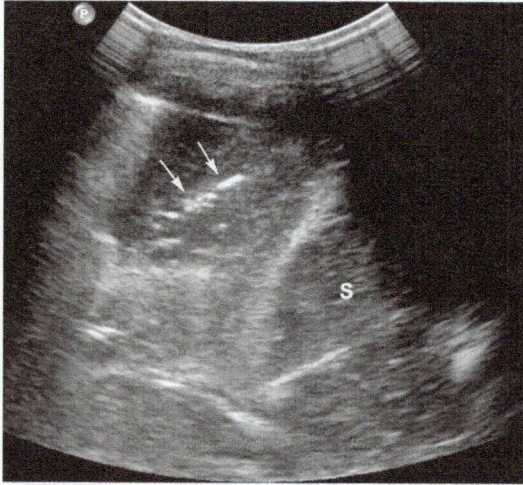

Fig. 5.1.3

Coronal ultrasound scans through the upper left abdomen are obtained in a 10-year-old boy with fever and chest pain. Above the spleen (*S*), the left lobe of the lung has a solid appearance. Small bright dots and echogenic linear branching structures (*arrows*) can be seen within the lung. A small, hypoechoic pleural effusion (*arrowheads*) can be seen between the diaphragm and the lower boundary of the lung (Figs. 5.1.1, 5.1.2, and 5.1.3).

Case Presentation and Imaging Findings

Parasternal and intercostal approaches can be used for exploring lung, pleura, and anterior mediastinum. Also, subxiphoid and transdiaphragmatic approaches, using the liver as the acoustic window, can be useful to explore the lower areas of lung, pleura, and posterior mediastinum. Suprasternal and supraclavicular approaches facilitate the evaluation of the lung apexes.

Comments

In lung diseases associated to consolidation, like pneumonia or atelectasis, the air disappears from the parenchyma, and there is a through transmission of the ultrasound beam. In these cases, the lung presents a "solid" appearance instead of the bright reflections of the aerated lung. The airless lung is similar in echogenicity and echotexture to the liver and spleen. However, the lung does not appear always homogeneous: multiple bright dot-like and, especially, branching linear structures are usually seen within the solid-appearing area. These findings represent air in the bronchi and residual air in the alveoli. This finding is termed a sonographic air bronchogram, which is the equivalent to the air bronchogram seen in alveolar pattern on chest radiographs.

Occasionally, the bronchial tree can appear filled with fluid rather than air. In these cases, a branching pattern of anechoic or hypoechoic tubular structures can be seen on ultrasound in the consolidated lung. This sign is the sonographic fluid bronchogram and is also a specific indicator of pulmonary parenchymal consolidation.

Ultrasound is an excellent tool to differentiate pleural fluid or thickening from pulmonary parenchymal lesions. This is important because distinction between both lesion types is not always easy at chest radiography, especially when both pulmonary and pleural lesions are present.

Case 2: Pulmonary Hydatid Cyst

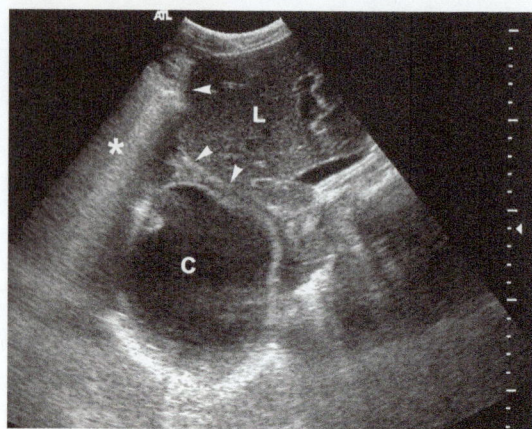

Fig. 5.2.1

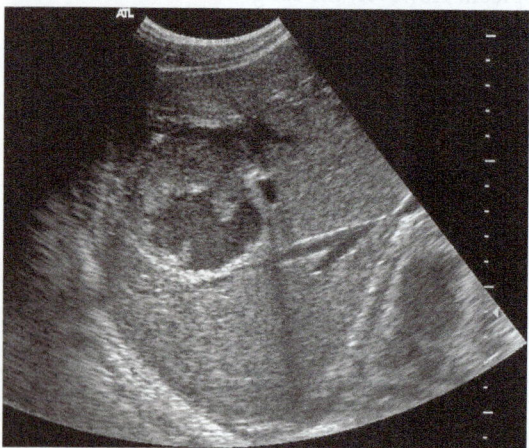

Fig. 5.2.2

Fig. 5.2.3

A 22-year-old North African male consulted because of fatigue and abdominal pain. A blood test was performed demonstrating altered liver function tests. An ultrasound exam was indicated. The images correspond to sagittal (Fig. 5.2.1) and axial (Figs. 5.2.2 and 5.2.3) planes through the right lobe of the liver. Both Figs. 5.2.1 and 5.2.2 show a spherical, well-delimited, anechoic lesion (*C*) located beyond the diaphragm (*arrowheads*). Both the right lobe of the liver (*L*) and the dirty shadowing caused by the air in the lung (*) can also be seen, each one in a different side of the diaphragm. In Fig. 5.2.3, corresponding to an axial section below the level of Fig. 5.2.2, another spherical, well-delimited, anechoic lesion can be seen in segment VIII of the liver.

The hydatid cyst is a zoonosis caused by the larval state of the taeniae *Echinococcus granulosus* and *Echinococcus multilocularis*. This infection appears in many parts of the world, especially in South America, Africa, and the Middle East. Humans who are intermediary hosts, like sheep, acquire the parasite by drinking water or vegetables contaminated by dog feces. The dog is the final host. The dog is contaminated by ingesting contaminated viscera of sheep or any other intermediate host.

After crossing the intestine, the parasite reaches an organ where it forms the hydatid cyst. Liver is the most frequently involved organ, being lung the second in frequency (15 % of the hydatid cysts) and the most common in children. Lung involvement can occur after hematogenous spread of the parasite or as a consequence of transdiaphragmatic migration of a previous hydatid disease from the liver, like in the case presented here. Transdiaphragmatic migration is common in hydatid cysts located in posterior segments of the right hepatic lobe, probably due to the lack of peritoneal coverage in this area (bare area), resulting in decreased resistance to cyst migration. Transdiaphragmatic migration from other segments of the liver is less common.

Cough, hemoptysis, and chest pain are the most common clinical symptoms. Cyst may rupture to bronchium, causing expectoration of cyst fluid, membranes, and scolices. Allergic episodes may also develop after cyst rupture.

Although the diagnosis is usually made after a radiograph, ultrasound can help confirm the presence of hepatic hydatid disease and demonstrate pleural effusion. However, the diaphragmatic defect is difficult to demonstrate. And, sometimes a pulmonary hydatid cyst can be detected on an ultrasound exam, especially when this cyst is the result of the transdiaphragmatic migration of a hepatic disease.

Case 3: Pleural Rhabdomyosarcoma

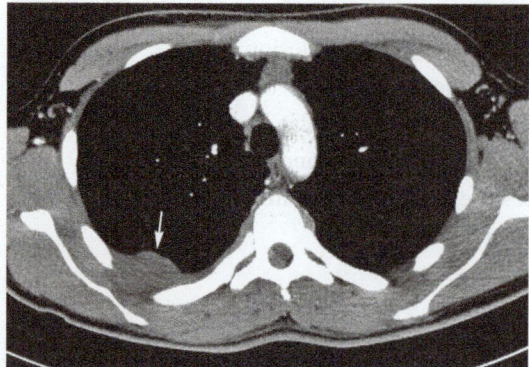

Fig. 5.3.1

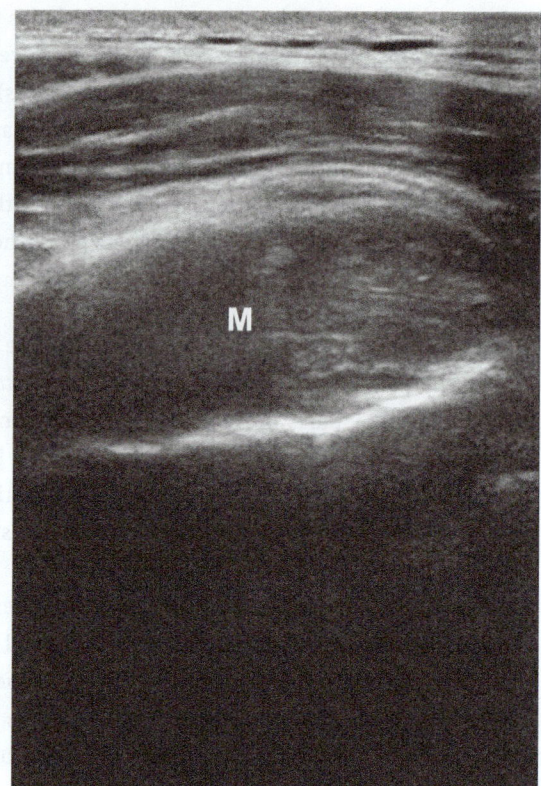

Fig. 5.3.2

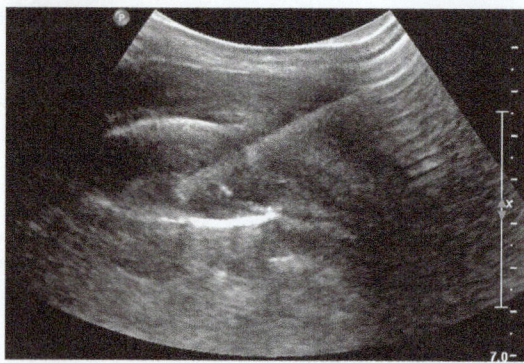

Fig. 5.3.3

On a chest radiograph obtained in a 16-year-old boy after an episode of fever and cough, a suspicious opacity in the right hemithorax was incidentally discovered. A CT performed (Fig. 5.3.1) detected a focal pleural thickening in the right hemithorax (*arrow*). An ultrasound was carried out in the precise area of the thorax where the lesion had been identified (Fig. 5.3.2) and a focal thickening of the pleura (*M*) was identified. A pleural tumor was suspected, and an ultrasound-guided biopsy was thus performed (Fig. 5.3.3). The result of the biopsy was pleural rhabdomyosarcoma.

Rhabdomyosarcoma is the most frequent soft tissue sarcoma in children and young adults. Although it may occur at any site, primary tumors are more common in head and neck. Location in thorax is rare, being pleural rhabdomyosarcoma exceptional with only a few cases reported.

Thoracic rhabdomyosarcoma is scarcely symptomatic until it reaches a big size, and thus it is frequently diagnosed late. The most common symptoms at the onset are cough and fever. Spontaneous pneumothorax and pleural effusion may appear too. Pleural rhabdomyosarcoma has a bad prognosis.

In pleural rhabdomyosarcoma, imaging is necessary for diagnosis and staging. Since chest X-ray is usually nonspecific, ultrasound can be an excellent tool for imaging the tumor. Ultrasound has gained a progressive acceptation as a highly useful tool in the evaluation of pleural diseases, and it has become the most sensitive technique in the detection of pleural fluid. Also, it is highly accurate to differentiate between pleural effusion and thickening. This is important because distinction between these two conditions on chest radiography, is not always easy especially when both are simultaneously present.

Differential diagnosis of pleural rhabdomyosarcoma includes Ewing's sarcoma, chest wall and pleural metastase, pleuropulmonary blastoma, and lymphoma. Pleural mesothelioma has similar features too, but it appears in older patients. Rhabdomyosarcomas generally do not destroy the ribs. Diagnosis should be confirmed by biopsy of the tumor, and ultrasound plays a role here too because it is the best technique to help guide the biopsy.

Case 4: Supraclavicular Schwannoma

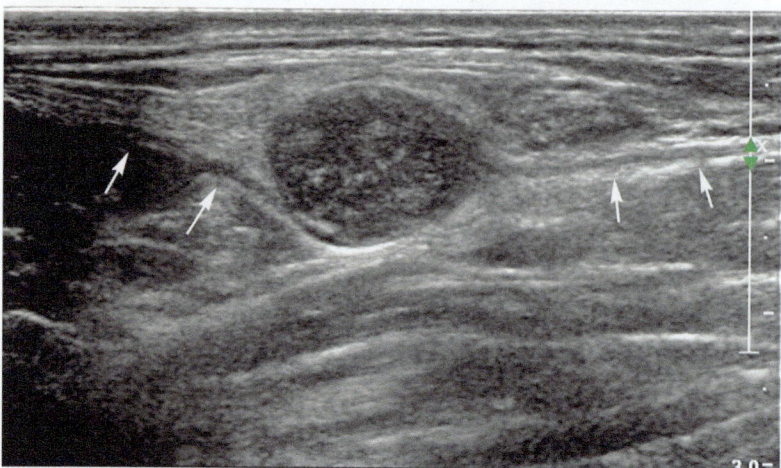

Fig. 5.4.1

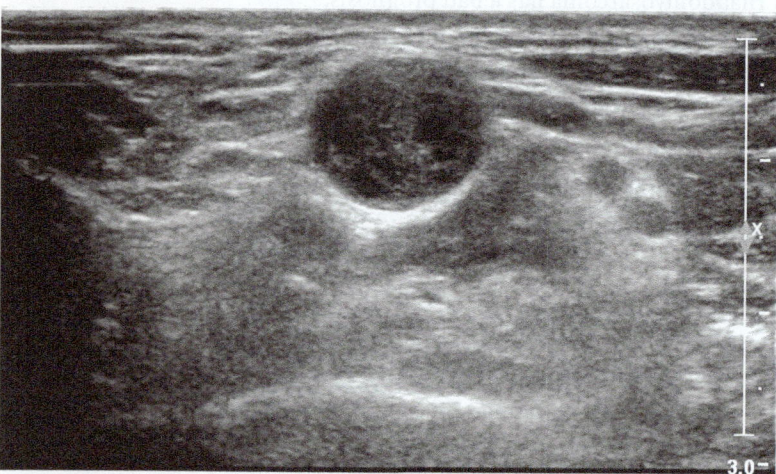

Fig. 5.4.2

A 35-year-old woman consults for a left supraclavicular palpable tumor. On palpation, the tumor was hard and not fixed to the deep layers. A sonography of the supraclavicular fossa was performed. The images show longitudinal (Fig. 5.4.1) and transverse (Fig. 5.4.2) sonograms of the lesion. A well-delimited homogeneous fusiform hypoechoic mass with posterior acoustic enhancement is shown. A direct continuity of the tumor with a nerve (*straight arrows*) can be observed also.

Case Presentation and Imaging Findings

High-frequency transducers are an excellent tool for the imaging of peripheral nerves. Thus, sonography has become the primary technique for imaging peripheral nerve pathology because it is widely available and allows quick, detailed imaging of most of the entire length of them. Sonography can diagnose any kind of diseases that affects nerves: entrapment syndromes, traumatic lesions, or tumors.

Comments

Usually, peripheral nerve sheath tumors are discovered in sonographic exams performed to evaluate a palpable soft tissue mass. The most common tumors are the schwannoma and the neurofibroma. Schwannomas are encapsulated tumors that grow eccentrically along the nerve, within the epineurium. Neurofibromas may present as a solitary mass or as multiple masses as part of neurofibromatosis.

Schwannomas represent approximately 5 % of benign soft tissue neoplasms. They appear especially in 20–40-year-old patients. Most are solitary and present as a slowly growing, painless soft tissue mass. The symptoms appear usually as a consequence of the compression of the adjacent nerve.

On ultrasound, schwannomas appear as discrete, homogeneous fusiform, hypoechoic masses, with posterior acoustic enhancement. Direct continuity with a healthy nerve can be observed at the fusiform proximal and distal aspects of the mass and is a key finding to diagnose a soft tissue mass as a nerve sheath tumor.

Sonography is unreliable in distinguishing between schwannomas and neurofibromas, although some features can help differentiate them. An eccentric lesion or the presence of cystic degeneration favors schwannoma rather than neurofibroma. This differentiation is important to decide the therapeutic management because schwannoma is generally separable from the underlying nerve fibers, thus often allowing the tumor to be surgically excised without loss of neurologic function, whereas neurofibromas are not. Ultrasound-guided biopsy of the tumor can be used to distinguish between both tumors.

Further Reading

Agarwal PP, Seely JM, Matzinger FR, MacRae RM, Peterson RA, Maziak DE, Dennie CJ (2006) Pleural mesothelioma: sensitivity and incidence of needle track seeding after image-guided biopsy versus surgical biopsy. Radiology 241:589–594

El Bari S, Chellaoui M (2010) Primary pleural rhabdomyosarcoma: a case report and literature review. Eur J Radiol 76:e55–e57

Kim OH, Kim WS, Kim MJ, Jung JY, Suh JH (2000) US in the diagnosis of pediatric chest diseases. Radiographics 20:653–671

Lin J, Martel W (2001) Cross-sectional imaging of peripheral nerve sheath tumors: characteristic signs on CT, MR imaging, and sonography. AJR Am J Roentgenol 176:75–82

Pedrosa I, Saíz A, Arrazola J, Ferreirós J, Pedrosa CS (2000) Hydatid disease: radiologic and pathologic features and complications. Radiographics 20:795–817

Reynolds DL Jr, Jacobson JA, Inampudi P, Jamadar DA, Ebrahim FS, Hayes CW (2004) Sonographic characteristics of peripheral nerve sheath tumors. AJR Am J Roentgenol 182:741–744

Stuart RM, Koh ES, Breidahl WH (2004) Sonography of peripheral nerve pathology. AJR Am J Roentgenol 182:123–129

Targhetta R, Chavagneux R, Bourgeois JM, Dauzat M, Balmes P, Pourcelot L (1992) Sonographic approach to diagnosing pulmonary consolidation. J Ultrasound Med 11:667–672

Pediatrics

Fermín Sáez, Elena Elizagaray, and José Martel

Introduction

The danger for patient's health posed by imaging techniques using radiations is especially high in children because of their greater sensitivity to the effects of radiation and also to their longer life expectancy. The risk that a radiological exploration causes a cancer is multiplied almost by ten in children compared to adults.

The reduced ossification of the children in the first months of life makes that some anatomical areas like central nervous system or hip, which are not accessible in the adult, can be studied by ultrasound in newborns and infants.

Children are also thinner and have less fat than adults. This makes most of their anatomy to be within the scope of scanning probes. Virtually any part of the anatomy of a child can be explored with high-resolution ultrasound probes, especially in the lower ages.

In this context, ultrasound has become the primary image technique of choice for the study of children, when the studied area is accessible to ultrasound. However, being a dynamic exploration, ultrasound requires specific skills by the operator in the management of pediatric patients, given that they do not follow the instructions as adults and require a different treatment.

Due to its high availability and easy access to the abdominal structures in the young child, ultrasound is also the most appropriate technique for the study of acute abdominal diseases of children such as intussusception or hypertrophic pyloric stenosis.

J.L. del Cura et al. (eds.), *Learning Ultrasound Imaging*, Learning Imaging,
DOI 10.1007/978-3-642-30586-3_6, © Springer-Verlag Berlin Heidelberg 2012

Case 1: Infantile Hypertrophic Pyloric Stenosis

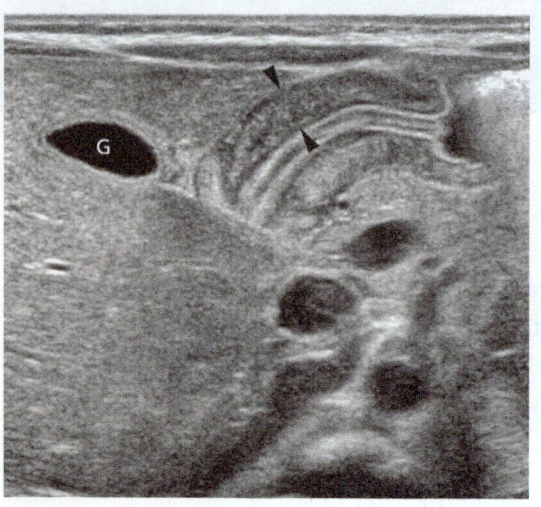

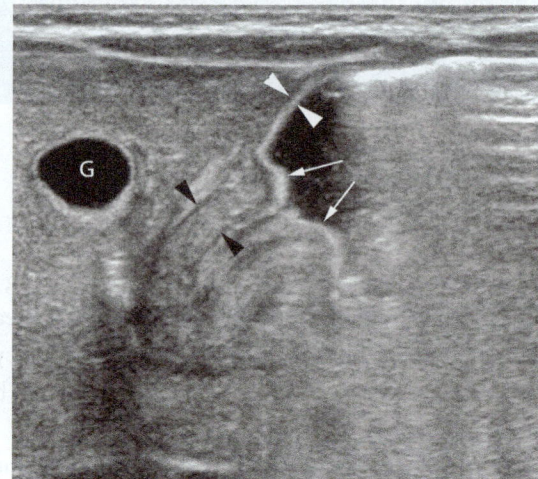

Fig. 6.1.1   **Fig. 6.1.2**

Case Presentation and Imaging Findings

A 3-week-old male with repeated vomiting. Figures 6.1.1 and 6.1.2 show a coronal US of the pyloric channel. The pylorus is close to the gallbladder (*G*). Its muscle layer (between *black arrowheads*) is markedly thickened (>4 mm), in contrast to the normal thickness of the gastric antrum (between *white arrowheads*). The length of the channel is more than 20 mm. There is shouldering effect (*arrows*) of the hypertrophic pylorus on the antrum. A redundant mucosa, slightly protruding into the antrum, is seen in Fig. 6.1.2.

Comments

Infantile hypertrophic pyloric stenosis is a common cause (frequency, 3 in 1,000 live births) of gastric outlet obstruction in infancy. The pyloric muscle is markedly hypertrophied (thickness of 3 mm or more) and elongated (15–22 mm), and the lumen is filled with compressed and redundant mucosa, which protrudes into the gastric antrum. The etiology is unknown, but environmental and genetic causes (siblings have five times more incidence) have been proved in some cases. It is postulated that an obstructing event at the gastric outlet may initiate a feedback cycle, leading to obstruction that resolves once the obstruction is relieved surgically and normal gastric activity resumes.

Typical presentation is an infant male (ratio male to female, 4:1) between 3 and 8 weeks, with repeated projectile nonbilious vomiting which can lead, if untreated, to dehydration and metabolic alkalosis, with hyponatremia and hypokalemia. A palpable mass (so-called olive) may be felt, especially after vomiting. In the classic case with an experienced clinician, no other diagnostic procedure is needed, and the patient may undergo surgery (pyloromyotomy).

Some cases, however, are more difficult to diagnose, and imaging can be of help. Upper gastrointestinal barium examination was the standard imaging test before the advent of US. However, radiation, lack of direct visualization of the pyloric muscle, and long examination times make barium examination a second-line procedure for a few selected cases, being ultrasound the preferred method. Sensitivity and specificity of US are close to 100 %.

A linear high-frequency transducer (6–12 MHz) is recommended, although a sector transducer may be of help in case of limited window access to the pylorus (especially when the infant is placed in the oblique right-side-down position to allow fluid filling of the gastric antrum). The elongation of the pylorus displaces it to a location very close to the gallbladder, which serves as a useful anatomical reference. Despite the vomiting, the stomach is usually overdistended. Gravity-aided maneuvers are very helpful in difficult cases.

Thickened muscle layer and elongated pyloric canal, together with a hypertrophied-redundant mucosa, are the hallmarks of this condition.

On cross section, a target sign may be seen (hypoechoic ring of hypertrofied pyloric muscle surrounding the echogenic redundant mucosa). Indentation of muscle mass on fluid-filled antrum on longitudinal section makes a so-called cervix sign or shoulder configuration.

The redundant mucosa protrudes into the gastric antrum (antral nipple sign). There are exaggerated peristaltic gastric waves. The main diagnostic criteria are a muscle layer thickness >3 mm, elongated pyloric canal >17 mm, and the pylorus does not open/relax during the whole examination. A tiny string of gastric content may pass through the closed pyloric canal (the so-called string sign in barium examination).

Clinical differential diagnosis of nonbilious vomiting includes infantile pylorospasm, milk allergy, gastroesophageal reflux, and eosinophilic gastroenteritis. From the imaging point of view, the main condition to differentiate is infantile pylorospasm. In pylorospasm (reversible condition; it is postulated that it may progress to hypertrophic pyloric stenosis), the muscle thickness varies between 1.5 and 3 mm, with some elongation of the pyloric canal (<15 mm). If the canal opens during the examination, hypertrophic pyloric stenosis can be ruled out. Infants in whom the muscle is 2–3 mm thick and does not relax/open throughout the examination warrant follow-up clinical and/or ultrasound examinations, until the vomiting resolves or until a definite diagnosis of hypertrophic pyloric stenosis can be made.

Case 2: Ileocolic Intussusception

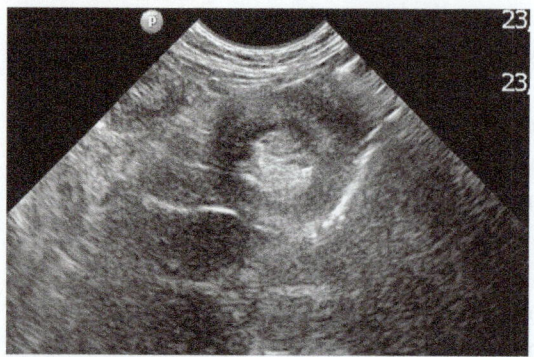

Fig. 6.2.1

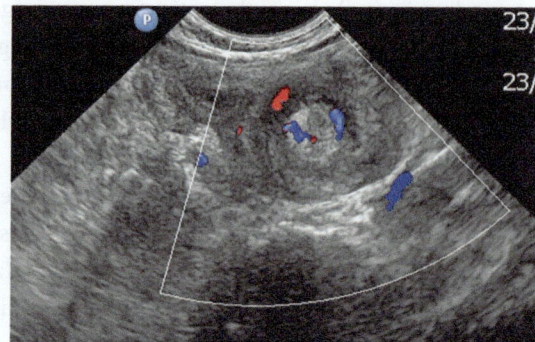

Fig. 6.2.2

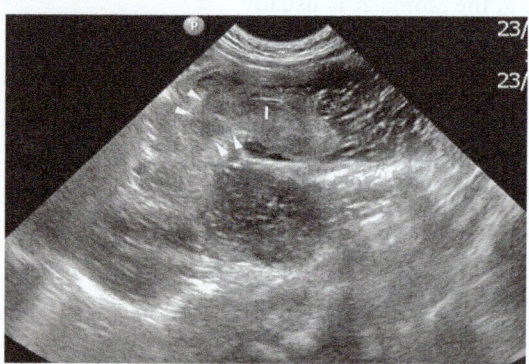

Fig. 6.2.3

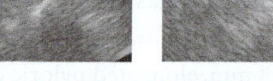

Fig. 6.2.4

Case Presentation and Imaging Findings

A 9-month-old boy with nausea, vomiting, and abdominal pain

Figure 6.2.1 Characteristic doughnut pattern of ileocolic intussusception. The external ring is mainly formed by the everted returning limb of intussusceptum (the part of the bowel that prolapses into the other), with smaller component of the intussuscipiens (the part that receives the intussusceptum). The hyperechoic crescent-shaped center corresponds to the mesentery accompanying the entering limb of the intussusceptum.

Figure 6.2.2 Normal Doppler color flow is visualized.

Figure 6.2.3 After water enema, the intussusception (*I*) is being pushed backwards through the ileocecal valve (*arrowheads*).

Figure 6.2.4 Open edematous ileocecal valve. The intussusception has been solved.

Comments

Intussusception is a common cause of abdominal pain and acute abdomen in infants and young children (especially between 3 months and 2 years of age). It is a medical condition in which a portion of the digestive tract has invaginated into the adjacent bowel segment. This can often result in an obstruction. Common symptoms are nausea, vomiting, abdominal pain, and eventually rectal bleeding (black currant jelly). Most cases are idiopathic, with no leading point. Early diagnosis and effective nonsurgical treatment (enema) lead to successful reduction in more than 80 % of the cases. Conversely, long-standing intussusception increases the likelihood of bowel ischemia and necrosis, requiring surgical resection. The main clinical differential diagnosis is acute gastroenteritis.

Ultrasound is the best method for diagnosing the intussusception, as plain abdominal films show useful signs (soft tissue mass, meniscus sign, and target sign) in only 40–50 % of the cases. Intussusception appears on ultrasound as a target-like or doughnut sign of 25–50 mm in diameter, most frequently located in the transverse colon. Some cases show the presence of a crescent of fluid within the intussusception, representing trapped peritoneal fluid. Doppler interrogation may show flow within the walls of the intussusceptum. The absence of flow is related to low reduction rate. Dilated bowel loops are visualized in long-standing obstruction. Although most intussusceptions are idiopathic, with no leading point other than lymph nodes, ultrasound can show the pathological lead points. Transient small bowel intussusceptions are frequently visualized on ultrasound and CT, but are smaller in size (diameter less than 25 mm), and usually resolve spontaneously.

Once diagnosed, intussusception must be treated with enema, unless the patient presents definite contraindications: shock not readily corrected and signs of perforation/peritonitis (small amounts of free peritoneal fluid are seen in up to 50 % of intussusceptions and do not contraindicate the enema). Absence of Doppler flow and trapped peritoneal fluid within the intussusception are related to ischemia and low rate of reducibility, but do not contraindicate the enema attempt.

Sedation before and during the enema is controverted.

The type of enema (barium, air, or saline/warm water) and imaging method (fluoroscopy or ultrasound) depends on the experience of the radiologist, with similar success reduction and perforation rates for any of these types of enemas. US with saline or warm water is the preferred method, due to the lack of ionizing radiation and the good control of the intussusception and potential related complications: perforation and residual ileoileal intussusception. The enema bag is filled with 1–2 l of saline or tepid water, starting at a height of 60 cm and increasing gradually this height up to 150 cm. The head of the intussusception is monitored until its passage through the ileocecal valve. Several attempts can be performed in case of partial reduction. A delayed attempt of at least 30 min after the initial partial resolution increases the rate of reduction in about 15 %. Approximately 5–10 % of the infants with successful reduction recur within 24 h.

Urgent surgery should be performed in case of nonreduction or perforation.

Case 3: Enteric Duplication

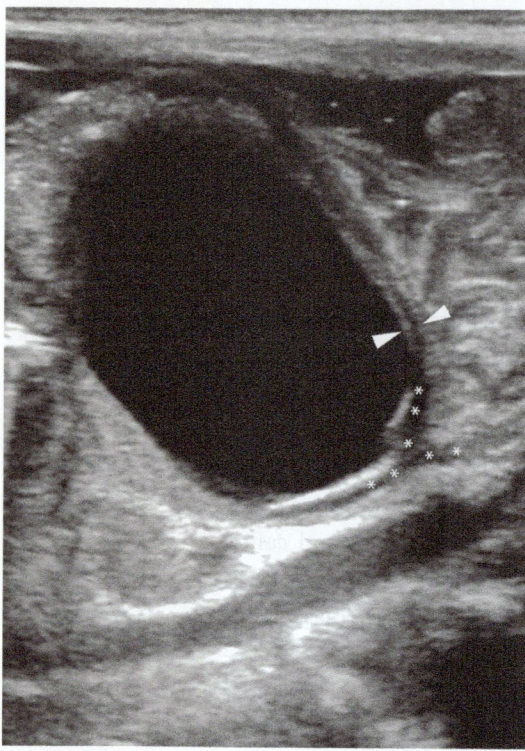

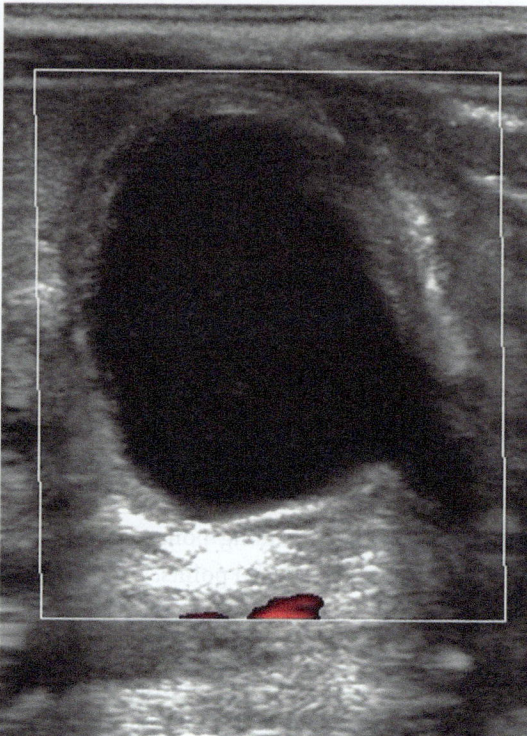

Fig. 6.3.1

Fig. 6.3.2

A 2-week-old boy with prenatal diagnosis of an abdominal cyst

Figure 6.3.1 A 30 × 22 mm ovoid cyst is shown in the right flank/iliac fossa, inferior to the liver, but separate from it, and unattached to any solid viscera. A double layer (hyperechoic gastrointestinal mucosa/submucosa and hypoechoic smooth muscle) is demonstrated (between *arrowheads*). An area of split hypoechoic muscularis propria layer, resulting in a Y configuration, is also seen (*asterisks*).

Figure 6.3.2 Color Doppler. No color flow is identified in the wall.

Mesenteric and/or omental cysts are classified by their lining: enteric duplication (mucosa and muscle layers), lymphangioma (endothelial lining), enteric cyst (mucosa, but no muscle layer), mesothelial cyst (mesothelial lining), and nonpancreatic pseudocyst (fibrous lining).

Gastrointestinal duplications are rare congenital lesions that can develop anywhere along the mesenteric side of the alimentary tract, but are more frequent (30–40 %) at the ileum. They may be spherical (more common) or tubular, and they rarely communicate with the bowel lumen. The etiology is not known.

They may be asymptomatic or may present during the first year of life with vomiting and pain due to obstruction (internal secretions cause them to increase in size). Rectal bleeding is uncommon, but, when present, poses a differential diagnosis with Meckel's diverticulum, colitis, and intussusception.

Ultrasound is the initial examination for a child with an abdominal mass. Enteric duplication usually presents as a well-defined anechoic unilocular cystic lesion. Occasionally, debris may be present inside the cyst. The wall is double layered, with an echogenic inner rim (mucosa/submucosa) and an outer thick hypoechoic layer (muscularis propria), similar to a normal bowel wall (gut signature). However, the mucosa may be extensively ulcerated so that the hyperechoic inner rim is no longer present. The muscle layer may split in a Y configuration in a localized area of the lesion, where the muscle layer is shared by the cyst and the normal related bowel. The gut signature, together with this Y configuration, is virtually diagnostic of enteric duplication. Less often, five sonographic layers are identified, reflecting superficial mucosa, deep mucosa, submucosa, muscularis propria, and serosa. Meckel's diverticulum presents also the gut signature, but its lining is usually more irregular, and lacks the Y configuration of the muscle layer.

Doppler interrogation usually does not show flow within the wall of the duplication. On the other hand, Meckel's diverticulum, especially when inflamed, shows hypervascular color flow.

Treatment is surgical: the cyst is removed together with the related bowel.

Differential diagnosis include, apart from the above-mentioned Meckel's diverticulum, lymphangioma, mesenteric cyst, pancreatic pseudocyst, choledochal cyst, exophytic hepatic or renal cysts, and cystic tumors. Ovarian cyst must be ruled out in a baby girl. All these cystic lesions do not usually present the gut signature.

Case 4: Neutropenic Colitis

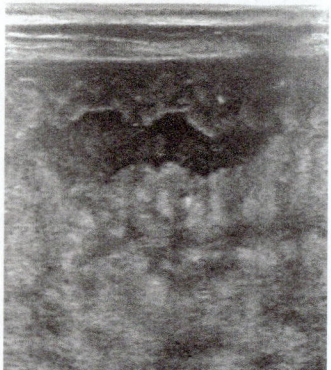

Fig. 6.4.1

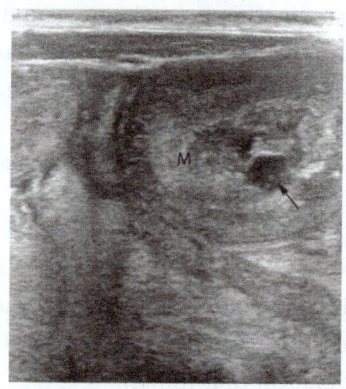

Fig. 6.4.2

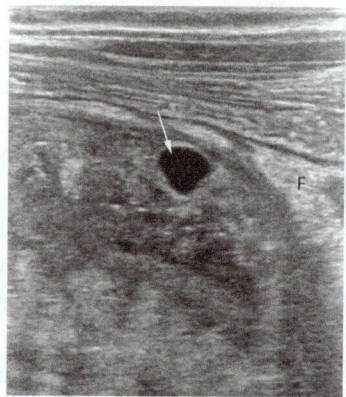

Fig. 6.4.3

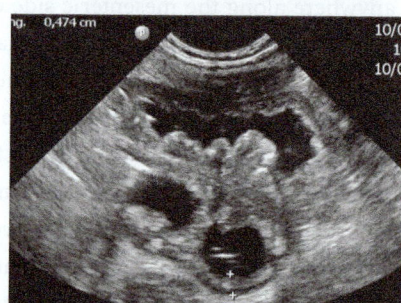

Fig. 6.4.4

Case Presentation and Imaging Findings

A 12-year-old boy with acute myeloid leukemia on intensive chemotherapy treatment, with an absolute neutrophil count of 250. Figures 6.4.1, 6.4.2, and 6.4.3 Sonographs of the colon. Marked mural thickening (8 mm from mucosa to serosa) is demonstrated in the ascending (Fig. 6.4.1) and transverse colon (Figs. 6.4.2 and 6.4.3). The mucosa of the ascending colon is thin and shows many small ulcers/erosions. However, there are areas of the transverse colon with markedly thickened, sphacelous mucosa (*M*) which presents cystic areas (*arrow*). More cystic lesions are seen deeply within the colonic wall (*arrow* in Fig. 6.4.3). Inflamed (hyperechogenic) pericolic fat (*F*) is also seen. Figure 6.4.4 Follow-up after 1 month. There is only mild thickening (4 mm) of the colonic wall. The cystic lesions are no longer visualized. The child was discharged from hospital.

Comments

Neutropenic colitis is an uncommon (1–3 % in children treated for neoplasia) acute life-threatening condition in a neutropenic child (absolute neutropenic count <500/mm³) undergoing prolonged (10–20 days) chemotherapy for malignancy, most frequently acute leukemia, who presents with RLQP, fever, diarrhea, and sometimes clinical signs of peritonitis. The mechanism of this disease is not well understood; implicated factors are mucosal injury, neutropenia, and impaired immune response to pathogen infiltration, leading to hemorrhage and necrosis of the bowel wall and eventually perforation.

The cecum is most frequently involved (typhlitis), probably due to ease of distensibility, relative stasis of bowel contents, and decreased vascularity relative to remainder of colon. However, our case showed more involvement of the ascending and transverse colon than the cecum.

Uncomplicated disease is treated with total parenteral nutrition, IV fluids, and broad-spectrum antibiotics; in cases of peritonitis, perforation, or gastrointestinal bleeding, surgical management with resection of the affected segment is indicated. Mortality rate is very high with a wide range (20–80 %), due to transmural necrosis, perforation, and sepsis.

Pathological features include loss of mucosa, marked edema of the submucosa, hemorrhage, ulceration, and transmural necrosis (eventually perforation) without significant inflammatory reaction. Frequently, the deeper portions of the bowel wall are infiltrated by fungi and gram-negative bacteria.

Imaging plays an important role in the diagnosis and follow-up of this condition. Plain films, usually nonspecific or even normal, may show right lower abdominal mass density, paralytic ileus, obstruction, pneumatosis intestinalis, and, in case of perforation, pneumoperitoneum. However, ultrasound and CT are much more precise and are considered the imaging methods of choice. Concerns about radiation, paucity of abdominal fat, and portability make ultrasound, with high-frequency probes (7–14 MHz), the preferred method for neutropenic colitis in children in most settings. The whole abdomen is studied with the graded compression technique. The process has a predilection for the terminal ileum and cecum, but any segment of the bowel can be involved.

Ultrasound shows mural nonstratified thickening and hyperemia on color Doppler interrogation. The mucosa may have a pseudopolypoid sphacelous appearance, or may present as a very thin layer, with erosions/ulcers. Our case showed these two different mucosal appearances and several cysts, both in the mucosa and deep within the wall, a finding that has not been described, to our knowledge. There is absence of colonic gas and peristalsis, and there may be signs of pneumatosis (hyperechoic reverberant echoes within the bowel wall). The pericolonic mesentery may be hyperechogenic, due to the transmural inflammation. A thickness of the wall (from mucosa to serosa) greater than 3 mm is considered abnormal. The degree of thickening has a prognostic value, with reported mortality rates as high as 60 % when the wall measures more than 10 mm. Good clinical response correlates with progressive normalization of the bowel wall.

CT findings include cecal distention, circumferential wall thickening with areas of low attenuation secondary to edema or necrosis, and inflammatory stranding of the adjacent mesenteric fat. The presence of pneumatosis, pneumoperitoneum, and pericolic fluid collections can be recognized, and they may indicate complications such as necrosis and perforation that require urgent surgery.

Differential diagnosis includes appendicitis, gastroenteritis, inflammatory bowel disease, acute megacolon, and pseudomembranous colitis. History of treatment for malignancy, clinical and laboratory data, and imaging findings usually lead to the right diagnosis.

Case 5: Partial Absence of Septum Pellucidum and Intracranial Hemorrhage

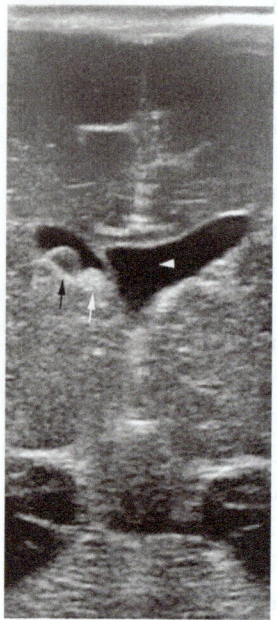

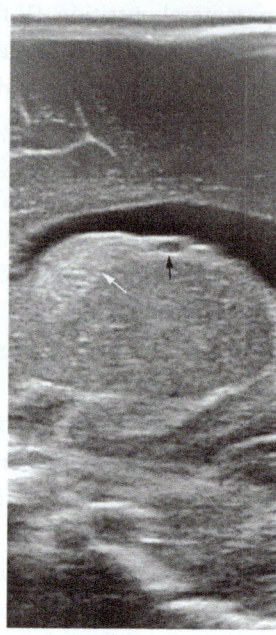

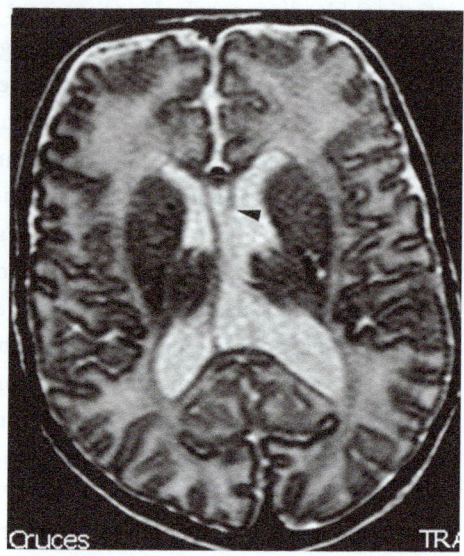

Fig. 6.5.1   **Fig. 6.5.2**   **Fig. 6.5.3**

Case Presentation and Imaging Findings

Preterm neonate, 1-week-old boy

Coronal (Fig. 6.5.1) and sagittal (Fig. 6.5.2) sonograms of the brain show two areas of evolutive grade 1 hemorrhage at the caudothalamic groove: a cyst (*black arrow*) and a hyperechoic nodule (*white arrow*). There is partial absence of the left leaflet of the septum pellucidum (*arrowhead*). The frontal horn of the left lateral ventricle assumes a characteristic square or boxlike appearance.

On coronal T2-weighted MRI performed at the age of 2 months (Fig. 6.5.3), the grade 1 hemorrhage is no longer identified. The absence of a portion of the left leaflet of the septum pellucidum (*arrowhead*) is again demonstrated. No other associated central nervous system anomalies were seen.

Comments

Isolated absence of the septum pellucidum is a rare congenital anomaly. Some sort of dysgenesis of the septum pellucidum occurs in 2–3 per 100,000 births, and it is often associated with other anomalies such as holoprosencephaly, schizencephaly, agenesis of corpus callosum, and septo-optic dysplasia. When septal leaflet agenesis is an isolated central nervous system finding, outcomes range from asymptomatic to severe pituitary or psychiatric abnormalities. It is postulated that, in some cases, the absence of septum pellucidum may be secondary to hydrocephalus with eventual destruction of the septal leaflets. Our case showed no associated central nervous system anomalies, apart from grade 1 intracranial hemorrhage, which disappeared in the follow-up MRI.

Subependymal and intraventricular hemorrhage are frequent complications of the high-risk preterm infant (most common in neonates <32 weeks gestation and <1,500 g). These hemorrhages start in the subependymal germinal matrix of the caudothalamic groove (grade 1) and may extend into the lateral ventricle (grade 2); when the intraventricular hemorrhage produces acute dilatation because of flooding of 50 % or more of one or both lateral ventricles, it is classified as grade 3. Hemorrhagic extension into brain tissue is grade 4 (most researchers regard grade 4 hemorrhages to be venous hemorrhagic infarctions, due to the compression of the venous outflow by the subependymal hemorrhage). Prognosis is generally good for grades 1 and 2; grades 3 and 4 have variable long-term deficits. Hydrocephalus is a common complication and may require ventriculoperitoneal shunting.

Cerebral ultrasound is the initial examination in a high-risk preterm infant.

In the acute phase, intracranial hemorrhage presents as hyperechoic foci (similar to the normal choroid plexus), changing to iso- and hypoechoic/anechoic, cystic appearance, with time. Our case shows a grade 1 hemorrhage with two different age bleedings (hyper- and anechoic foci), which disappeared on the follow-up MRI (usual outcome).

There was also partial absence of the left leaflet of the septum pellucidum, with squaring of the left frontal horn. The septum pellucidum leaflets and cavum septum pellucidum (anechoic cavity between the leaflets) should always be visualized between 18 and 37 weeks gestation. Failure to detect the cavum septum pellucidum, and/or the septal leaflets, within this time interval is abnormal. A thorough ultrasound scanning must be performed to rule out common associated anomalies: corpus callosum dysgenesis, optic nerve hypoplasia, schizencephaly, and holoprosencephaly. MRI is the examination of choice to fully confirm if we are dealing with an isolated anomaly, as in our case, or a more severe central nervous system dysgenesis.

Case 6: Lymphatic Malformation

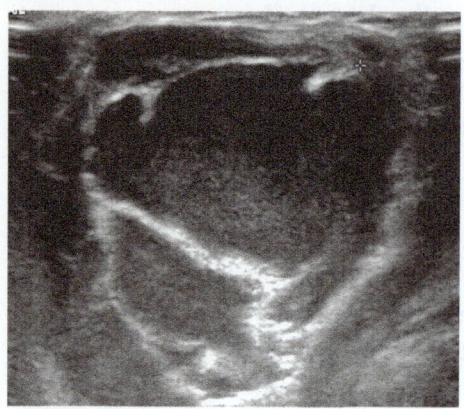

Fig. 6.6.1

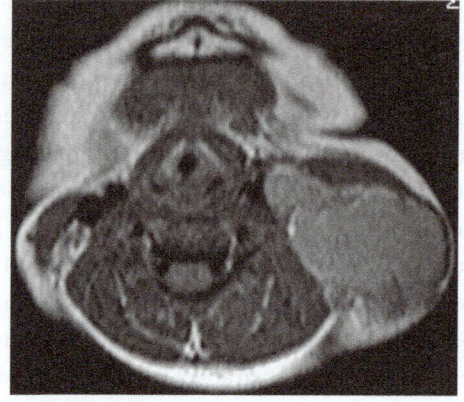

Fig. 6.6.2

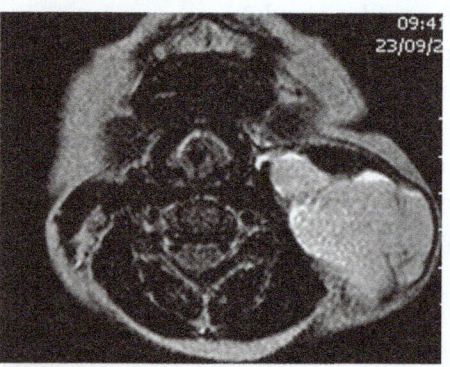

Fig. 6.6.3

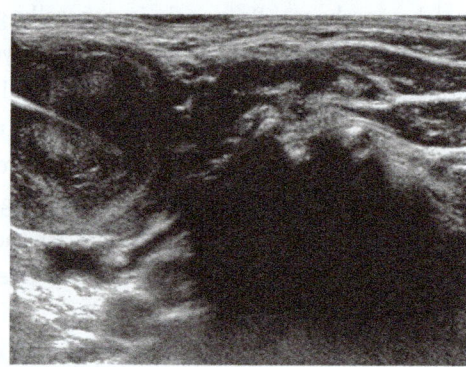

Fig. 6.6.4

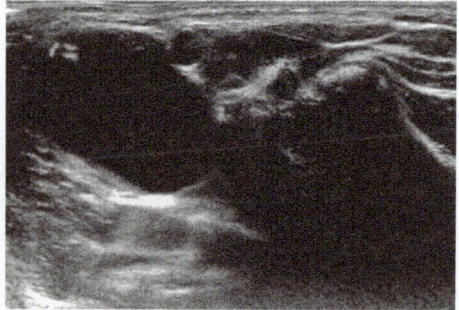

Fig. 6.6.5

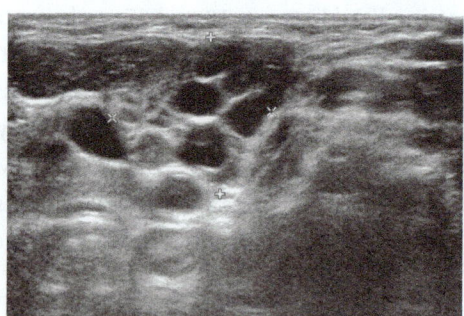

Fig. 6.6.6

Case Presentation and Imaging Findings

A 2-year-old girl with a slowly growing soft mass on the left side of the neck with no other symptoms other than the esthetic problem

Ultrasound showed a cystic multiloculated mass with markedly echogenic fluid within the cysts (Fig. 6.6.1). No Doppler flow was identified (not shown). MRI confirmed the macrocystic multiloculated nature of the lesion, which showed hyperintense signal on both T1 (Fig. 6.6.2) and T2 (Fig. 6.6.3), suggestive of sub-acute hemorrhage. There was no enhancement after IV contrast, other than in the periphery of the lesion. A low-flow lymphatic malformation (macrocystic) with internal hemorrhage was diagnosed.

Treatment of the bigger cyst (27×30 mm) with US-guided injection of Picibanil (0.1 mg of Picibanil in 10 cc of saline) was undertaken. A hemorrhagic fluid was aspirated (Fig. 6.6.4) through an 18-gauge needle (note the hyperechoic fluid), and the same amount of Picibanil (Fig. 6.6.5) was injected (now the fluid is anechoic). A follow-up examination 6 months after the treatment shows disappearance of the treated, bigger cyst. The whole lesion, with several small cysts, measures now 17 mm (Fig. 6.6.6) and no longer constitutes an esthetic problem.

Comments

Vascular anomaly describes two abnormal vascular conditions: the congenital vascular malformation (CVM) and vascular tumor, most commonly represented by the neonatal or infantile hemangioma. Vascular anomalies are common, with an estimated prevalence of 4.5 %.

Congenital vascular malformations are malformed vessels that result from developmental arrest during embryogenesis and are always present at birth, although it may not become clinically evident. It continues to grow commensurate with the patient, and it never involutes. Infantile or neonatal hemangioma, on the other hand, is a true vascular tumor that originates from endothelial cells. It usually appears in the early neonatal period. Unlike congenital vascular malformations, hemangiomas undergo self-limited growth followed by subsequent involution that usually occurs before the age of 5–10 years in the majority of cases.

Congenital vascular malformations are classified into different types based on its predominant vascular component: capillary, arterial, venous, arteriovenous, lymphatic, and combined vascular malformation (the most common combined or mixed malformation is the venolymphatic). They can be divided into two groups depending on their hemodynamic and lymphodynamic characteristics: low-flow and high-flow malformations. Low-flow lesions include capillary, venous, and lymphatic malformations or a combination of these elements. High-flow lesions include arterial malformations and arteriovenous malformations.

Lymphatic malformations may be further classified into macro- and micro-cystic, based on the size of the cystic spaces. Lymphatic malformations may be complicated by hemorrhage or infection and compression to adjacent vital structures. They involve most frequently the head and neck area (61.2 %).

US shows cystic macro- or microcystic multiloculated masses, with no evidence of high arterial flow on Doppler. Combined venolymphatic malformations may have a solid component.

Macrocystic lymphatic malformations respond to treatment with sclerosing agents (alcohol, bleomycin, etc.). We prefer using OK-432 (Picibanil), which induces an inflammatory response eventually leading to cystic involution. The injection can be repeated, in case of treatment failure or progression of the other cysts.

Case 7: Developmental Dysplasia of the Hip

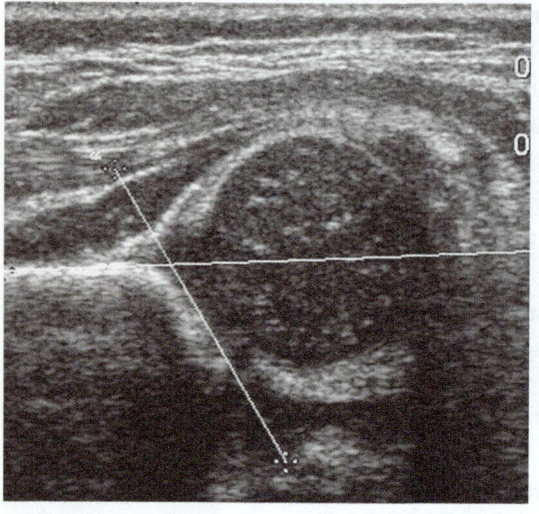

Fig. 6.7.1

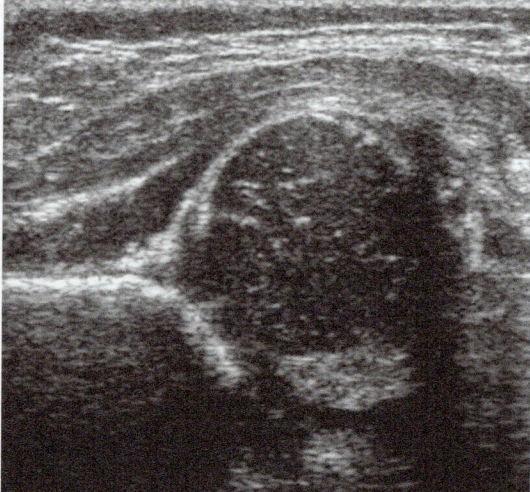

Fig. 6.7.2

Case Presentation and Imaging Findings

Newborn with uneven skin folds on the thigh and positive Ortolani and Barlow maneuvers. A hip ultrasound is performed.

On static coronal view (Fig. 6.7.1), the iliac baseline is straight, the ischium is visualized, and the scan displays the maximum diameter of the femoral head. Alfa angle is >60°. Acetabular roof is concave. Femoral head appear round. Acetabular margin is sharp. Femoral head cover is >50 %. Thus, static exploration is normal.

Although anatomically normal, the hip is unstable under stress maneuvers (Fig. 6.7.2). The percentage of femoral head cover drops to 35 %.

Comments

Developmental dysplasia of the hip (DDH) refers to a continuum of abnormalities in the immature hip that can range from subtle dysplasia to dislocation. Developmental dysplasia of the hip occurs in about 1–1.5 out of 1,000 births.

The cause is unknown. It may be unilateral (80 %) or bilateral (20 %). When unilateral, it involves more frequently the left hip. Risk factors include:

- First born children
- Female to male ratio is about 80 %:20 %
- Intrauterine packaging problems such as clubfoot and congenital torticollis
- Breech position during pregnancy
- Oligoamnios
- Family history of the disorder

The condition may be asymptomatic, but it may present with uneven skin folds on the thigh, reduced abduction, and shorter leg on the side of the hip dysplasia. The physical exam usually shows positive Ortolani and Barlow maneuvers.

Radiographs of newborns with suspected developmental dysplasia of the hip are of limited value because the femoral heads do not ossify until 4–6 months of age. Ultrasound is best suited for the evaluation of morphology, femoroacetabular relationship, and stability of the joint in infants below the age of 6 months. The ossification of the femoral head makes the visualization of the acetabulum and ischion difficult after that age, and plain films are generally preferred. It is advisable to perform the ultrasound at 4–6 weeks of age. Ultrasonography has documented its ability to detect abnormal position, instability, and dysplasia not evident on clinical examination.

Examination technique is paramount for an adequate diagnosis. With a high-resolution linear array, the infant is examined in the lateral decubitus position, with the hip in a 90° flexed position. The examiner must obtain a correct coronal plane, as reported by Graf. The alpha angle (normal when 60° or more) and the percentage of femoral head cover (normal when >50 %) should be analyzed. The stability of the joint is also assessed by performing the Barlow maneuver (adduction of the femur and push backwards with the hip flexed at 90°) while scanning in the transverse and coronal planes. Stress maneuvering may reveal instability (slight movement of the head inside the socket), subluxation, or dislocation.

Treatment decisions are often made on the basis of measurements of Graf angles and percentage of femoral head cover (static and under stress).

There are other ancillary findings associated with instability: notched acetabular margin, flat or even convex acetabular roof, and flattening of the femoral head.

The use of ultrasonography is recommended as an adjunct to the clinical evaluation. It is the technique of choice for clarifying a physical finding, assessing a high-risk infant, and monitoring developmental dysplasia of the hip as it is observed or treated. Used in this selective capacity, it can guide treatment and may prevent overtreatment.

Case 8: Subperiosteal and Intraosseous Abscesses

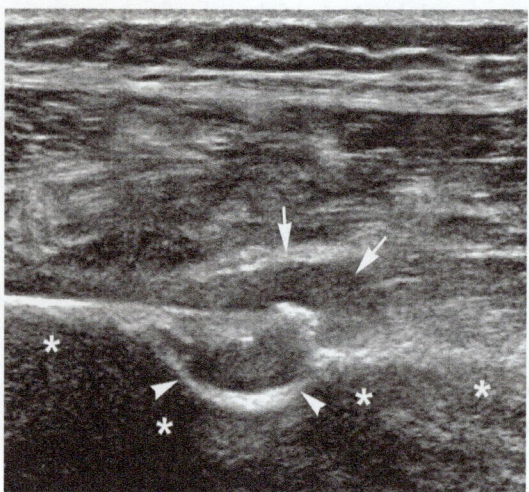

Fig. 6.8.1

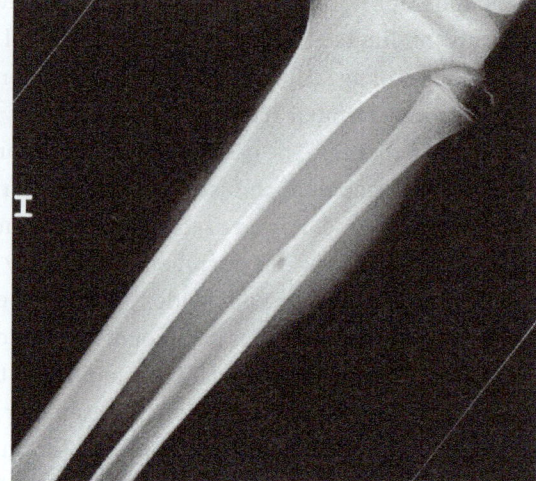

Fig. 6.8.2

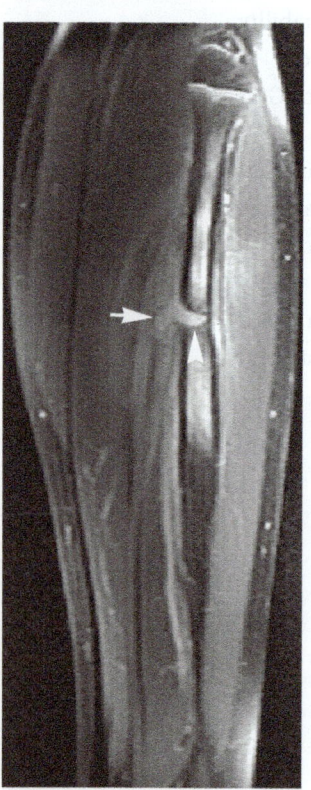

Fig. 6.8.3

Figure 6.8.1 Longitudinal US image of the diaphysis of the fibula (*asterisks*) that demonstrates a cortical defect in the bone (*arrowheads*) and anechoic fluid immediately above the bony lesion (*arrows*).

Figure 6.8.2 On X-ray, a small lytic lesion is seen in the fibula.

Figure 6.8.3 Sagittal fat-suppressed T1-weighted MRI shows periosteal abscess (*white arrow*), cortical bone defect, and intraosseous abscess (*arrowhead*).

Imaging Findings

Osteomyelitis is one of the most common invasive bacterial infections in children leading to hospitalization and prolonged antibiotic administration. By far the most common bacterial pathogen causing osteomyelitis in children of any age is *Staphylococcus aureus*. In most cases, infection spreads hematogenously to the bone and characteristically arises in the metaphysis of long bones.

A multimodality approach is often needed to establish the diagnosis. Plain radiographs early in the clinical course usually show soft tissue swelling and obliteration of tissue planes, but bone abnormalities, such as periosteal elevation or lytic lesions, are not identified until 10–14 days after the start of the disease. Bone scintigraphy is also frequently used.

Sonography is excellent for children. Its main strength lays in its ability to depict periosteal elevation of the infected bone and deep soft tissue inflammation. The sonographic criterion for the diagnosis of osteomyelitis is an abnormal collection of fluid adjacent to the bone without soft tissue involvement. The differential diagnosis includes serous effusions, septic arthritis, and subcortical hematoma.

More useful yet is the possibility of using ultrasound to guide needle aspiration of the subperiosteal pus to obtain a sample for culture. This allows a quick diagnosis and treatment.

MRI is now the most sensitive modality for detecting changes in bone consistent with acute osteomyelitis. Bone marrow edema is seen as low signal intensity (dark) on T1-weighted images and high signal intensity (bright) on T2-weighted images. Abscesses are best demonstrated with intravenous gadolinium contrast on the fat-suppressed T1-weighted images.

Antibiotic treatment is the cornerstone of the treatment of osteomyelitis. Drainage is indicated when a subperiosteal or intraosseous abscess is present in patients with acute hematogenous osteomyelitis. Sometimes, the drainage can be performed using interventional radiology techniques.

Comments

Further Reading

American Academy of Pediatrics, Committee on Quality Improvement, Subcommittee on Developmental Dysplasia of the Hip (2000) Clinical practice guideline: early detection of developmental dysplasia of the hip. Pediatrics 105:896–905

Averill LW, Hernandez A, Gonzalez L, Peña AH, Jaramillo D (2009) Diagnosis of osteomyelitis in children: utility off at-suppressed contrast-enhanced MRI. Am J Roentgenol 192:1232–1238

Baud C, Saguintaah M, Veyrac C, Couture A, Ferran JL, Barneon G, Veyrac M (2004) Sonographic diagnosis of colitis in children. Eur Radiol 14:2105–2119

Beek E, Groenendaal F. Neonatal brain ultrasound. http://www.radiologyassistant.nl/en/440c93be7456f. Accesed on Aug 8th 2012

Berrocal T, del Pozo G (2008) Imaging in pediatric gastrointestinal emergencies. In: Devos AS, Blickman JG (eds) Radiological imaging of the digestive tract in infants and children. Springer, Berlin, pp 36–46

Cartoni C, Dragoni F, Micozzi A, Pescarmona E, Mecarocci S, Chirletti P, Petti MC, Meloni G, Mandelli F (2001) Neutropenic enterocolitis in patients with acute leukemia: prognostic significance of bowel wall thickening detected by ultrasonography. J Clin Oncol 19:756–761

Cheng G, Soboleski D, Daneman A, Poenaru D, Hurlbut D (2005) Sonographic pitfalls in the diagnosis of enteric duplication cysts. AJR Am J Roentgenol 184:521–525

Daneman A, Navarro O (2004) Intussusception. Part 2: an update on the evolution of management. Pediatr Radiol 34:97–108

Del-Pozo G, Albillos JC, Tejedor D et al (1999) Intussusception in children: current concepts in diagnosis and enema reduction. Radiographics 19:299–319

Greene AK (2012) Current concepts of vascular anomalies. J Craniofac Surg 23:220–224

Gruber H, Peer S (2009) Ultrasound diagnosis of soft tissue vascular malformations and tumours. Curr Med Imaging Rev 5:55–61

Hernanz-Schulman M (2003) Infantile hypertrophic pyloric stenosis. Radiology 227:319–331

Jamieson D, Stringer DA (2000) Small bowel. In: Stringer DA, Babyn PS (eds) Pediatric gastrointestinal imaging and intervention, 2nd edn. BC Decker Inc, London, pp 348–353

Kaplan SL (2005) Osteomyelitis in children. Infect Dis Clin North Am 19:787–797

Keller MS (2005) Musculoskeletal sonography in the neonate and infant. Pediatr Radiol 35:1167–1173

Ogita S et al (1996) OK-432 therapy for lymphangiomas in children: Why and How does it work? J Pediatr Surg 31:477–480

Sansgiri RK, Estroff JA, Mehta TS et al (2011) Outcome of fetuses with cerebral ventriculomegaly and septum pellucidum abnormalities. AJR Am J Roentgenol 196:W83–W92

Supprian T, Sian J, Heils A, Hofmann E, Warmuth-Metz M, Solymosi L (1999) Isolated absence of the septum pellucidum. Neuroradiology 41:563–566

Wesley JR, DiPietro MA, Coran AG (1990) Pyloric stenosis: evolution from pylorospasm? Pediatr Surg Int 5:425–428

BLANCA PAÑO AND PEDRO SEGUÍ

Real-time assessment of the flow patterns of the vessels, especially in peripheral ones, can be done very accurately and noninvasively using Doppler ultrasound. The Doppler Effect is the change in frequency of a wave due to movement of the source or observer. The ultrasound beam reflected by moving red blood cells show an increase in frequency when the blood flow is directed toward the transducer, and a decrease in frequency as it moves away. Frequency changes are interpreted as different flow velocities and directions.

There are several types of Doppler image.

Introduction

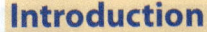

- Pulsed Doppler
  The transducer operates like in conventional ultrasound, as transmitter and receiver of ultrasound, transmitting very short pulses with a specific frequency called Pulse Repetition Frequency. A new pulse cannot be emitted until having received the previous one. Time interval between transmission and reception determines the depth at which the Doppler shift occurs. Pulsed Doppler obtains in vascular flow a spectrum of velocities, or spectral Doppler. The combination of spectral Doppler and B-mode image is known as duplex Doppler.

- Color Doppler
  This technique overlaps a color image on the conventional gray-scale real-time sonographic image. The speed and direction are color coded. Usually, red is used to represent the flow directed towards the transducer and blue the flow flowing away. The brighter colors correspond to higher speeds and darker shades to lower speeds.

- Power Doppler
  Alternative way of color Doppler in which a sum of the power or amplitude of the received signal is obtained, representing the signal power at each point in the examination area. It will be directly proportional to the number of erythrocytes present in it.

It does not represent changes in frequency or speed, but in the Doppler signal power. Therefore, it is more sensitive, and the image is less angle dependent than color Doppler, and no aliasing phenomenon appears.

J.L. del Cura et al. (eds.), *Learning Ultrasound Imaging*, Learning Imaging,
DOI 10.1007/978-3-642-30586-3_7, © Springer-Verlag Berlin Heidelberg 2012

Case 1: Carotid Artery Stenosis

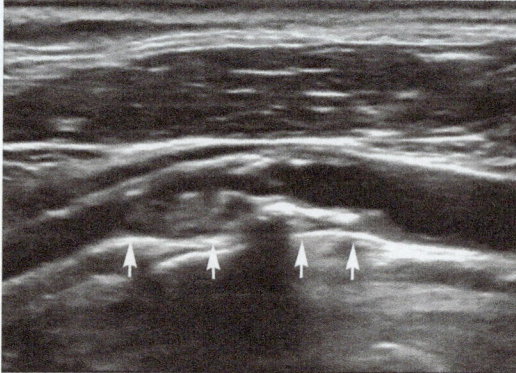

Fig. 7.1.1

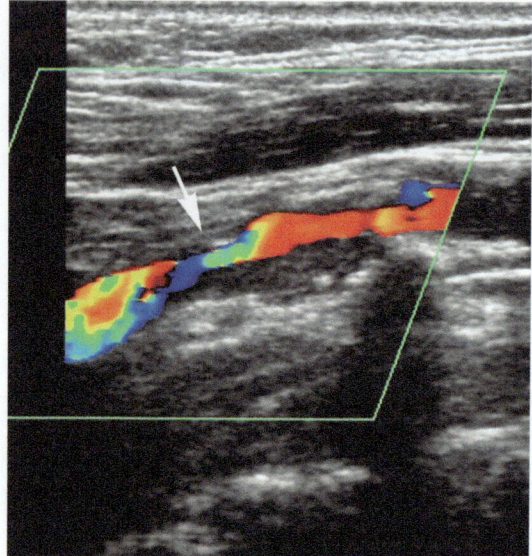

Fig. 7.1.2

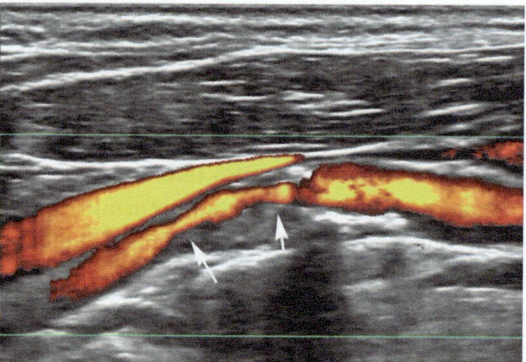

Fig. 7.1.3

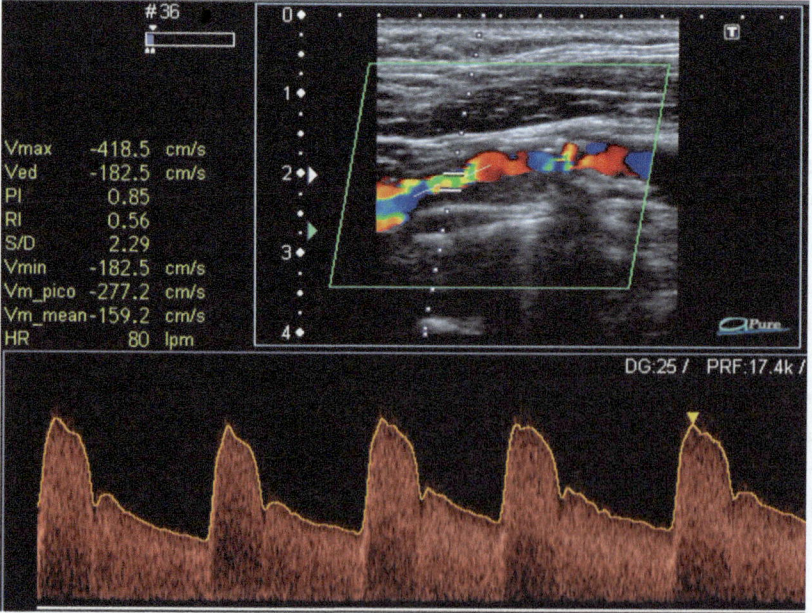

Fig. 7.1.4

A 67-year-old man presented with dysarthria of 2 month's duration. CT was performed and no findings were detected. Magnetic resonance of the brain showed bilateral small infarcts in both cerebral hemispheres. A Doppler ultrasound of the carotid arteries was scheduled.

Longitudinal US image (Fig. 7.1.1) of right common carotid artery (*C*) and internal carotid artery (*I*) showed a large heterogeneous plaque at the origin of the internal carotid artery with calcified and fibrolipoid components (*arrows*).

Longitudinal color Doppler (Fig. 7.1.2) and power Doppler (Fig. 7.1.3) US images showed a heterogeneous plaque with apparent severe luminal narrowing (*arrows*) at internal carotid artery origin. Note color aliasing at the point of maximal stenosis (*arrow* in Fig. 7.1.2).

Duplex Doppler image (Fig. 7.1.4) showed a peak systolic velocity of 418 cm/s at the point of maximal stenosis. This velocity represents severe stenosis (more than 70 %). Two centimeter distal to the stenosis, duplex Doppler (Fig. 7.1.5) showed a peak systolic velocity of 82 cm/s, within normal limits, but with turbulent flow features.

Digital angiography (Fig. 7.1.6) confirmed a severe stenosis in the proximal internal carotid artery (*arrow*). An endovascular stent was placed.

Case Presentation and Imaging Findings

Stroke is the third most important cause of death in developed countries and one of the most common causes of disability. The most well-known risk factor for the development of cerebrovascular events is internal carotid artery stenosis. Three large-scale, multicenter, randomized trials, published between 1991 and 1995, recommended carotid endarterectomy in symptomatic patients with >60 % stenosis of the internal carotid artery and in asymptomatic patients with >70 % stenosis. In recent years, stent implantation in the carotid artery has been shown to be safe and effective and seems to be a minimally invasive alternative to endarterectomy. Digital subtraction angiography is the standard imaging modality for quantifying the degree of stenosis, but it is an invasive examination. Duplex ultrasound is an excellent noninvasive examination for detecting stenosis and is a widely accepted technique for screening patients with extracranial artery stenosis due to atheromatous disease. Other noninvasive tests are MR angiography and CT angiography.

Ultrasound examinations of the internal carotid artery should be performed with gray-scale, color, and spectral Doppler in a standardized fashion. The Doppler waveform should be obtained with an angle of insonation less than or equal to 60°. As stenotic lesions increase in severity, they perturb carotid artery blood flow patterns. Stenosis over 50 % of diameter narrowing will increase peak systolic velocity (PSV) and make the blood flow profile more turbulent at the point of maximal narrowing. Peak systolic velocities remain elevated for varying distances that typically extend for 1–2 cm beyond the stenosis. Care should be taken to position the sample volume within the

Comments

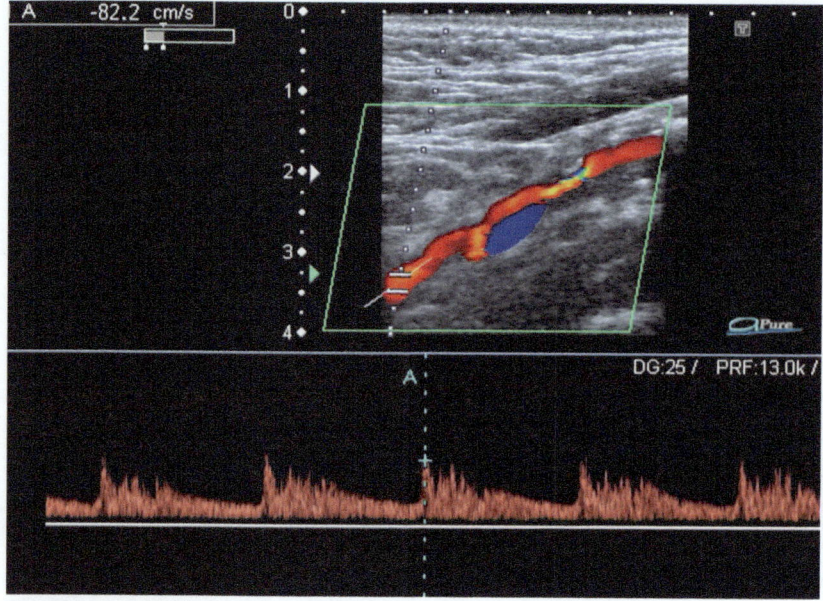

Fig. 7.1.5

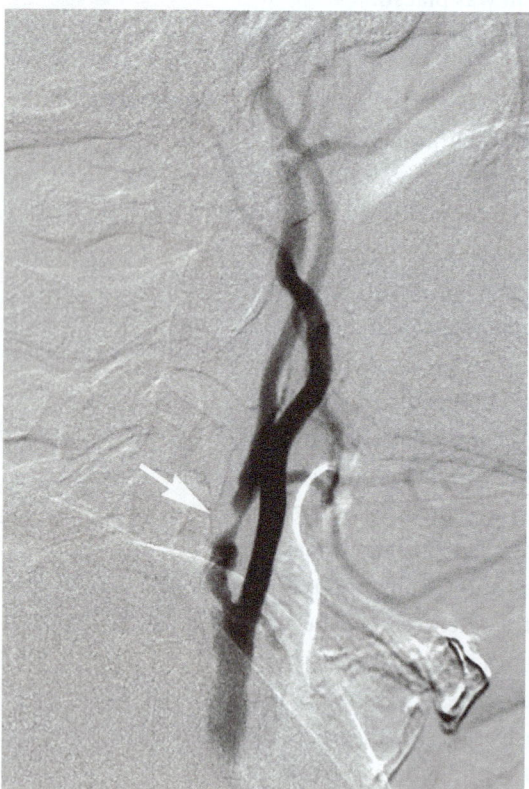

Fig. 7.1.6

area of greatest stenosis. Color Doppler serves as a guide for the sonographer: sites of aliasing are likely to have elevated peak velocities and correspond to areas or high-grade stenosis that must be further interrogated with Doppler waveform analysis.

Doppler ultrasound cannot be used to predict a certain percentage of stenosis. Expert consensus recommends stratification of the degree of stenosis into the following:

- *Normal* (no stenosis) when internal carotid artery PSV is less than 125 cm/s and no plaque is visible sonographically.
- <50 % stenosis when internal carotid artery PSV is less than 125 cm/s and plaque is visible.
- *50–69 % stenosis* when internal carotid artery PSV is 125–230 cm/s.
- *70 % stenosis or more but less than near occlusion* when the internal carotid artery PSV is greater than 230 cm/s, with visible plaque and luminal narrowing at gray-scale and color Doppler US.
- *Near occlusion* the velocity parameters are not applied here: this diagnosis is established by demonstrating a markedly narrowed lumen at color or power Doppler ultrasound.
- *Complete occlusion* should be suspected when there is no flow in spectral, power, and color Doppler ultrasound.

Two additional parameters, ICA/CCA PSV ratio and internal carotid artery end diastolic velocity (EDV), are useful when internal carotid artery PSV may not be representative of the extent of the disease owing to technical or clinical factors (tandem lesions, contralateral high-grade stenosis, discrepancy between visual assessment of plaque and internal carotid artery PSV, elevated common carotid artery PSV, or low cardiac output).

Case 2: Carotid Artery Dissection

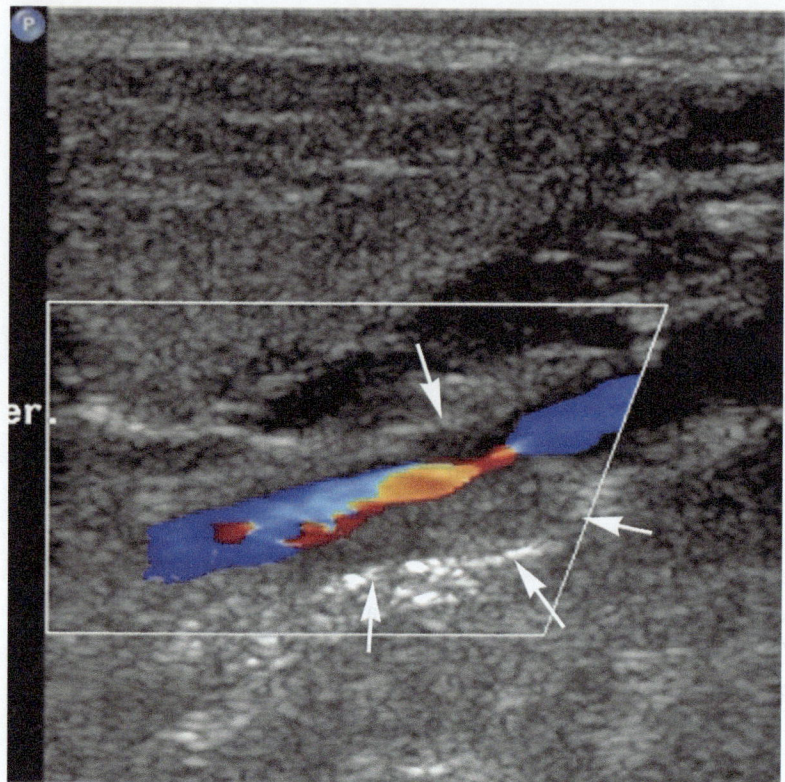

Fig. 7.2.1

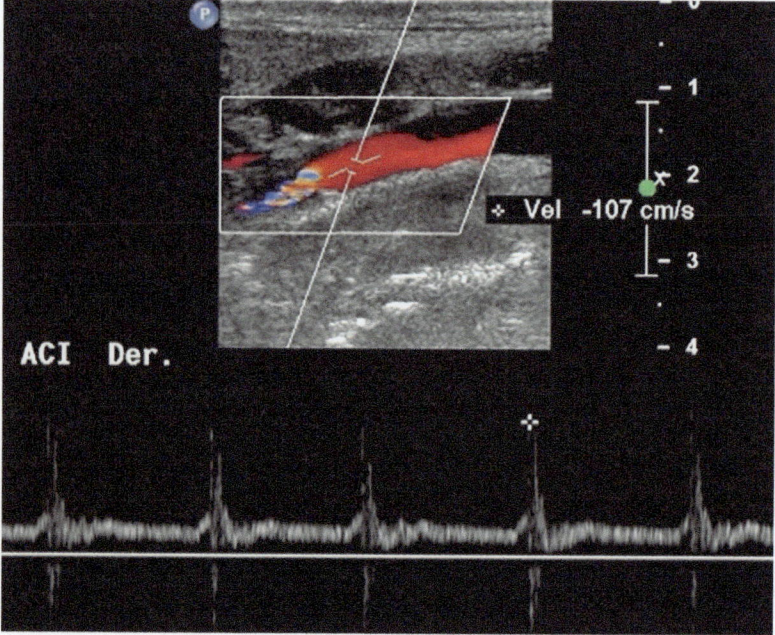

Fig. 7.2.2

A 17-year-old male presented to the emergency department with a 2-day history of left lower-extremity weakness and paresthesia. Two weeks before, he had an accidental fall from an amusement park ride, and after this event, he had right-sided neck pain for 1 day. Physical examination revealed left hemiparesis. Cranial magnetic resonance showed some ischemic foci in the right cerebral hemisphere. A Doppler ultrasound was performed.

Figure 7.2.1 Longitudinal color Doppler ultrasound of the right internal carotid artery demonstrating a low-reflective intramural hematoma (*arrows*) compressing the true lumen of the internal carotid artery 2 cm cranially from the bulb. These findings are strongly suggestive of internal carotid artery dissection with intramural hematoma.

Figure 7.2.2 Color and spectral Doppler ultrasound of internal carotid artery immediately proximal to the lesion shows a high-resistance triphasic waveform.

Figure 7.2.3 Spectral Doppler at the point of maximal lumen stenosis shows a very high peak systolic velocity (4 m/s).

Figure 7.2.4 Digital angiography confirmed an irregular stenosis (*arrowheads*) starting 2 cm distal to the carotid bulb.

The patient was treated with anticoagulants and showed good clinical evolution.

Extracranial carotid artery dissection is a relatively uncommon cause of cerebrovascular symptoms and accounts for about 1 % of all ischemic strokes; however, it accounts for 10–25 % of strokes in young adults. Although the classification of internal carotid artery dissection as traumatic or spontaneous may be apparent clinically, there are no angiographic differences between both groups. External trauma may be minimal in the former group, and spontaneous dissection may be linked in a few cases with an underlying arteriopathy such as fibromuscular dysplasia. The mechanism of dissection is thought to be either a tear in the intima, which allows intraluminal blood to dissect along the layers of the vessel wall or, alternatively, direct hemorrhage from the vasa vasorum of the media. The hematoma dissects longitudinally along the media. When the hematoma lies beneath the intima, luminal narrowing or occlusion occurs. If the hematoma dissects beneath the adventitia, a pseudoaneurysm is formed. When blood reenters the true lumen, a false lumen appears. This false lumen may remain patent, resolve completely, or thrombose and cause narrowing of the true lumen.

The typical patient with carotid dissection presents with pain on one side of the head, face, or neck, accompanied by a partial Horner's syndrome and followed hours or days later by cerebral or retinal ischemia. This triad of symptoms is found in less than one-third of patients. Cerebral infarcts are reported in 50 % and transient ischemic attacks in 20 % of patients with internal carotid artery dissection.

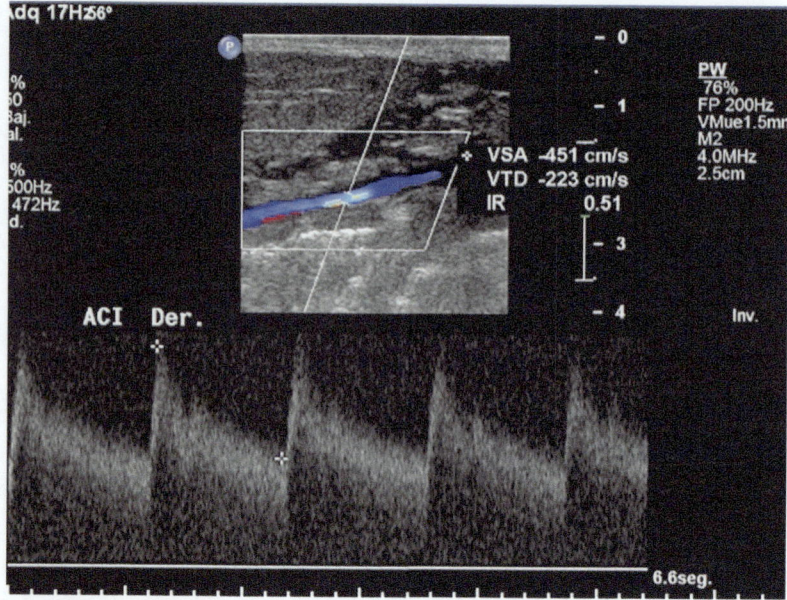

Fig. 7.2.3

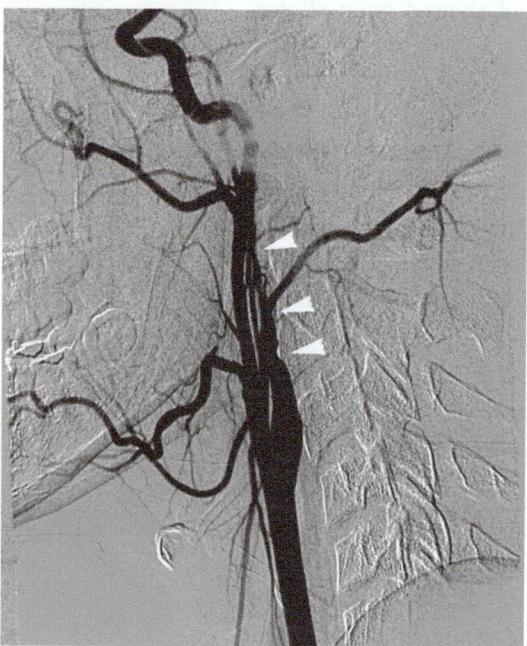

Fig. 7.2.4

The commonest location for a spontaneous internal carotid artery dissection is the cervical segment 2–3 cm distal to the carotid bulb. Dissections extend for a variable length, but they rarely reach the point of entry of the internal carotid artery into the petrous temporal bone. Recurrent dissection is rare in absence of arteriopathy.

Angiography has long been the gold standard in the diagnosis of dissections, but it is increasingly being replaced by noninvasive imaging techniques. Angiography does not allow direct visualization of the vessel wall when there is a thrombus in the false lumen. Nowadays, the diagnosis of carotid dissection is essentially established with cervical MR and MR angiography. The former can provide direct visualization of an intramural hematoma, which is the hallmark of a dissection, and the later allows noninvasive visualization of blood vessels. However, MR is often not available around the clock, and many centers use ultrasound to assess carotid dissection.

Ultrasound allows a direct visualization of the pathological findings, hemodynamic information, flow direction, and velocity data and enables evaluation of the vessel wall and lumen patency. The commonest gray-scale finding is the presence of a hypoechoic thrombus (corresponding to intramural hematoma or thrombosed false lumen) 2–3 cm cranially from the bulb, with or without true lumen narrowing. The presence of an arterial luminal flap (membrane) in the longitudinal and axial view is pathognomonic, but this finding is uncommon. The commonest spectral Doppler US finding is a high-resistance pattern or absence of signal in cases of total occlusion. Another, less common spectral pattern is a damped spectral waveform (lower amplitude with biphasic pattern). Visualization of intramural hematoma combined with high-resistance flow strongly suggests dissection. The diagnostic sensitivity of ultrasound decreases if an internal carotid artery dissection results in a low-grade stenosis, and gray-scale and spectral findings can be normal in these cases. Ultrasound is less reliable for dissections located in the subpetrous segment and the carotid canal.

Case 3: Carotid Intrastent Stenosis

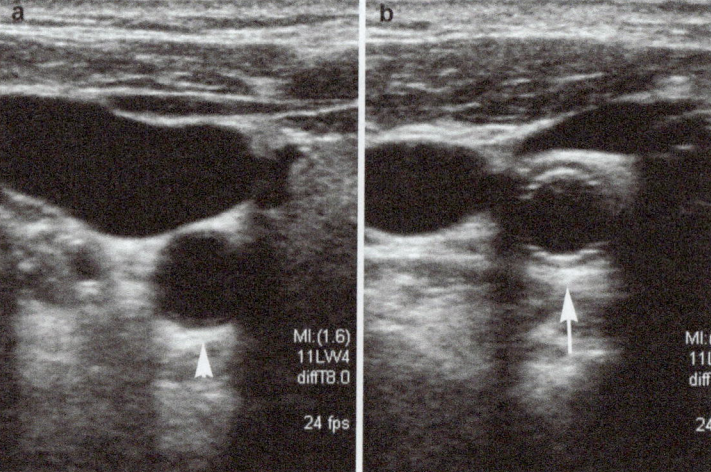

Fig. 7.3.1

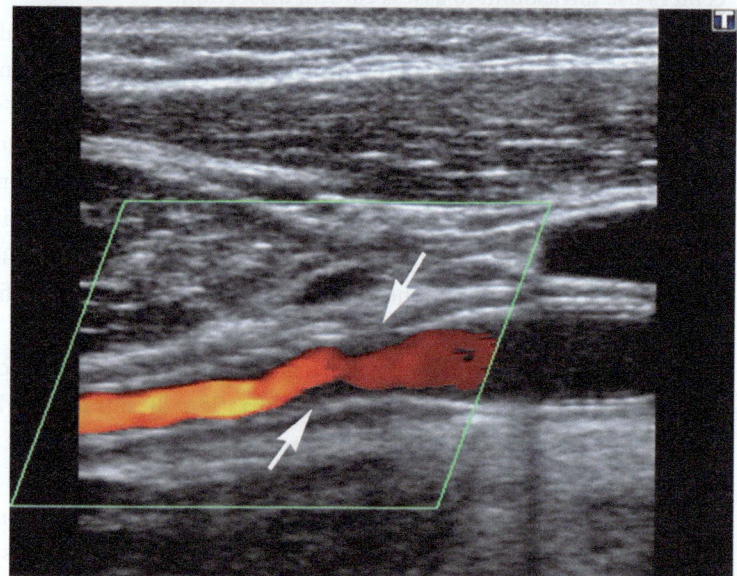

Fig. 7.3.2

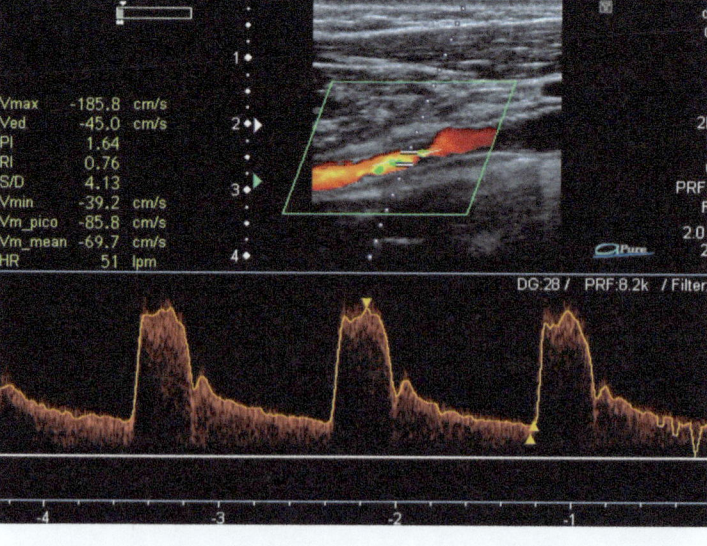

Fig. 7.3.3

A 79-year-old male, asymptomatic, with a history of stent placement in right carotid artery 2 years ago. A routine Doppler ultrasound follow-up was performed.

Figure 7.3.1 Transverse ultrasound images of common right carotid artery. Left image (a) shows common carotid artery proximal to the stent (*arrowhead*). Right image (b) shows distal common carotid artery with stent (*arrow*).

Figure 7.3.2 Longitudinal color Doppler ultrasound image of the stent at distal common carotid and proximal internal carotid arteries shows moderate stenosis at the origin of internal carotid (*arrows*), probably due to intimal hyperplasia.

Figure 7.3.3 Spectral Doppler ultrasound image shows peak velocity flow of 1.85 m/s at the stenosis. This velocity represents stenosis in 50–69 % range.

Carotid angioplasty with stent placement has become a common and standardized procedure for the treatment of symptomatic carotid stenosis. Doppler ultrasound is the procedure that is most frequently used to follow-up the stent. In the untreated carotids, the Doppler is a well-validated and standardized method, with well-established threshold velocities for the different grades of stenosis. On the contrary, in the carotids with stent, the thresholds for each grade of stenosis are not well established. Neither is agreement about the clinical consequences of the restenosis in patients with carotid stent. In the stent, the cause of the stenosis is generally intimal hyperplasia, instead of atherosclerotic plaque. An alternative technique to the Doppler for the follow-up of stents is CT angiography. MR angiography is not appropriate for this purpose given the artifacts caused by the metallic components of the stent.

Incidence of restenosis after placement of the stent is quite variable in the published studies, but in general it ranges between 3 % and 5 % at 6 months of follow-up for 70 % stenosis. Other possible complications such as intrastent thrombosis, occlusion, or dissection are much less frequent, below 1 % at 6 months.

An artery with stent presents less elasticity than an artery without a stent. For this reason, the artery with stent is going to present some peak systolic velocities higher than those of an untreated artery for the same degree of stenosis. In both cases, the peak systolic velocity (PSV) is going to be the best marker to quantify the severity of the stenosis, but with different cutoff points. Among the PSV values most accepted as cutoff points are 1.75–2.99 m/s for stenosis of 50–69 % and >3 m/s for stenosis over or equal to 70 %, but up to now, based on very limited studies. It is important to obtain a basal Doppler study after the placement of the stent in order to avoid overestimating the grade of stenosis. The appropriate schedule for performing ultrasound follow-ups is not standardized either, although the most common is to carry them out at 6 and at 12 months. Subsequently, a routine annual ultrasound follow-up can be enough. Also, a new exploration is indicated in case of clinical suspicion of recurrence.

Case 4: Temporal Arteritis

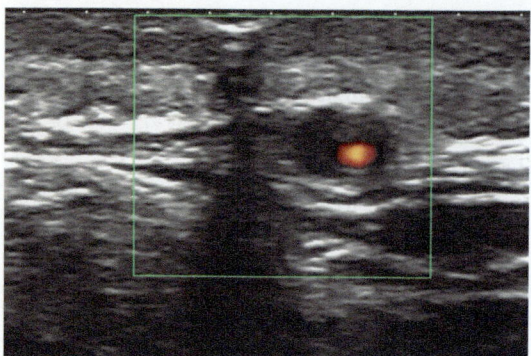

Fig. 7.4.1

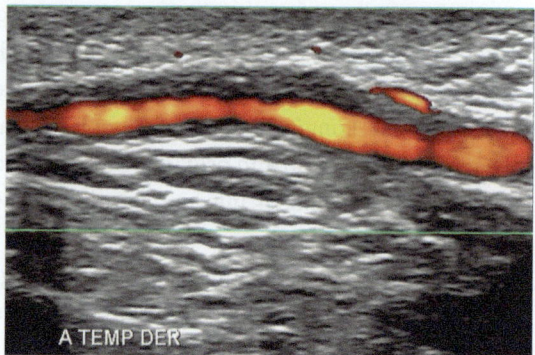

Fig. 7.4.2

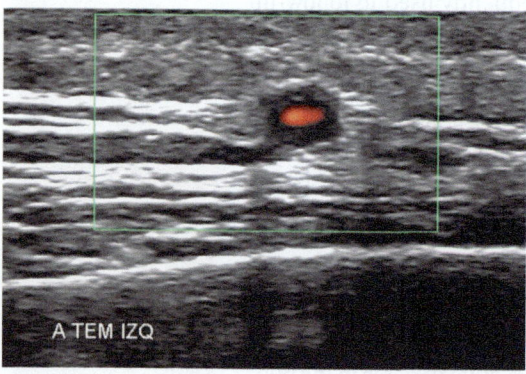

Fig. 7.4.3

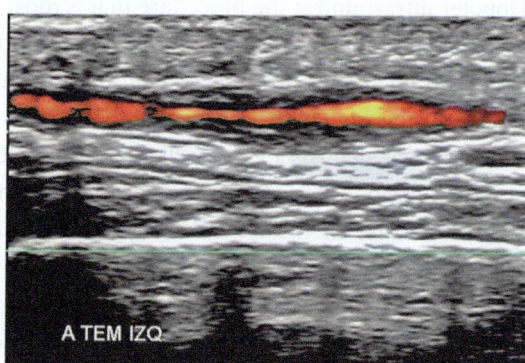

Fig. 7.4.4

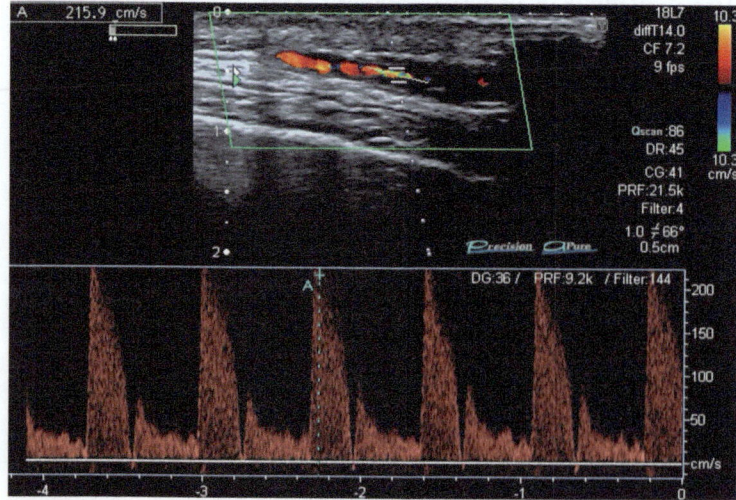

Fig. 7.4.5

A 66-year-old male was admitted to the hospital for weight loss, headache, and jaw soreness. Blood analysis revealed elevation of inflammatory parameters. In the physical examination, a decrease of pulses in both temporal arteries was noted. An ultrasound was performed.

Transverse (Fig. 7.4.1) and longitudinal (Fig. 7.4.2) ultrasound images of right temporal artery show a hypoechoic halo in the artery wall (halo sign).

Transverse (Fig. 7.4.3) and longitudinal (Fig. 7.4.4) ultrasound images of left temporal artery also show the halo sign. Note also stenosis of the arterial lumen.

Flow velocity in left temporal artery (Fig. 7.4.5) is increased over 2 m/s due to stenosis.

Bilateral temporal arteritis was diagnosed. Symptoms of the patient improved and ultrasound findings disappeared after corticosteroid treatment.

Also called giant-cell arteritis, temporal arteritis typically affects the branches of the external carotid (among them the temporal artery) and is histologically characterized by transmural inflammation, intimal thickening, and edema. Giant cells are frequently observed. To diagnose this condition, three of five criteria must be met according to the American College of Rheumatology (ACR):

- Over 50 years of age
- Localized cephalea of recent onset
- Discomfort upon temporal palpation
- High sedimentation speed (> 50 mm/h)
- Temporal artery biopsy that shows vasculitis

A biopsy of the temporal artery with the described histological findings is diagnostic, but the sensitivity of this procedure is around 60 %. Takayasu arteritis presents identical histological characteristics, but generally appears in younger patients and typically affects other vessels such as the thoracic aorta, the proximal left subclavian artery, and the carotid or the renal artery.

In recent years, high-resolution B-mode ultrasound and Doppler ultrasound have been used as diagnostic tools to substitute the biopsy of the temporal artery. The most specific finding is the presence of a concentric mural thickening in the form of a hypoechogenic halo, interpreted as mural edema. The halo sign must be demonstrated in the longitudinal plane as well as the cross section of the vessel. This halo sign has above 80–90 % specificity, but the sensitivity is below 70 %, not very far from those of the temporal biopsy.

The finding of stenosis or occlusion in the artery is more sensitive, but the specificity is low, given that atherosclerosis can also involve these vessels. In summary, the presence of a halo sign is practically diagnostic in the presence of compatible symptoms, but its absence does not rule out vasculitis. Ultrasound findings can be uni- or bilateral. It must be taken into account that ultrasound findings disappear in about 2 weeks after the onset of treatment with corticosteroids.

Case 5: Deep Venous Thrombosis

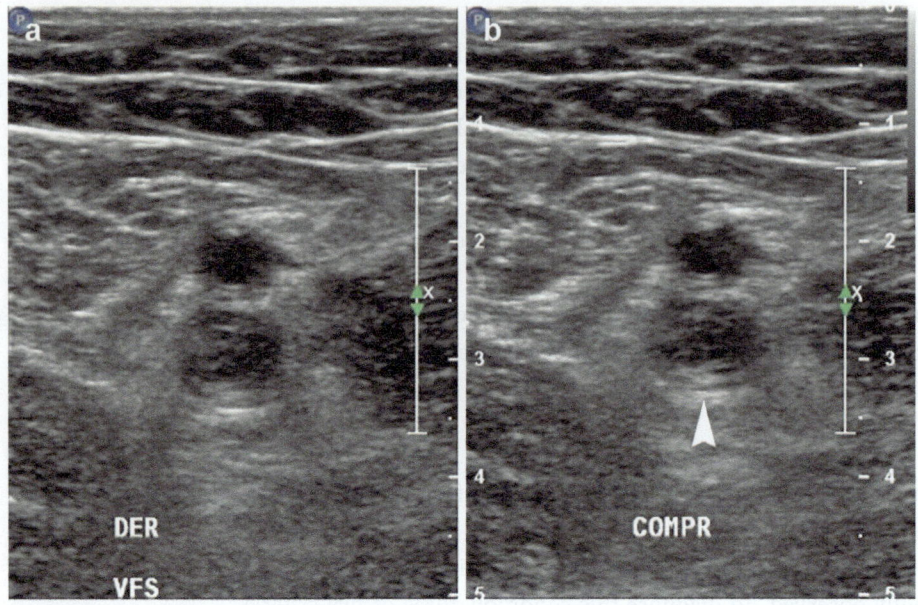

Fig. 7.5.1

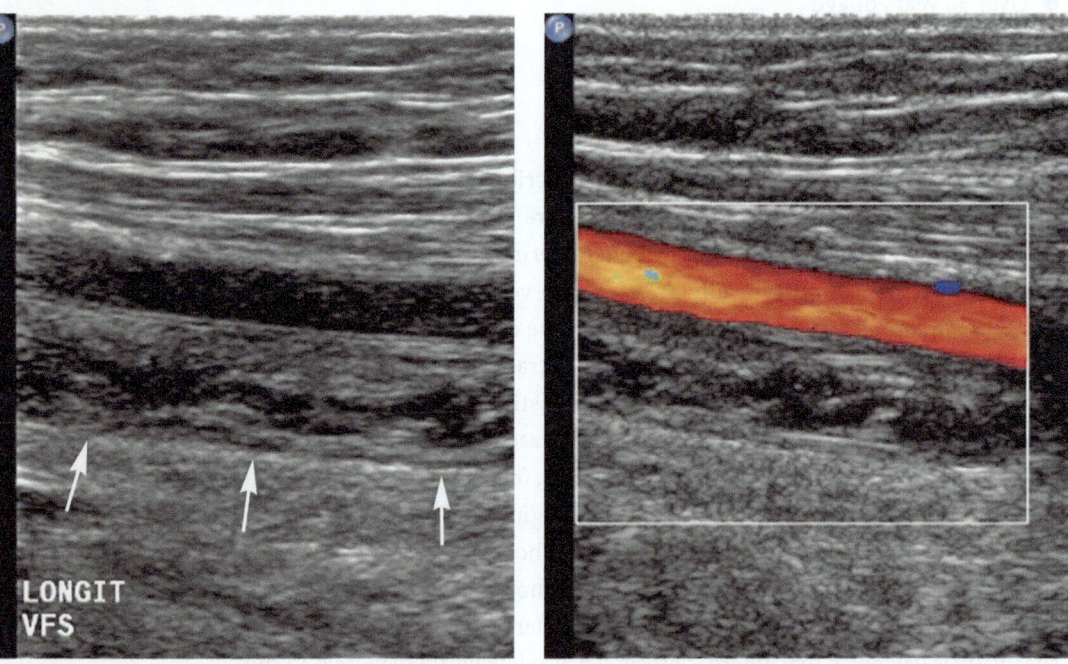

Fig. 7.5.2   **Fig. 7.5.3**

Case Presentation and Imaging Findings

A 51-year-old man experienced a gradual onset of pain and swelling in his right calf 5 days before admission. The patient has been immobilized for 3 weeks because of an ankle strain.

A venous US scan of the right leg was performed (Fig. 7.5.1). Transverse ultrasound uncompressed (a) and compressed (b) images show a noncompressible superficial femoral vein (*arrowhead*).

Longitudinal ultrasound image (Fig. 7.5.2) shows the distended vein (posterior to the artery) with intraluminal clot (*arrows*).

Color Doppler longitudinal image (Fig. 7.5.3) shows normal flow in the superficial femoral artery and no flow in the superficial femoral vein. A deep venous femoropopliteal thrombosis was diagnosed. Anticoagulant treatment was initiated.

Comments

Deep venous thrombosis (DVT) is a common problem in the emergency room. Commonly, DVT begins in the veins of the calf and progresses proximally over time. Less than 20 % of patients with confirmed DVT have thrombi limited to the calf veins. While the thrombus is exclusively located in the iliofemoral region in only approximately 10 % of patients with lower-extremity DVT, this is a common presentation of DVT during pregnancy, usually in the left side. The more central the thrombus, the greater is the risk of pulmonary emboli. About 50 % of the patients with DVT develop pulmonary emboli, although many of these may be subsegmental and undiagnosed. Patients with acute calf-popliteal-vein thrombosis usually present with symptoms of unilateral pain and swelling in the calf, and this condition may be associated with warmth, redness, and tenderness. The clinical signs and symptoms of DVT are notoriously unreliable, so a noninvasive screening test is usually necessary.

Compression ultrasonography is the diagnostic procedure of choice for the assessment of patients with suspected DVT. It has been shown to be highly sensitive and specific for the diagnosis of DVT, particularly in the lower extremities in symptomatic patients. Sensitivity and specificity are near 100 % in the femoropopliteal segment. Sensitivity decreases in isolated calf thrombi and in asymptomatic patients.

Compression ultrasonography of the deep venous system of the lower extremities is performed with the patient in the supine position, with the leg externally rotated and slightly flexed at the knee. To assess the popliteal fossa, patients should be placed prone or in the sitting position if there is difficulty in identifying the calf veins. A linear transducer with a frequency in the 5–12-MHz range is used. The transducer is placed transversely, moving down the leg following the common femoral vein, superficial femoral vein, and popliteal vein. The value of performing compression ultrasonography of the calf veins when proximal veins are normal remains controversial.

Gentle pressure is applied to the vessels with the transducer at 1-cm intervals. In absence of DVT, the lumen of the vein should collapse. In the presence of DVT, the lumen does not collapse, and this is the more sensitive and specific sign of DVT. In acute DVT, the thrombosed vein is distended and clot echogenicity is variable. Duplex and color Doppler are not required but can be helpful. In case of complete occlusion, no spectral or color flow can be demonstrated, and phasic response is lost in the segment distal to the thrombosis.

Case 6: Femoral Artery Pseudoaneurysm

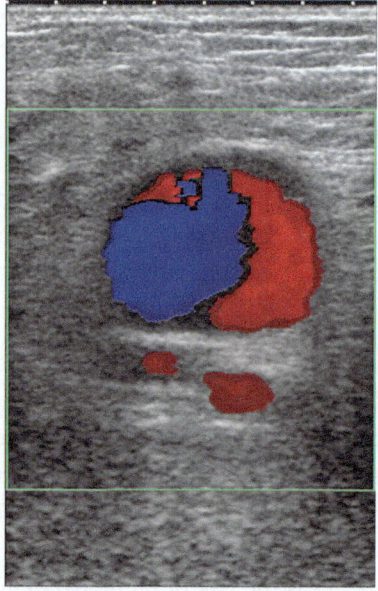

Fig. 7.6.1

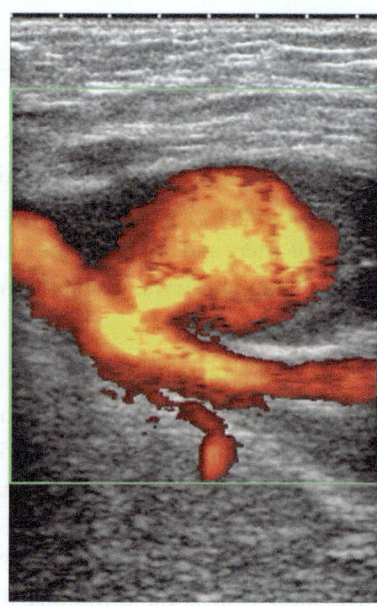

Fig. 7.6.2

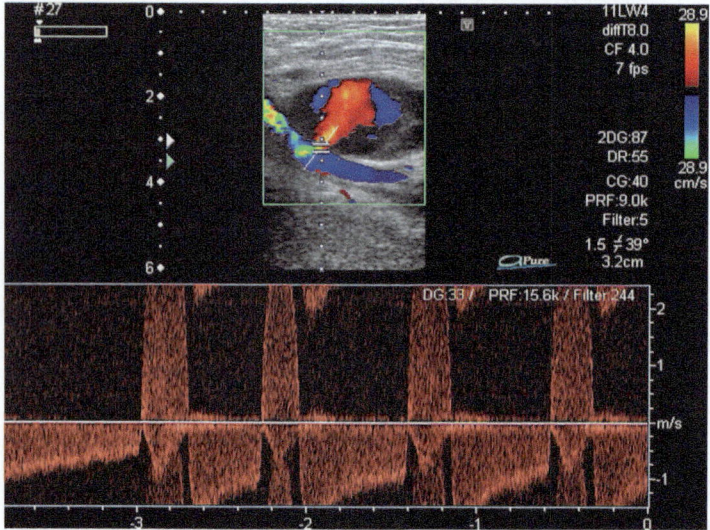

Fig. 7.6.3

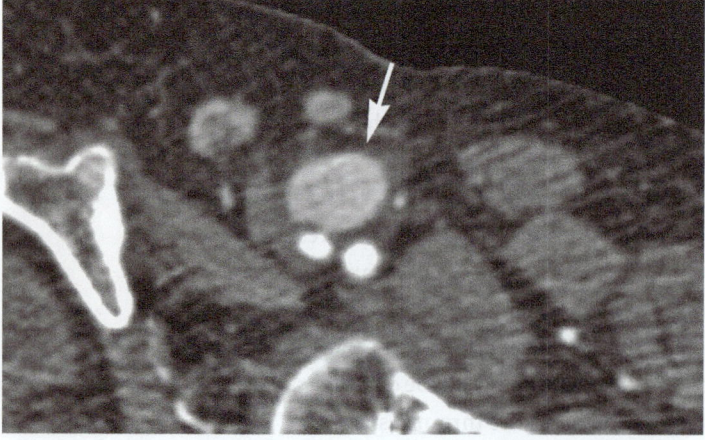

Fig. 7.6.4

A 83-year-old female patient consults for a left inguinal mass, painful to palpation, a few days after a cardiac catheterization via femoral artery.

Color Doppler ultrasound image (Fig. 7.6.1) demonstrates "to-and-fro" flow within a simple pseudoaneurysm sac (ying-yang sign). On power Doppler ultrasound image (Fig. 7.6.2), pseudoaneurysm sac communicates via a short neck with the common femoral artery. Duplex Doppler image (Fig. 7.6.3) shows "to-and-fro" pulsatile flow in the neck.

Axial contrast-enhanced CT image (Fig. 7.6.4) shows the pseudoaneurysm superficial to the left common femoral artery (*arrow*).

Case Presentation and Imaging Findings

Pseudoaneurysm is the most common complication of catheterization of the femoral artery. It is an outflow of blood through the arterial puncture orifice, forming a cavity (false lumen) with a neck communicating to the artery though which the flow "enters and exits." This pseudoaneurysm does not have a true wall and is only contained by hematoma and the adjacent tissues. This complication can occur in any percutaneously accessed artery, but the common femoral artery is the most frequently used. Among risk factors for this complication are the bore of the material used, anticoagulation or antiaggregation treatments, an inadequate compression after the procedure, and the puncture of the superficial femoral artery instead of the common femoral artery. The clinical presentation is usually as a painful pulsatile inguinal mass in a patient after femoral catheterization.

Comments

Ultrasound is the method of choice when suspecting this complication, with sensitivity near 100 %. It usually appears as a hypoanechoic collection adjacent to the femoral artery and communicated with the artery through a small neck. Color Doppler will show a swirling flow inside the collection (ying-yang pattern), and in the neck, a pulsating to-and-fro flow will be detected with the spectral Doppler. This flow in the neck can reach very high velocities. When exploring a pseudoaneurysm, it is also necessary to describe the number of loculations (whether it is simple or complex), diameter and volume of the cavity, and length and width of the neck.

Although most pseudoaneurysms below 2 cm in diameter will spontaneously thrombose before 4 weeks, it is generally preferred to treat them before to resolve the symptoms and to avoid follow-up. The usual treatment is US-guided thrombin injection (see Case 8 in Chap. 9).

Case 7: Renal Artery Stenosis

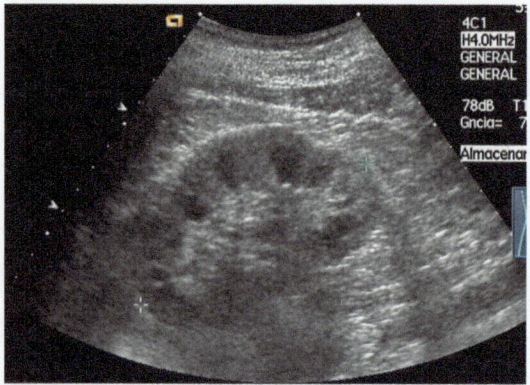

Fig. 7.7.1

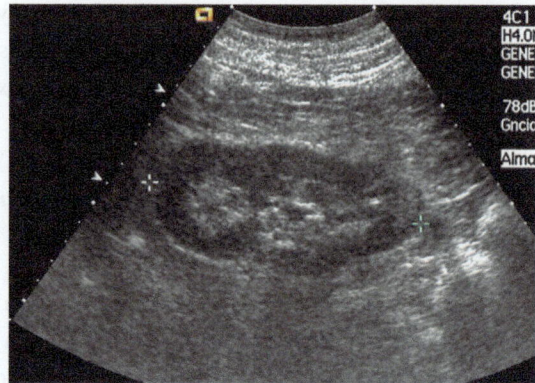

Fig. 7.7.2

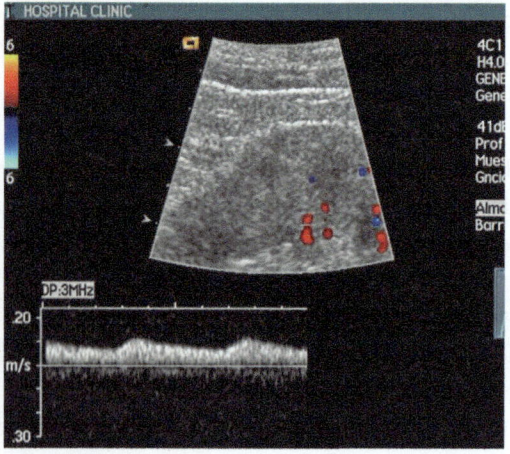

Fig. 7.7.3

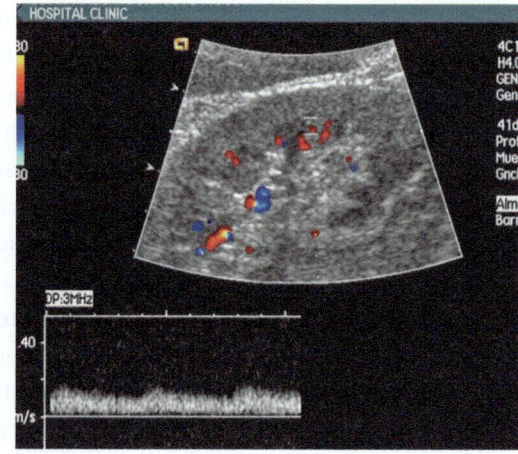

Fig. 7.7.4

A 55-year-old woman with hypertension not properly managed using three antihypertensive drugs. Doppler ultrasound was indicated.

Right (Fig. 7.7.1) and left (Fig. 7.7.2) kidneys did not show abnormalities on gray-scale US. Doppler waveform in interlobar arteries, shown in the middle (Fig. 7.7.3) and lower (Fig. 7.7.4) part of the right kidney, presented a typical damped parvus-tardus waveform with a low acceleration index and a long acceleration time suggesting significant renal artery stenosis.

Doppler spectrum from the proximal right renal artery (Fig. 7.7.5) shows increase velocities (peak systolic velocity = 5 m/s) compatible with significant renal artery stenosis.

Angiography (Fig. 7.7.6) confirmed the presence of significant proximal right renal artery stenosis (*arrow*).

Significant renal artery stenosis is the cause of 4–5 % of the cases of hypertension in adults. The most common cause of renal artery stenosis is atherosclerotic disease, accounting for about 80 % of cases and usually affecting the proximal renal artery. The second most common cause is fibromuscular dysplasia, accounting for about 15 % of cases and affecting the mid and distal renal artery of young to middle-aged patients. Imaging modalities should be reserved for the subgroup of hypertensive patients that fulfill well-established clinical criteria for renal artery stenosis. In this respect, Doppler ultrasound is widely considered the first imaging technique to be performed in these cases. Doppler ultrasound of the renal arteries is one of the most challenging ultrasound studies because of the technical difficulties to visualize the entire renal arteries due to bowel gas interposition or their deep location in obese patients. However, Doppler ultrasound is successfully performed in most patients when performed with gold standard US equipments. Two main Doppler methods can be used to diagnose renal artery stenosis. The direct and more accurate method is the detection of increased velocities in the stenotic arterial segment associated to turbulent blood flow just downstream the stenosis. Several Doppler indexes have been evaluated to identify significant stenosis, but the most accepted one is the peak systolic velocity (PSV) in the stenotic segment. Every center should have their own values of reference, but it is widely accepted that PSV values higher than 180–200 cm/s represent significant stenosis. The ratio between the renal artery and the aorta PSV is also a useful parameter in doubtful cases. The indirect method to diagnose renal artery stenosis is based on changes on the intrarenal arterial Doppler waveforms secondary to the hemodynamic changes related to reduction of blood flow to the kidney. A normal arterial waveform in the interlobar arteries of a healthy kidney shows a low-resistance waveform with an early systolic peak and continuous flow through diastole. When there is a significant renal artery stenosis, a dampened and rounded waveform called "parvus-tardus" with decreased acceleration

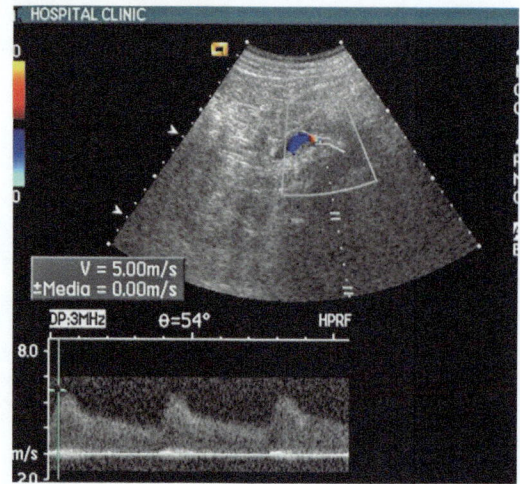

Fig. 7.7.5

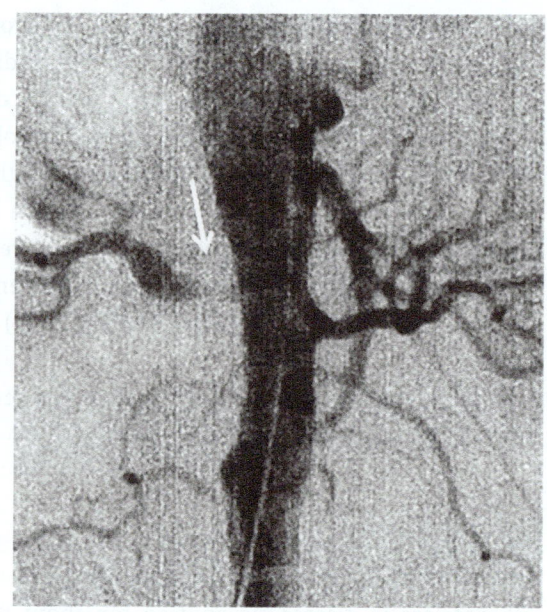

Fig. 7.7.6

index (<3 ms^{-2}) and increased acceleration time (>0.07 s) is detected. However, intrarenal indexes are affected only in cases of severe renal artery stenosis, so it is advisable to use them combined with the information obtained in the main renal artery or especially when the renal artery has not been successfully visualized. The intrarenal Doppler waveform can be also used as an indicator of the response to interventional treatment. It has been described that kidneys with a resistive index (RI) > 0.8 in the interlobar arteries have a poor response, while most kidneys with a RI < 0.8 show improvement in blood pressure after treatment.

Case 8: Portal Vein Thrombosis

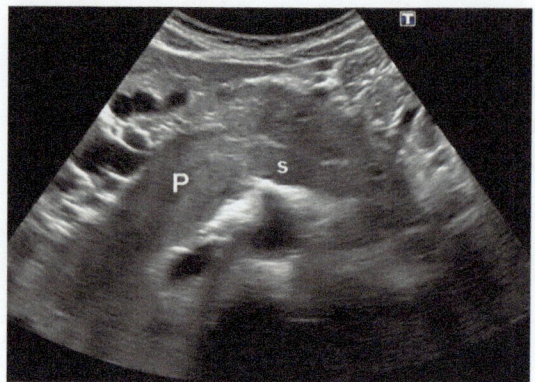

Fig. 7.8.1

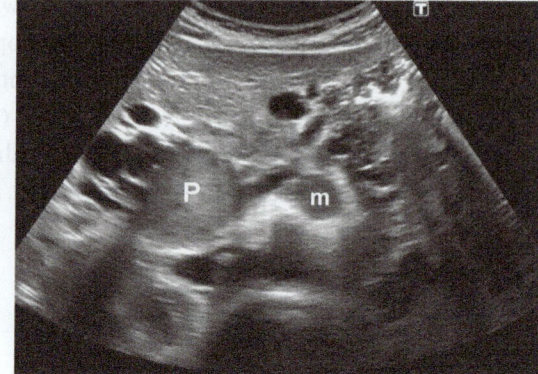

Fig. 7.8.2

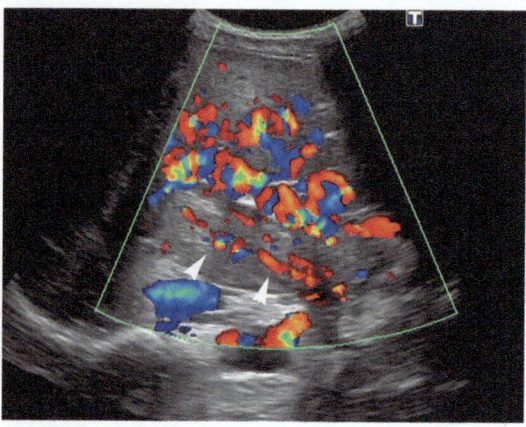

Fig. 7.8.3

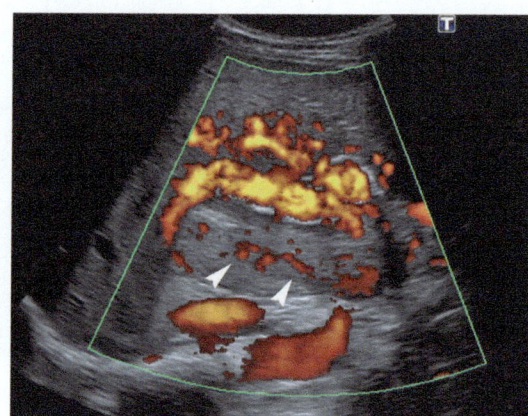

Fig. 7.8.4

A 37-year-old female is being studied for abdominal pain and pancytopenia.

Transverse US sonograms of the upper abdomen (Fig. 7.8.1 is 2 cm above to Fig. 7.8.2) show a solid, homogeneous thrombus occluding the main portal (*P*) and splenic (*s*) veins and the cranial superior mesenteric vein (*m*).

Color Doppler (Fig. 7.8.3) and power Doppler (Fig. 7.8.4) sonograms show small flow signals within the thrombus (*arrowheads*). Extensive collateral periportal flow is also present. Spectral Doppler sonogram (Fig. 7.8.5) shows arterial flow signals within the thrombus, a sign of tumoral thrombosis.

Sagittal US sonogram of right hepatic lobe (Fig. 7.8.6) shows a 12-cm heterogeneous hepatic mass, corresponding to HCC.

A malignant portal vein thrombus was diagnosed. A core biopsy of the mass in right hepatic lobe was performed, with the result of hepatocellular carcinoma.

Case Presentation and Imaging Findings

The thrombosis of the portal vein and/or of some of its branches can occur in cirrhotic and noncirrhotic patients and in both cases may or may not be associated to malignancy; that is, it can be a tumoral thrombus or a bland thrombus. The tumoral invasion of the portal vein occurs more frequently in hepatocellular carcinoma (HCC) and in pancreatic carcinoma, although it can also appear in a metastatic liver of any origin and in the primary leiomyosarcoma of the portal vein. In cirrhotic patients, the thrombosis can be produced by the stagnation of fluid, although in these cases, great attention must always be paid to rule out HCC. In noncirrhotic patients and without evidence of malignancy, the thrombosis can be associated to states of hypercoagulability (among them, pregnancy) or other predisposing factors (abdominal infections, surgery), but in a significant number of cases no associated cause can be found. The symptoms can be quite nonspecific, with pain or abdominal distension or appearance of ascites.

The most usual ultrasound findings in acute-phase portal thrombosis are the presence of echogenic material in the principal portal vein or its branches, the increase in the caliber of the portal vein, and the absence of detectable flow with Doppler US. The very recent thrombi can be almost anechoic and can go unnoticed if attention is not paid and the Doppler US is not used. Occasionally, the portal vein thrombosis is partial and flow can be detected with Doppler US in the peripheral area of the vessel. The thrombus can extend to the splenic or upper mesenteric veins. Within weeks, partial recanalization may be detected in the thrombus, whatever the origin. The detection of arterial-type (pulsating) signal in the thrombus is very suggestive of tumoral-type thrombus, but this sign has a sensitivity of only 60 %. Other finding suggestive of tumoral thrombus is the increase in the diameter of the thrombus in the follow-up, the disruption of the vessel wall, and of course the presence of a mass or infiltration of parenchyma adjacent to the thrombosed vessel.

Comments

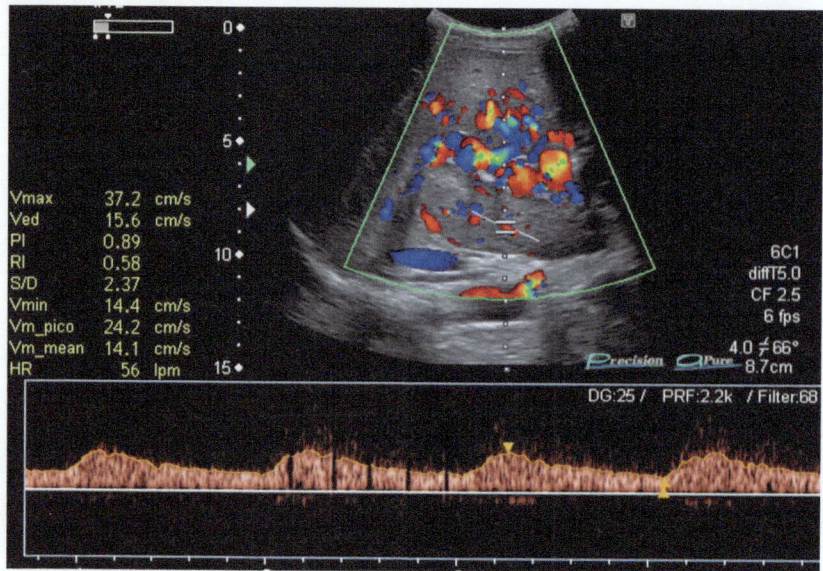

Fig. 7.8.5

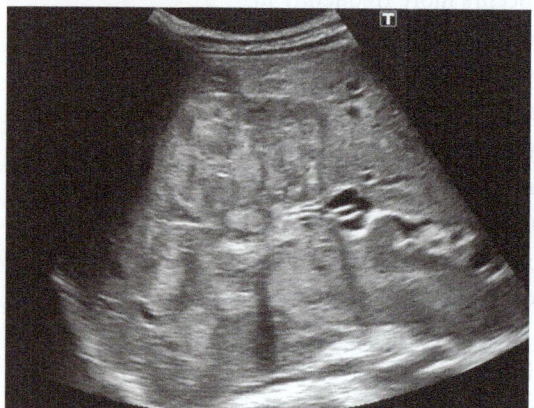

Fig. 7.8.6

Some authors state that a thrombosed portal vein of large caliber in the initial diagnosis (over 23 mm) should warn of the possibility of tumoral thrombus. The evolution of the thrombi not associated to malignancy is quite variable: in up to a third of the cases, the thrombus can resolve itself through complete recanalization, but in the majority of the cases, the thrombosed portal vein will fibrose, progressively decreasing in diameter until being almost indistinguishable, and in a few cases, it will become calcified. When thrombus is not rechanneled, a tangle of collateral vermiform periportal vessels, called portal cavernomatosis, will develop in the hepatic hilum in months after the onset of the thrombosis.

Further Reading

Ahmad F, Turner SA, Torrie P (2008) Iatrogenic femoral artery pseudoaneurysms – a review of current methods of diagnosis and treatment. Clin Radiol 63:1310–1316

Ball EL, Walsh SR, Tang TY (2010) Role of ultrasonography in the diagnosis of temporal arteritis. Br J Surg 97:1765–1771

Flis CM, Jager HR, Sidhu PS (2007) Carotid and vertebral artery dissections: clinical aspects, imaging features and endovascular treatment. Eur Radiol 17: 820–834

Fraser JD, Anderson DR (2004) Venous protocols, techniques, and interpretations of the upper and lower extremities. Radiol Clin North Am 42:279–296

Gaitini D, Soudack M (2005) Diagnosing carotid stenosis by Doppler sonography: state of the art. J Ultrasound Med 24:1127–1136

Grant EG, Benson CB, Moneta GL et al (2003) Carotid artery stenosis; gray-scale and Doppler US diagnosis – society of radiologist in ultrasound consensus conference. Radiology 229:340–346

Hamper UM, DeJong MR, Scoutt LM (2007) Ultrasound evaluation of the lower extremity veins. Radiol Clin North Am 45:525–547

House MK, Dowling RJ, King P, Gibson RN (1999) Using Doppler sonography to reveal renal artery stenosis: an evaluation of optimal imaging parameters. AJR Am J Roentgenol 173:761–765

Jamadar DA, Jacobson JA, Theisen SE et al (2002) Sonography of the painful calf: differential considerations. AJR Am J Roentgenol 179:709–716

Li JC, Jiang YX, Zhang SY, Wang L, Ouyang YS, Qi ZH (2008) Evaluation of renal artery stenosis with hemodynamic parameters of Doppler sonography. J Vasc Surg 48:323–328

Middleton WD, Dasyam A, Teefey SA (2005) Diagnosis and treatment of iatrogenic femoral artery pseudoaneurysms. Ultrasound Q 21:3–17

Nederkoorn PJ, Brown MM (2009) Optimal cut-off criteria for duplex ultrasound for the diagnosis of restenosis in stented carotid arteries: review and protocol for a diagnostic study. BMC Neurol 9:36

Pipitone N, Versari A, Salvarani C (2008) Role of imaging studies in the diagnosis and follow-up of large-vessel vasculitis: an update. Rheumatology (Oxford) 47: 403–408

Radermacher J, Chavan A, Bleck J, Vitzthum A, Stoess B, Gebel MJ, Galanski M, Koch KM, Haller H (2001) Use of Doppler ultrasonography to predict the outcome of therapy for renal-artery stenosis. N Engl J Med 344:410–417

Ripollés T, Aliaga R, Morote V, Lonjedo E, Delgado F, Martínez MJ, Vilar J (2001) Utility of intrarenal Doppler ultrasound in the diagnosis of renal artery stenosis. Eur J Radiol 40:54–63

Rodallec MH, Marteau V, Gerber S (2008) Craniocervical arterial dissection: spectrum of imaging findings and differential diagnosis. Radiographics 28:1711–1728

Setacci C, Chisci E, Setacci F (2008) Grading carotid intrastent restenosis: a 6-year follow-up study. Stroke 39:1189–1196

Tahmasebpour HR, Buckley AR, Cooperberg PL et al (2005) Sonographic examination of the carotid arteries. Radiographics 25:1561–1575

Tantino L, Francica G, Sordelli I (2006) Diagnosis of benign and malignant portal vein thrombosis in cirrhotic patients with hepatocellular carcinoma: color Doppler US, contrast-enhanced US, and fine-needle biopsy. Abdom Imaging 31:537–544

Tublin ME, Dodd GD, Baron RL (1997) Benign and malignant portal vein thrombosis: differentiation by CT characteristics. Am J Roentgenol 168:719–723

Contrast Ultrasound

8

Teresa Fontanilla, Carlos Nicolau, Javier Minaya, Rafael Pérez-Arangüena, and Blanca Paño

Introduction

Ultrasound contrasts are exogenous substances that increase the echo signal after intravenous or intracavitary administration. They are composed of gas-filled microbubbles surrounded by a capsule stabilizer which allows them to persist more time. Most microbubbles are smaller than red blood cells. So they can cross the pulmonary capillaries, though not the endothelium, remaining intravascular. Contrast-enhancement shows vessels and microvessels, providing information of macroscopic vascularization and parenchymal perfusion.

When the microbubbles are submitted to an ultrasound beam, a potentiation of the Doppler signal appears. Also, if a low mechanical index is used, an oscillation occurs in the microbubbles, with compression and expansion phases, and a nonlinear response rich in harmonic frequencies. Specific ultrasound contrast image techniques are required to detect the signals from the contrast media. The techniques currently used are based on pulse inversion (pulse inversion and amplitude modulation).

Ultrasound contrast is especially used in the characterization of focal liver lesions, follow-up after percutaneous treatment of tumors, characterization of complex renal cysts and assessment of parenchymal perfusion of different organs in trauma, infection, or ischemia. Also in ultrasonography of the cerebral vascularization, and complicated pyelonephritis. It is also used endocavitary to detect vesicoureteral reflux in children.

Contraindications are few. It must not be used during pregnancy or lactation or intravenously in children. It is also contraindicated in patients with severe cardiovascular disease, especially in recent acute coronary syndrome, unstable ischemic heart disease, acute heart failure, and serious heart rhythm disorders.

J.L. del Cura et al. (eds.), *Learning Ultrasound Imaging*, Learning Imaging,
DOI 10.1007/978-3-642-30586-3_8, © Springer-Verlag Berlin Heidelberg 2012

Case 1: Hepatic Hemangioma

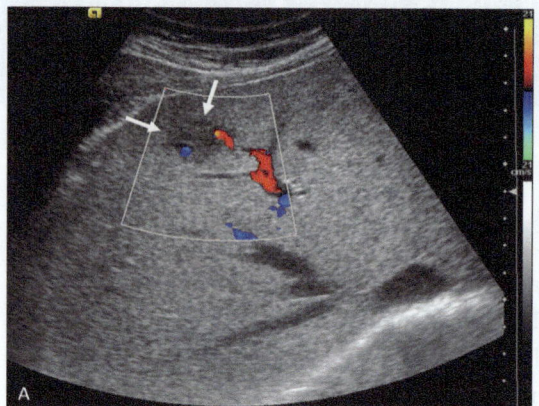

Fig. 8.1.1

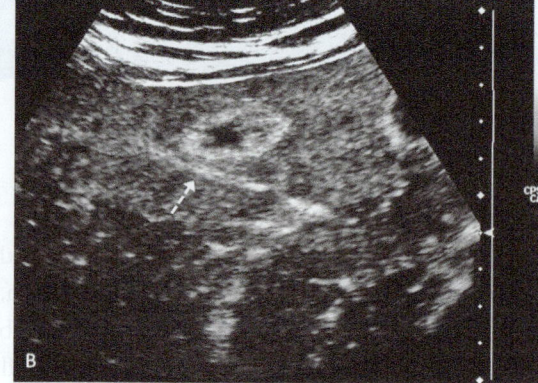

Fig. 8.1.2

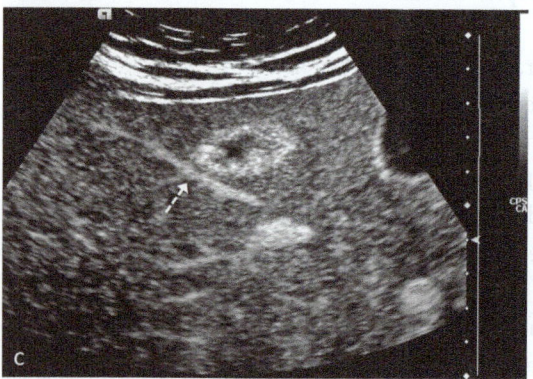

Fig. 8.1.3

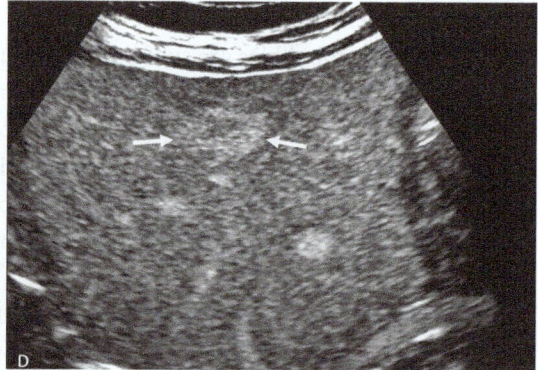

Fig. 8.1.4

A 40-year-old man with epigastric pain

Figure 8.1.1 Subcostal transversal gray-scale ultrasound and color Doppler image shows small hypoechoic nonspecific hepatic focal lesion (*arrows*) with some peripheral vascularization in a slightly echogenic liver, probably due to fatty liver.

Figure 8.1.2 17-s contrast-enhanced ultrasound image shows that the lesion enhances earlier and more intensely than the adjacent hepatic parenchyma. The periphery of the lesion is enhanced, in a nodular fashion. The *discontinuous arrow* shows branch of the hepatic vein.

Figure 8.1.3 30-s contrast-enhanced ultrasound image shows progressive centripetal enhancement of the lesion, which is typical for hemangioma, and progressive parenchymal enhancement.

Figure 8.1.4 2-min contrast-enhanced ultrasound image shows complete enhancement of the lesion (*arrows*) with no washout.

The finding of incidental lesions during ultrasound is very common. Most of them are benign, usually hemangiomas or cysts, also focal nodular hyperplasia. When their appearance is not typical, other imaging methods are needed to characterize them. In the case shown, an experienced radiologist would probably guess looking at the gray-scale ultrasound that this is an angioma with an atypical hypoechoic appearance in comparison to the surrounding echogenic fatty liver; but this cannot be assured. Concern is raised especially in those patients with an oncologic history. Second-generation ultrasound contrast agents, such as sulfur hexafluoride, are blood pool agents that permit a real-time demonstration of the timing of enhancement and washout of lesions and of the spatial pattern and direction of enhancement, which are valuable to characterize lesions. The manipulation of the mechanical index (MI) during the explorations permits to reevaluate the arterial phase enhancement, after total or partial rupture of the contrast microbubbles, which may be useful in the case of small- or rapid-filling lesions, such as high-flow hemangiomas. Generally speaking, most common solid benign lesions enhance during the arterial and portal phases and show no washout, except abscesses and sometimes adenomas. On the other hand, most common malignant lesions that enhance during the arterial phase show washout (for instance metastases).

The contrast-enhanced ultrasound findings in this case show enhancement typical for hemangioma, similar to that of CT and MR: Initial peripheral nodular enhancement with progressive centripetal enhancement until all or most of the lesion is enhanced, with no washout. In this patient, no further imaging work-up is required, so he can be spared from CT-associated radiation and from the potential adverse effects or toxicity of other contrast media and also from cumbersome and more expensive explorations, such as MR.

Case 2: Hepatic Abscess

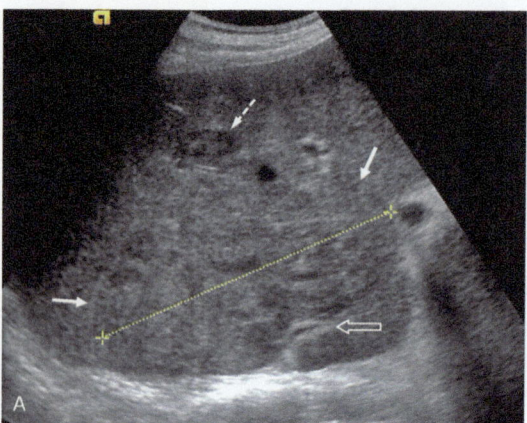

Fig. 8.2.1

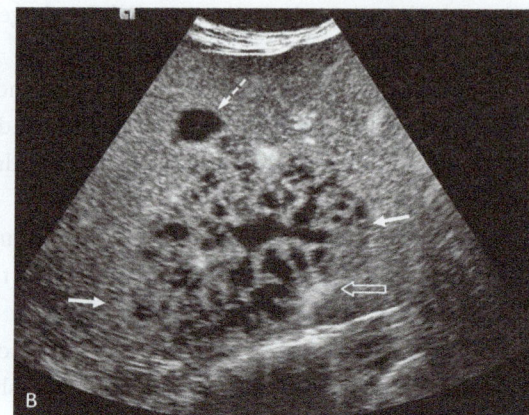

Fig. 8.2.2

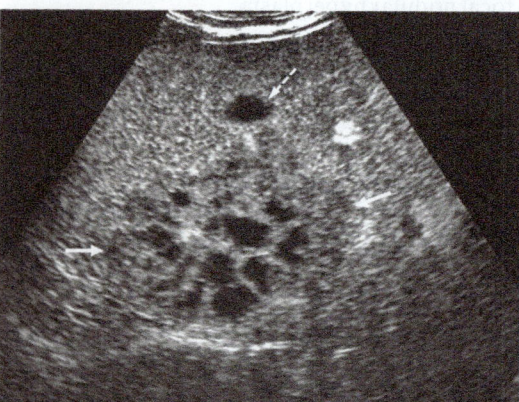

Fig. 8.2.3

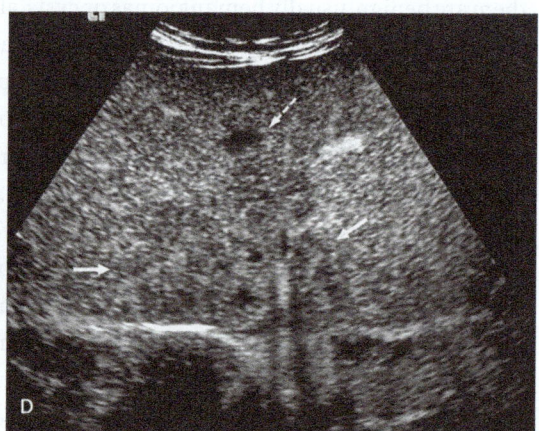

Fig. 8.2.4

Case Presentation and Imaging Findings

A 50-year-old male that seeks attention in the emergency unit because of fever and right upper quadrant pain

Figure 8.2.1 Gray-scale US transversal image of the liver shows 14-cm mass (*white arrows*) which involves mostly the right hepatic liver lobe but also part of the left hepatic lobe and which abuts the inferior vena (*open arrow*). The lesion is isoechoic to the surrounding parenchyma, although heterogeneous. A satellite lesion (*discontinuous arrow*) is seen.

Figure 8.2.2 Contrast-enhanced ultrasound image, 50 s after contrast injection shows confluent nonenhancing areas and enhancing periphery and septa. Satellite lesion is nonenhancing. The enhanced components showed progressive slow washout throughout the exploration (not shown). These findings are very suggestive of partially liquefied hepatic abscess.

Figure 8.2.3 Follow-up 15 days later, after antibiotic treatment. Fifty-second contrast-enhanced ultrasound image shows that the lesion is smaller, nonenhancing areas are fewer, and contrast enhancement is diminished. These data suggest good response to treatment.

Figure 8.2.4 Follow-up contrast-enhanced ultrasound 35 days later. Fifty-second image shows lesion size reduction, almost disappearance of nonenhancing areas, and diminishment of contrast enhancement.

Many hepatic masses are nonspecific on gray-scale ultrasound, as happens in this case in which an apparently solid hepatic lesion was found. In such circumstance, other imaging technique is needed to characterize the lesion. Contrast-enhanced ultrasound enables to characterize them in the ultrasound suite, in the same radiologic act. In this case, contrast-enhanced ultrasound revealed the partially liquefied nature of the lesion, with confluent nonenhancing areas. The ultrasound and contrast-enhanced ultrasound appearance of abscesses depends on the degree of liquefaction and on the timing of imaging if the patient is under antibiotic treatment. The classic abscess is mostly liquefied, and gray-scale ultrasound typically shows an anechoic or hypoechoic round or geographic lesion with increased through transmission, sometimes with gas inside. Less liquefied abscesses may show a nonspecific image; moreover, even if the abscess is mostly liquefied, the gray-scale appearance may be nonspecific, with a "solid" appearance due to the presence of numerous interfaces, because of the presence of dense cellularity and debris. Contrast-enhanced ultrasound reveals the internal structure of the abscess and enables to evaluate the size of the liquefied area, the presence and number of septa, and the thickness of the wall. Liquefied areas lack enhancement, because they are necrotic areas with pus and debris, with no vessels. Septa among these areas and the periphery of the abscess enhance more than the adjacent parenchyma in arterial and early portal phases and show washout during the portal or late phase. If the liquefied area is bigger than 3 cm and most of the abscess is liquefied, drainage may be performed under ultrasound guidance. If not, contrast-enhanced ultrasound enables to follow up these lesions and to evaluate response to antibiotic treatment. Image resolution tends to be slow, even though the clinical course is satisfactory, and complete resolution of the lesion sometimes takes months to ensue.

Comments

Case 3: Hepatocarcinoma

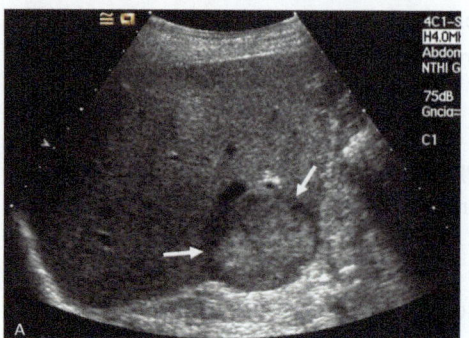

Fig. 8.3.1

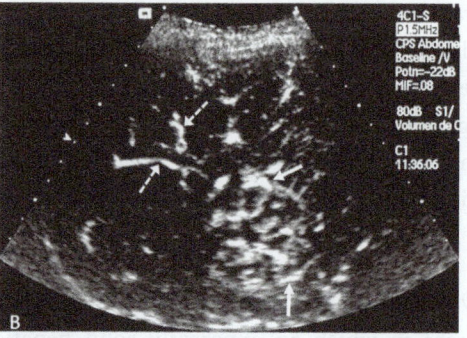

Fig. 8.3.2

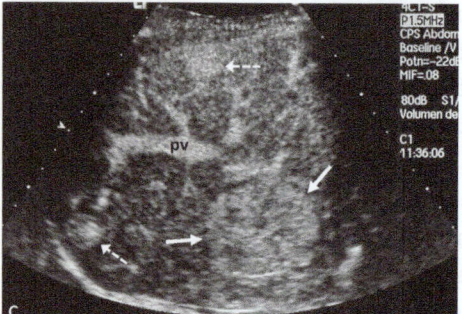

Fig. 8.3.3

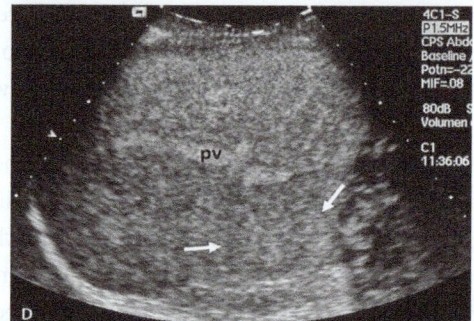

Fig. 8.3.4

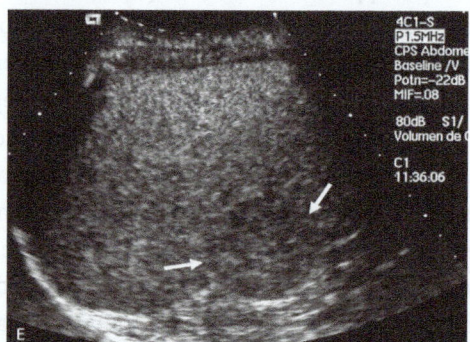

Fig. 8.3.5

Case Presentation and Imaging Findings

A 55-year-old man with chronic hepatitis C infection under ultrasound follow-up

Figure 8.3.1 Basal gray-scale ultrasound shows focal liver mass (*arrows*) in segment V and nodular liver borders which suggest chronic liver disease.

Figure 8.3.2 13-s contrast-enhanced ultrasound image (arterial phase) shows enhancement of arterial vessels (*discontinuous arrows*) without parenchymal enhancement. Two afferent arteries to the lesion are shown (*white arrows*) as well as dysmorphic tortuous vessels inside it, suggestive of neoplastic vessels.

Figure 8.3.3 21-s contrast-enhanced ultrasound image shows scarce parenchymal enhancement, initial portal enhancement (*pv*), and intense enhancement of the lesion (*white arrows*) and of two other lesions (*discontinuous arrows*).

Figure 8.3.4 1.5-min contrast-enhanced ultrasound image shows that the mass is now isoechoic to the surrounding parenchyma.

Figure 8.3.5 2.3-min contrast-enhanced ultrasound image shows contrast washout.

Comments

A nodule bigger than 1 cm in a hepatitis C chronic liver disease patient is considered a hepatocarcinoma (HCC) until proven otherwise. CT and MR are the imaging methods recommended by the AASLD guidelines to diagnose HCC through the demonstration of contrast uptake and washout, but contrast-enhanced ultrasound is able to demonstrate this too. Since ultrasound is the imaging method of surveillance for chronic liver disease, most nodules are detected by ultrasound. In our practice, when a nodule is found in such a setting, contrast-enhanced ultrasound is performed in the same radiologic act and is a rapid and nonexpensive imaging method that permits an initial evaluation of the enhancement pattern of the lesion so as to direct the following imaging strategy. If the nodule seems to be a HCC or cholangiocarcinoma, the next best imaging method probably will be MR; if it looks like metastases, CT will probably prove more useful; if it is a typical hemangioma, contrast-enhanced ultrasound follow-up will suffice.

In the case shown above, gray-scale ultrasound findings are nonspecific. Early and intense enhancement during the arterial phase, as happens in this case, is suggestive of HCC, but it is not definite, since other lesions, such as focal nodular hyperplasia, may show arterial intense enhancement. The demonstration of washout is of great importance to diagnose HCC; in this case, washout is evident during the late phase (2.3 m). Indeed, contrast-enhanced ultrasound washout in HCC may be early, but in the authors' experience, it tends to occur during the late phase and sometimes to be subtle. The timing of washout seems to be related to the histologic differentiation of HCC. Contrast-enhanced ultrasound real-time exploration permits to evaluate better than CT or MR the morphology of the vessels and the direction of enhancement, especially during the early arterial phase. The demonstration in this case of dysmorphic and tortuous arterial vessels and at least of two afferent arteries 13 s after contrast injection contributed to suggest HCC. Contrast-enhanced ultrasound sensibility is higher than that of basal US, as is demonstrated by this case in which two other nodules are seen, with the same pattern of enhancement and washout (not shown), thus suggesting multicentric HCC.

Case 4: Focal Nodular Hyperplasia

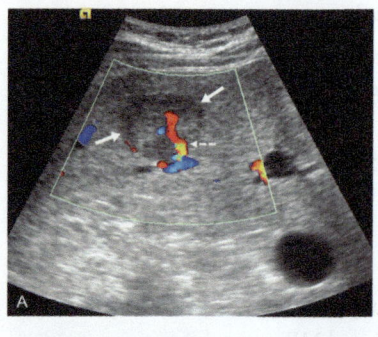

Fig. 8.4.1

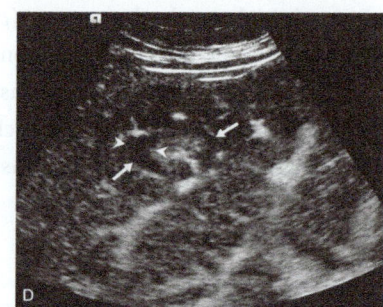

Fig. 8.4.4

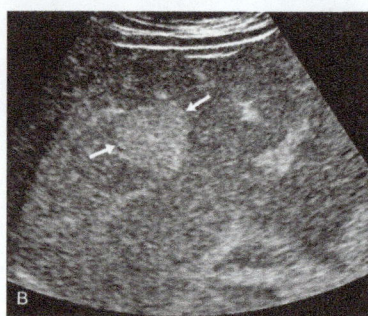

Fig. 8.4.2

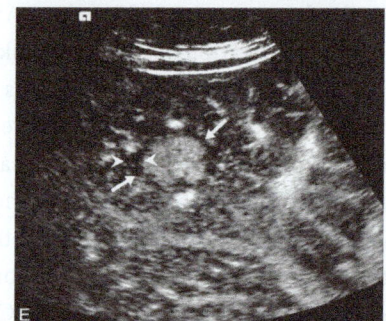

Fig. 8.4.5

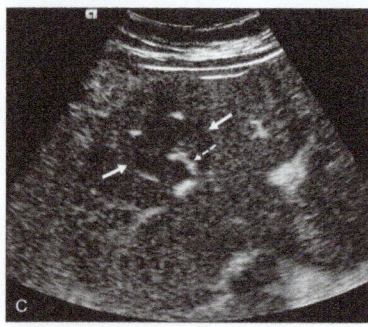

Fig. 8.4.3

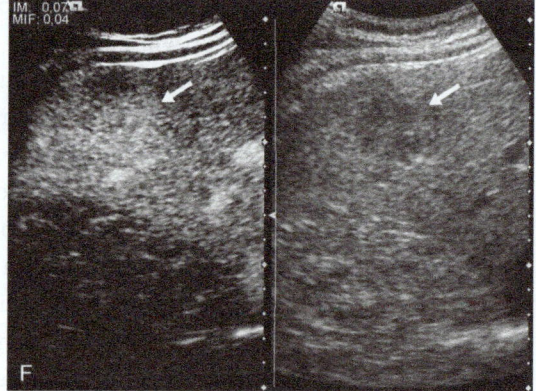

Fig. 8.4.6

Imaging Findings Figure 8.4.1 Gray-scale image and color Doppler show nonspecific hypoechoic 2.8-cm focal liver lesion (*arrows*) with a feeding vessel (*discontinuous arrow*) with arterial normal waveform and resistive index (not shown).

Figure 8.4.2 23-s contrast-enhanced ultrasound image shows hyperenhancing homogeneous lesion (*arrows*), but the fill-in was too fast so as to appreciate the vascular detail and the direction of the enhancement.

Figures 8.4.3, 8.4.4, and 8.4.5 Contrast-enhanced ultrasound arterial phase images after tailored adjustment of the mechanical index (MI) confirm the presence of a central feeding artery (*discontinuous arrow*). Real-time imaging demonstrated centrifugal progressive enhancement of the lesion (*arrows*), as is shown in the video frames (Figs. 8.4.3, 8.4.4, and 8.4.5). This pattern and the presence of a peripheral nonenhanced area (*arrowheads*) which narrows with time and ultimately disappears are typical for focal nodular hyperplasia (FNH).

Figure 8.4.6 Late-phase dual contrast-enhanced ultrasound image shows sustained contrast enhancement (no washout): The lesion (*arrow*) is slightly hyperenhancing, although hard to distinguish from the adjacent parenchyma. Dual imaging with a gray-scale window helps to maintain the lesion in the exploration window.

Comments

Doppler demonstration of a central feeding arterial vessel and of radial distribution of arterial vessels (spoke-wheel distribution) inside an otherwise nonspecific focal hepatic lesion is very suggestive of focal nodular hyperplasia (FNH). In this case, the radial arterial distribution is not conspicuous. The presence of a feeding artery without the stellate arterial sign must be cautiously analyzed, because afferent arteries may be shown in hepatocarcinoma and other lesions, and arterial encasement may occur in different tumors such as cholangiocarcinoma. Contrast-enhanced ultrasound provides with information regarding the fill-in enhancement and washout and regarding the lesion's vascular distribution, which has been proven to be very useful to distinguish FNH from other hypervascular lesions. In the case shown, the initial contrast-enhanced ultrasound exploration suggested a benign lesion since a hypervascular lesion in arterial phase and no washout were demonstrated. However, the absence of a hypoechoic nonenhancing central scar (typical for FNH) and of the stellate arterial pattern did not allow a precise characterization. The detection rate of the central scar and spoke-wheel sign in FNH at contrast-enhanced ultrasound is dependent on lesion size, and these features are often missing in FNH smaller than 3 cm. The manual adjustment of the mechanical index (MI) during the real-time exploration tailored to each case provides an exquisite temporal and spatial display of the vascular distribution and of the fill-in direction which is extremely useful in some cases, especially in rapid fill-in lesions or small lesions. In this case, the MI was manually raised first, which allowed for controlled bubble rupture and was gradually lowered thereafter so as to obtain a controlled replenishment, which revealed the afferent central artery and the progressive centrifugal arterial enhancement of the lesion with the presence of a peripheral nonenhancing area that progresively was completely filled-in. This pattern is typical for FNH. In most of FNH, the combination of Doppler ultrasound and contrast-enhanced ultrasound demonstrates characteristic features, thereby allowing a confident diagnosis, with no further imaging required. Eventually, MR may provide a reliable tool for the characterization of those FNH still undiagnosed at contrast-enhanced ultrasound. Even in these cases, contrast-enhanced ultrasound is an excellent follow-up means.

Case 5: Renal Abscess in Complicated Acute Pyelonephritis

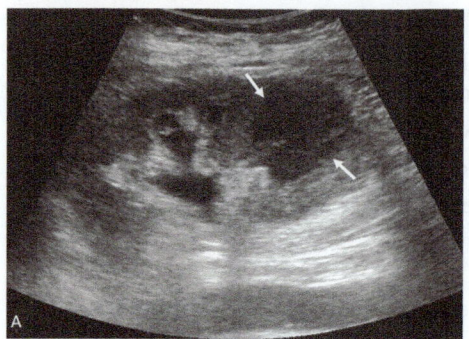

Fig. 8.5.1

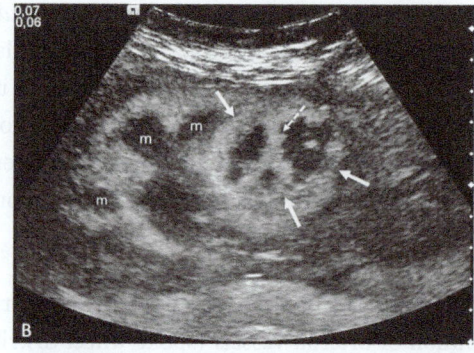

Fig. 8.5.2

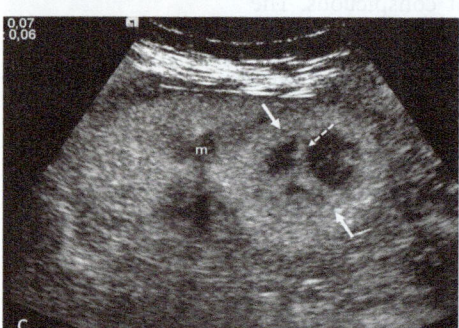

Fig. 8.5.3

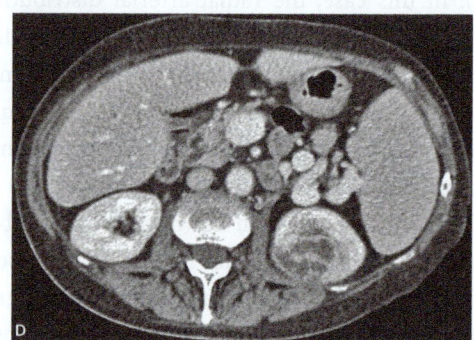

Fig. 8.5.4

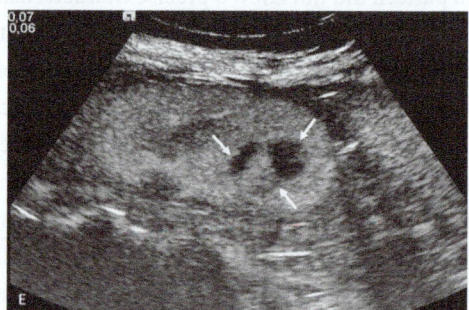

Fig. 8.5.5

Case Presentation and Imaging Findings

A 70-year-old female with transplanted liver presenting fever and left flank pain

Figure 8.5.1 A. Gray-scale sagittal ultrasound of the left kidney shows hypoechoic lower-pole cortical mass (*arrows*) and slight pyelocaliceal dilatation. Even though the clinical history suggests inflammatory mass, from an imaging standpoint, this mass is nonspecific.

Figures 8.5.2 and 8.5.3 Contrast-enhanced ultrasound sagittal views depict a round mass (*white arrows*) with central areas of no enhancement in all phases and peripheral rim and septal enhancement (*discontinuous arrow*), which is early and intense during the cortical phase (Fig. 8.5.2, 8 s), with washout during the parenchymal phase (Fig. 8.5.3, 50 s), in comparison to the adjacent cortex. These findings suggest partially liquefied renal abscess. *m*, medullae.

Figure 8.5.4 CT findings were coincidental with contrast-enhanced ultrasound findings. Axial image during nephrographic phase shows round mass which abuts into the sinus, with peripheral rim and septa and central nonenhancing areas.

Figure 8.5.5 15-day follow-up contrast-enhanced ultrasound 40-s sagittal image shows good response to antibiotic treatment with lesion size reduction but with persistence of liquefied nonenhancing areas (*arrows*).

Comments

In this case gray-scale findings show a nonspecific mass that needs further characterization. When complicated acute pyelonephritis is suspected, as happens in this case, contrast-enhanced ultrasound permits immediate diagnosis in the ultrasound suite, or bedside urgent diagnosis. If there is abscess, it is important to determine its size, internal structure (presence of septa), and extension to perirenal spaces. These data are clues to decide if other imaging modalities are needed or if drainage or surgery is indicated. Contrast-enhanced ultrasound findings of abscesses reflect the inflammatory activity and the presence of necrotic areas. As happens in the case shown, typically the wall and septa enhance early and more than the adjacent cortex in the cortical phase and show washout early in the parenchymal phase. Necrotic areas which contain pus and debris show lack of enhancement during the whole exploration. Contrast-enhanced ultrasound is an excellent means of obtaining imaging information concerning response to treatment and resolution of the lesion, avoiding exposure to ionizing radiation and to nephrotoxic contrast media. The length of the follow-up period and the follow-up schedule depends on the abscess size and on the clinical situation of the patient. Big abscesses tend to have a long course (frequently longer than a month); abscesses gradually turn smaller, and the wall and septa enhance less. Eventually, they disappear, but a focal scar with or without calcification may remain as a residual lesion. In focal pyelonephritis without abscess, contrast-enhanced ultrasound shows a focal wedge- or round-shaped hypoenhancing cortical or corticomedullary area, most conspicuous during the late (more than 1 m) parenchymal phase or early cortical phase. Other differential diagnoses include complex cystic masses Bosniak categories III and IV and partially necrotic neoplastic masses. In these cases, the washout of the solid components tends to occur later in the parenchymal phase, but most importantly, the size of inflammatory masses diminishes with time, whereas complex cystic masses or neoplastic masses remain the same size or grow.

Case 6: Cystic Renal Cell Carcinoma

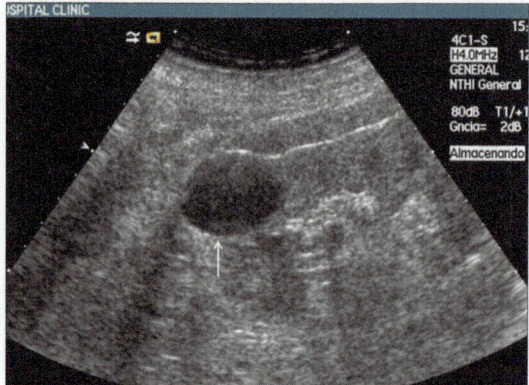

Fig. 8.6.1

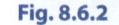

Fig. 8.6.2

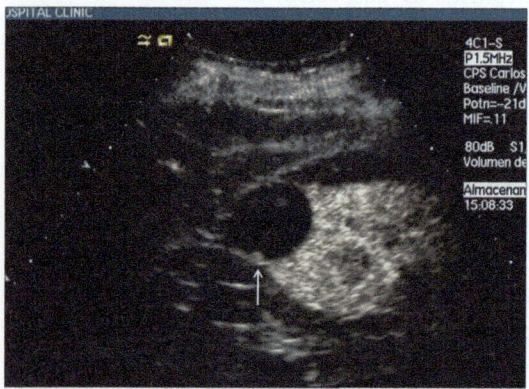

Fig. 8.6.3

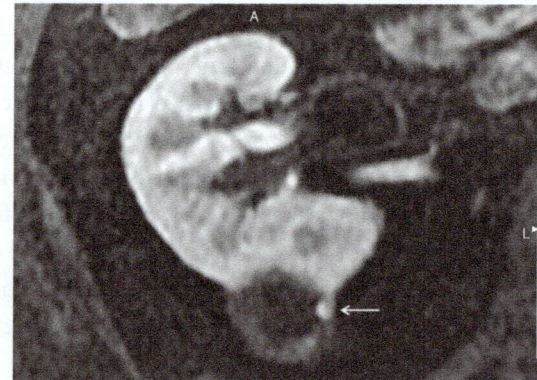

Fig. 8.6.4

A 66-year-old man with a 2-week history of nonspecific abdominal pain. An ultrasound examination was indicated.

Gray-scale ultrasound study (Fig. 8.6.1) showed a 2.8-cm cystic renal mass in the right kidney with focal intracystic, increased echoes (*arrow*) compatible with complex cyst. Arterial (Fig. 8.6.2) and venous (Fig. 8.6.3) phases of a contrast-enhanced ultrasound study that was indicated demonstrated enhancement of a very small soft tissue mass (*arrow*), compatible with cystic renal cell carcinoma. The small solid-enhancing nodule was confirmed (*arrow*) using enhanced MR imaging (Fig. 8.6.4).

Case Presentation and Imaging Findings

Renal cysts are the most common renal masses in adults. US features of simple cysts include a rounded or ovoid shape, smooth hairline-thin wall, absence of internal echoes, and absence of vascularization on color Doppler. Renal cell carcinoma has a complex appearance due to the presence of septa, wall thickening, internal echoes, or intracystic soft tissue lesions. Most complex cysts are benign and secondary to infection or hemorrhage and pus and debris cause the heterogeneous echo structure. When a complex cyst is detected, further investigation is necessary to rule out a renal cell carcinoma since 10 % of renal cell carcinomas may have a complex cystic appearance. On ultrasound, thick (>1 mm) or irregular septations or intracystic soft tissue masses are especially suspicious, but the detection of vascularity is the key, suggesting malignancy. Color Doppler US can be used to detect the presence of vascularity in septations and soft tissue nodules. Nonetheless, a negative color Doppler ultrasound study does not rule out the presence of vascularity, since color Doppler ultrasound shows low accuracy to detect tiny microvascularization; thus, further imaging techniques such as CT or MR after the administration of an intravenous contrast agent are required. Some criteria have been developed to assign a risk of malignancy using CT and MR imaging. In this respect, the most widely accepted are the Bosniak criteria. Contrast-enhanced ultrasound can be used to evaluate complex cysts, and Bosniak classification has been adapted to contrast-enhanced ultrasound. Type I cysts are simple cysts; type II cysts may have few hairline-thin septa with minimal thin enhancement; type IIf cysts may have multiple hairline-thin septa, smooth minimal thickening of the wall or septa, and absence of nodular enhancement; type III cysts may have thickening or irregularity of the wall or/and septa with enhancement; and type IV cysts may have soft tissue-enhancing masses independent of the wall or septa. Type III and IV cysts have a higher probability of malignancy, and surgery is recommended in such cases. On the contrary, if contrast-enhanced ultrasound does not show features of malignancy and a follow-up is necessary, this follow-up can be performed with contrast-enhanced ultrasound because of its high sensitivity to detect microvascularization of the wall and septa with the advantage of absence of radiation and absence of contrast-agent nephrotoxicity.

Comments

Further Reading

Ascenti G, Mazziotti S, Zimbaro G, Settineri N, Magno C, Melloni D, Caruso R, Scribano E (2007) Complex cystic renal masses: characterization with contrast-enhanced US. Radiology 243:158–165

Bartolotta TV, Taibbi A, Matranga D, Malizia G, Lagalla R, Midiri M (2010) Hepatic focal nodular hyperplasia: contrast-enhanced ultrasound findings with emphasis on lesion size, depth and liver echogenicity. Eur Radiol 20:2248–2256

Bhayana D, Kim TK, Jang HJ, Burns PN, Wilson SR (2010) Hypervascular liver masses on contrast-enhanced ultrasound: the importance of washout. AJR Am J Roentgenol 194:977–983

Catalano O, Sandomenico F, Raso MM, Siani A (2004) Low mechanical index contrast-enhanced sonographic findings of pyogenic hepatic abscesses. AJR Am J Roentgenol 182:447–450

Claudon M, Cosgrove D, Albrecht T, Bolondi L, Bosio M, Calliada F et al (2008) Guidelines and good clinical practice recommendations for contrast-enhanced ultrasound (CEUS) – update 2008. Ultraschall Med 29:28–44

Dietrich CF, Mertens JC, Braden B, Schuessler G, Ott M, Ignee A (2007) Contrast-enhanced ultrasound of histologically proven liver hemangiomas. Hepatology 45:1139–1145

Fontanilla T, Mendo M, Cañas T, Pérez Arangüena R, Velasco MJ, Cortes C (2009) Diagnosis and differential diagnosis of liver abscesses using contrast-enhanced (SonoVue) ultrasonography. Radiologia 51:403–410

Fontanilla T, Minaya J, Cortes C, Hernando CG, Aranguena RP, Arriaga J, Carmona MS, Alcolado A (2011) Acute complicated pyelonephritis: contrast-enhanced ultrasound. Abdom Imaging 37:639–646

Jang HJ, Kim TK, Burns PN, Wilson SR (2007) Enhancement patterns of hepatocellular carcinoma at contrast-enhanced US: comparison with histologic differentiation. Radiology 244:898–906

Kim TK, Jang HJ, Burns PN, Murphy-Lavallee J, Wilson SR (2008) Focal nodular hyperplasia and hepatic adenoma: differentiation with low-mechanical-index contrast-enhanced sonography. AJR Am J Roentgenol 190:58–66

Liu GJ, Lu MD, Xie XY, Xu HX, Xu ZF, Zheng YL et al (2008) Real-time contrast-enhanced ultrasound imaging of infected focal liver lesions. J Ultrasound Med 27:657–666

Mitterberger M, Pinggera GM, Colleselli D, Bartsch G, Strasser H, Steppan I, Pallwein L, Friedrich A, Gradl J, Frauscher F (2008) Acute pyelonephritis: comparison of diagnosis with computed tomography and contrast-enhanced ultrasonography. BJU Int 101:341–344

Nicolau C, Vilana R, Catala V, Bianchi L, Gilabert R, Garcia A et al (2006) Importance of evaluating all vascular phases on contrast-enhanced sonography in the differentiation of benign from malignant focal liver lesions. AJR Am J Roentgenol 186:158–167

Nicolau C, Bunesch L, Sebastia C (2011) Renal complex cysts in adults: contrast-enhanced ultrasound. Abdom Imaging 36(6):742–752

Park BK, Kim B, Kim SH, Ko K, Lee HM, Choi HY (2007) Assessment of cystic renal masses based on Bosniak classification: comparison of CT and contrast-enhanced US. Eur J Radiol 61:310–314

Wilson SR, Burns PN (2010) Microbubble-enhanced US in body imaging: what role? Radiology 257:24–39

Xu HX, Liu GJ, Lu MD, Xie XY, Xu ZF, Zheng YL et al (2006) Characterization of focal liver lesions using contrast-enhanced sonography with a low mechanical index mode and a sulfur hexafluoride-filled microbubble contrast agent. J Clin Ultrasound 34:261–272

Interventional Ultrasound

9

Jose Luís del Cura, Rosa Zabala, and Igone Korta

Introduction

Percutaneous procedures can be performed using any of the methods of imaging for guidance. Ultrasound has important advantages that make it preferable to guide procedures when the lesion is visible on sonography. Ultrasound is not expensive and, thus, is widely available. It does not use ionizing radiation, which is especially important in procedures that may be long. It allows real-time continuous monitoring of the position of the needle. The equipment can be moved, making ultrasound particularly suitable for procedures on patients in intensive care units or operating room. The time required for any ultrasound-guided procedure is always less than required when using other techniques for guidance. Finally, it is versatile and allows to select multiple paths to the lesion.

However, ultrasound also has limitations: the echo signal is attenuated with depth, limiting its use in deeply located lesions: ultrasound has a lower sensitivity in the detection of some lesions, and ultrasound does not pass through air or bone, limiting its use for guidance in some organs.

The technique consists in introducing a needle or a catheter following the plane of exploration with real-time control. The transducers more suitable for intervention in superficial tissues are linear high-resolution probes, whereas in deep lesions 3.5-MHz curved array probes are the best option.

Ultrasound guidance can be performed using devices attached to the probes or by freehand technique (holding the needle with one hand and the probe with the other). Performing ultrasound-guided procedures requires a careful planning, including hemostasis survey, asepsis, and appropriate anesthesia. The most common procedures include biopsies, percutaneous drainage, and injections.

J.L. del Cura et al. (eds.), *Learning Ultrasound Imaging*, Learning Imaging,
DOI 10.1007/978-3-642-30586-3_9, © Springer-Verlag Berlin Heidelberg 2012

Case 1: Percutaneous Biopsy

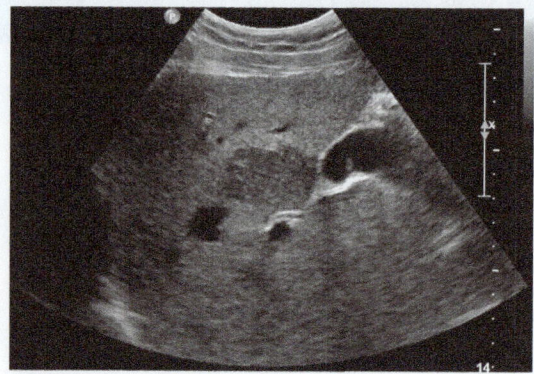

Fig. 9.1.1

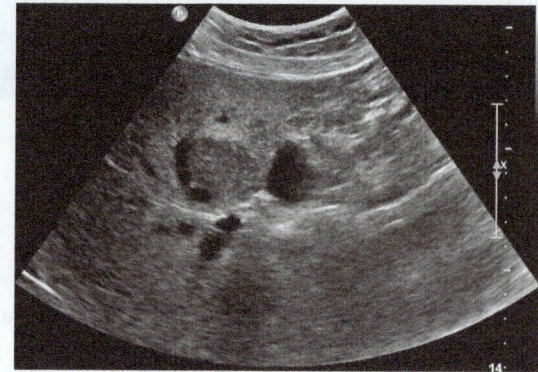

Fig. 9.1.2

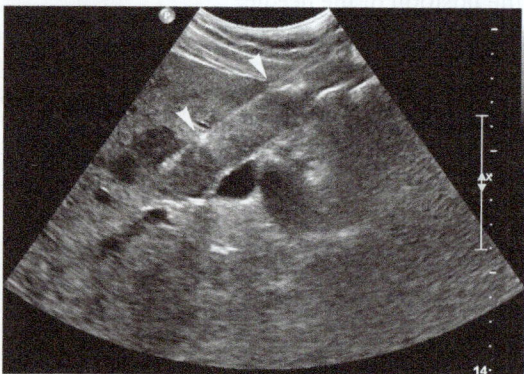

Fig. 9.1.3

In an ultrasound examination carried out because of a renal colic on a 41-year-old female, a hypoechoic lesion was discovered in segment IV of the liver (Figs. 9.1.1 and 9.1.2). The lesion was homogeneous, hypoechoic, and well delimited. After performing CT and MRI, a definitive diagnosis was not achieved. A biopsy of the lesion was indicated and performed with ultrasound guidance (Fig. 9.1.3). The image shows the needle (*arrowheads*) reaching the lesion. The pathological diagnosis was focal nodular hyperplasia.

Case Presentation and Imaging Findings

Percutaneous biopsy consists of placing a needle in the interior of the lesions to obtain cellular or tissue samples to identify its nature. Ultrasound guidance allows continuously monitoring and guiding the procedure. The needle is introduced up to its objective following the plane of exam of the ultrasound. It can be performed in nearly all the structures of the body, with the sole exception of the central nervous system. It is a very effective technique with low cost and minimum risk and can be used for any lesion visualized with ultrasound.

Comments

There are two techniques of percutaneous biopsy. Fine-needle biopsy uses fine needles (20–25 G) to obtain samples by aspiration for cytological analysis. Core-needle biopsy uses thicker needles (usually 14–18 G), spring-loaded or manual, to obtain small cylinders of tissue for histological analysis that include histochemical and immunohistochemical techniques. Core-needle biopsy is, as a general rule, more sensitive and specific than fine-needle biopsy. The rate of complications is very low, being hemorrhage the most frequent complication.

Percutaneous biopsy is a very sensitive technique for distinguishing between benign and malignant lesions with specificity near 100 %. However, as the samples are relatively scarce and they might not be representative of the whole tumor, pathological analysis of the samples poses some difficulties in typing and subtyping some tumors, especially when cytologic techniques are used.

To select where the samples should be taken, it is important to be aware that the center of many lesions is frequently occupied by necrotic tissue, not valid for histological analysis. Thus, the biopsy should be preferably performed on the periphery of the lesion. In adenopathies, it is the area farthest from the hilum the best election for sampling. In lesions with a cystic component, the solid areas must be chosen to sample. Enough representative samples of the whole lesion should be obtained to avoid sampling errors. This always means to perform several punctures in each lesion.

In lesions suspected of being pheochromocytomas, biopsy should be avoided because of the risk of a severe hypertensive crisis with cardiovascular complications. Also, biopsies should not be performed on lesions suspected of being hydatid cysts because of the risk of anaphylaxis. In the lesions located in the surface of the liver, a path should be selected to access the lesion through the healthy parenchyma of the organ, to avoid hemorrhages and tumor seeding.

Case 2: Drainage of a Hepatic Abscess

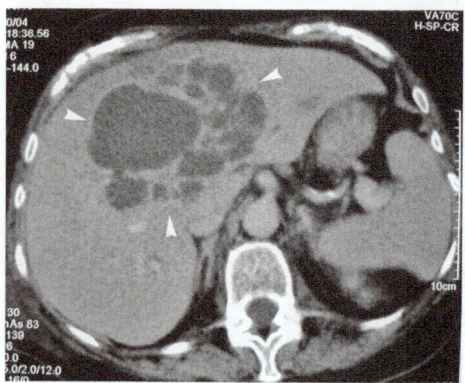

Fig. 9.2.1

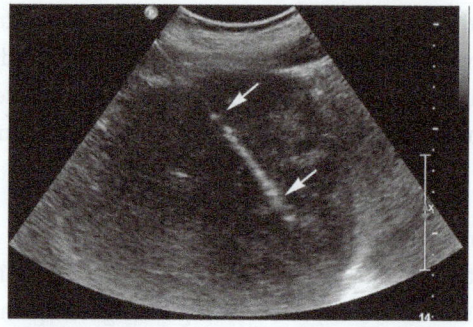

Fig. 9.2.3

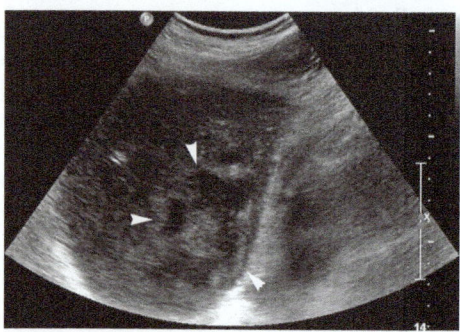

Fig. 9.2.2

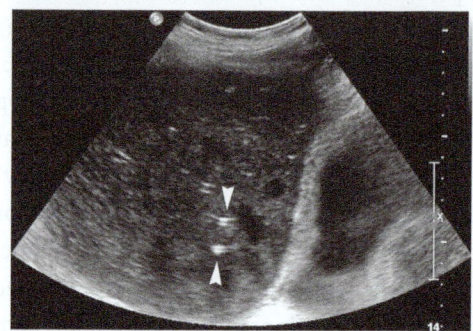

Fig. 9.2.4

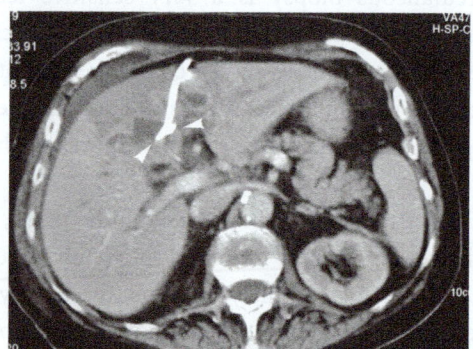

Fig. 9.2.5

Case Presentation and Imaging Findings

A 62-year-old man was admitted to the emergency room with high fever and abdominal pain. A CT was performed (not shown) and diverticulitis was diagnosed. The CT also discovered (Fig. 9.2.1) a multiloculated hypodense lesion in the liver (*arrowheads*) suggestive of hepatic abscess. On ultrasound (Fig. 9.2.2), the abscess appeared as an anechogenic anfractuous lesion (*arrowheads*).

A drainage catheter was immediately performed under ultrasound guidance (Fig. 9.2.3) using the trocar technique. The catheter can be seen in the image as a straight echogenic line (*arrows*) reaching the lesion. After a week, sonographic follow-up demonstrated, that the collection had disappeared (Fig. 9.2.4). The disappearance was confirmed on CT (Fig. 9.2.5). The distal pigtail of the catheter can be seen in both images (*arrowheads*). A week later, the drain was removed, and finally the patient was discharged. Surgery was not necessary.

Comments

Despite the effectiveness of antibiotherapy, abscesses pose a serious problem yet, and their treatment usually requires draining the pus. Because of receiving the blood of the portal system, the liver is one of the organs where abscesses are frequently found.

Given that it is easy to perform and have few complications, percutaneous drainage is currently the first choice of treatment in any symptomatic fluid collection, except when surgery is indicated due to other causes. It can be performed with a diagnostic purpose – to obtain fluid for cultures and analysis – or with therapeutic purposes – to cure the infection avoiding surgery.

Ultrasound is used less frequently than the CT to guide the drainage of collections, especially in the abdomen. However, ultrasound allows a more flexible approach to the collections, is faster and safer, and does not use ionizing radiations. So, when the collection is visible on ultrasound, we prefer to manage it using ultrasound guidance.

The collections can be drained by direct aspiration with a needle or by placement of drainage catheters. The aspiration with needle can be enough for the diagnosis or to treat small collections. However, most abscesses require the placement of a drainage catheter to be cured. These catheters have several holes in their distal part to allow the pus going out to the lumen of the catheter through them. The drains can be placed using two different techniques:

● Seldinger technique: a needle is introduced in the collection, and a guidewire is then advanced through the lumen of the needle. Then, the needle is withdrawn, and drainage tubes are passed over the guidewire.

● Trocar: the catheter is mounted over an inner rigid metallic sharp-pointed guide that gives it the shape of a spike allowing it to be directly introduced in the collection. It is faster and requires fewer steps to be carried out.

The most frequently used catheters have their distal end in the shape of a "pigtail," with the holes in its inner border to avoid being occluded by the walls of the collection once emptied. The catheter should be attached to the skin and connected to a bag or collector to allow the drainage of the pus.

The main complications of drainage are:

● Bacteriemia and sepsis. To prevent them, it is necessary to start antibiotic treatment before drainage.

● Hemorrhage.

● Lesions in adjacent organs.

Percutaneous drainage is highly effective and is successful in 85–90 % of the cases. Failure is more frequent in mycotic abscesses or collections with an associated fistula.

Case 3: Percutaneous Treatment of Severe Acute Pancreatitis

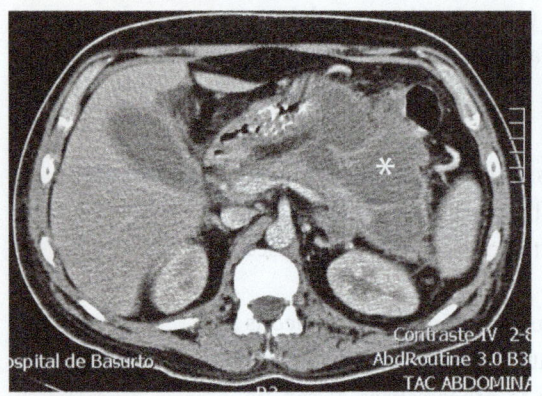

Fig. 9.3.1

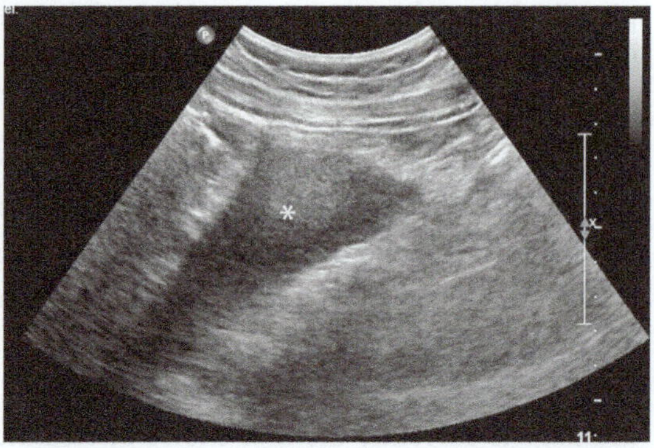

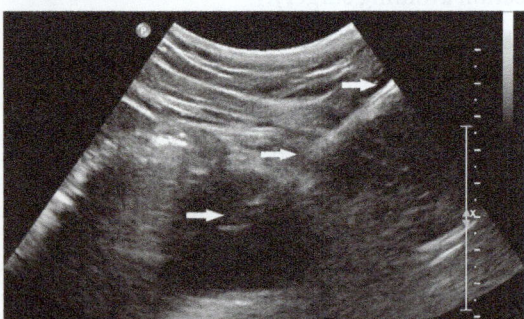

Fig. 9.3.3

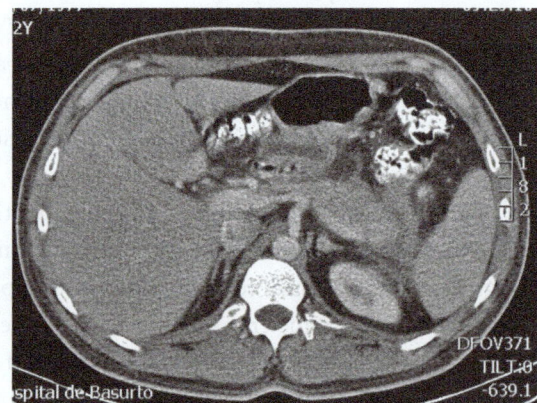

Fig. 9.3.2

Fig. 9.3.4

A 32-year-old male with acute abdominal pain was admitted to the emergency room where he was diagnosed with acute pancreatitis. His condition progressively worsened, being diagnosed with severe acute pancreatitis and translated 48 h later to an intensive care unit. There, after a week of treatment, he experienced a new clinical worsening. A CT scan was performed (Fig. 9.3.1) demonstrating peripancreatic fluid collections (*asterisk*), and a peripancreatic abscess was diagnosed. Drainage of the collections was indicated. As the collections (*asterisk*) were visible on ultrasound (Fig. 9.3.2), the drainage was performed using ultrasound guidance (Fig. 9.3.3), and a 10-F catheter (*arrows*) was introduced in the collection. The procedure was successful, and a follow-up CT scan demonstrated the disappearance of the collections (Fig. 9.3.4).

The patient improved gradually after drainage and was discharged from the ICU within a week. The drain was removed 3 weeks later, and the patient was eventually discharged home.

Case Presentation and Imaging Findings

Indications of ultrasound in the management of acute pancreatitis are currently limited. It is indicated as the initial image technique within 24 h of diagnosis of pancreatitis to rule out a biliary origin. Therefore, the main purpose of this initial exploration is the examination of the gallbladder and bile ducts and not the exploration of the pancreas. However, once a severe acute pancreatitis has been diagnosed, ultrasound can once again have a role as a technique to guide interventional procedures and especially for the drainage of collections, mainly peripancreatic abscesses.

In severe acute pancreatitis, percutaneous drainage is currently the first choice in case of symptomatic fluid collections. Two recent studies have shown that percutaneous management of fluid collections is superior to surgery in severe acute pancreatitis. Complicated fluid collections should therefore be managed initially by percutaneous drainage.

Drainage of collections associated with severe acute pancreatitis can be carried out using both CT and ultrasound to guide the procedure. Ultrasound has the advantage that it can be portable, allowing to perform the drainage without moving the patient from the intensive care unit. However, for planning the procedure is essential to have a recent previous CT scan.

The drainage of the collections has two effects. On the one hand, it allows eliminating infected collections. Also, it helps reduce abdominal volume and thus the intra-abdominal pressure, helping to avoid the abdominal compartment syndrome and, therefore, multiorgan failure. Other ultrasound-guided percutaneous procedures that may be useful in this context are pleural drains and paracentesis.

One of the drawbacks of percutaneous drainage in severe acute pancreatitis is the time the drains should be left in place. Sometimes, they can last for weeks or even months. This is especially true when there is a pancreatic fistula. If amylase is detected in the drained fluid treatment with octreotide is indicated to inhibit pancreatic secretion and help close the fistula.

Comments

Case 4: Percutaneous Treatment of Severe Acute Pancreatitis

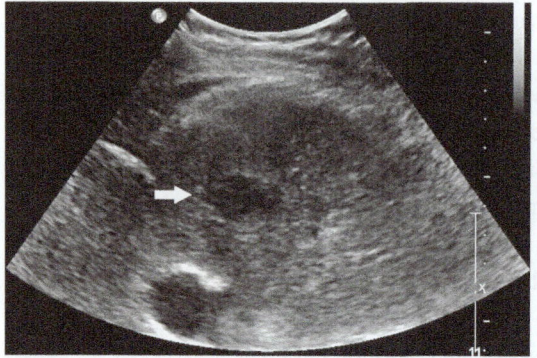

Fig. 9.4.1

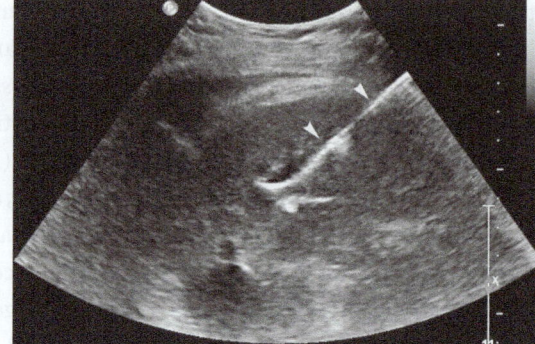

Fig. 9.4.2

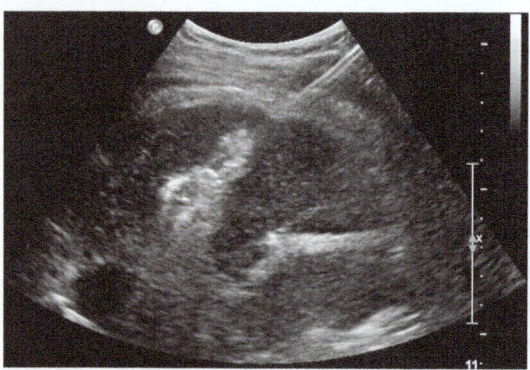

Fig. 9.4.3

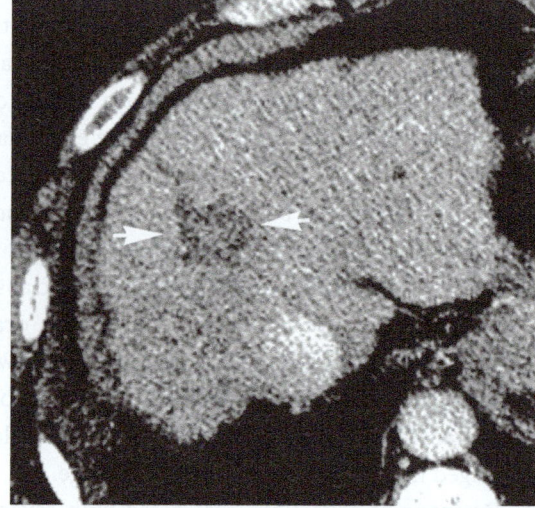

Fig. 9.4.4

Case Presentation and Imaging Findings

In a yearly US screening exam of a 68-year-old female patient with chronic hepatitis C infection and cirrhosis (Fig. 9.4.1), a 2-cm solitary hypoechoic liver nodule was detected (*arrow*). After CT and MRI exams, a hepatocellular carcinoma was diagnosed. The patient was not considered suitable for surgery due to co-morbidities, and a radiofrequency ablation was indicated.

The procedure was performed percutaneously, under sonographic guidance (Fig. 9.4.2). A multitined electrode (*arrowheads*) was inserted through the liver in the lesion. Some minutes after starting the ablation, echogenic gas bubbles progressively appear around the tip of the electrode (Fig. 9.4.3) as the ablation of the tumor progresses.

One month after the ablation, a follow-up TC (Fig. 9.4.4) showed a lack of enhancement of the liver in the area of the tumor (*arrows*), demonstrating that no residual tumor persisted and a successful treatment.

Liver resection is the treatment of choice with the best chance for long-term cure in patients with hepatocellular carcinoma or liver-only metastases. However, most patients are not candidates for resection. The tumors may be inoperable due to several factors such as size, tumor distribution within the liver or, especially, the presence of co-morbidities that preclude major surgery.

To overcome this limitation, ablative methods with less invasive approaches have been developed to allow a curative treatment in these cases increasing the number of patients who can be treated. Ablative techniques, used alone or in conjunction with resection, allow local treatment with lower morbidity and mortality and can be used in patients requiring otherwise extensive liver resection or with concurrent co-morbidities.

Radiofrequency is the most extensively used ablative technique. It induces a thermal injury to the tumor through electromagnetic energy deposition. The procedure consists in inserting a needle-shaped electrode in the tumor. This electrode is connected to an electric generator which creates an alternating electric field in the range of high frequency (200–1,200 kHz). The patient becomes a part of an electric circuit that includes the generator, grounding pads attached to the skin of the patient, and the electrode needle.

When the generator is switched on, the ions in the tissue that surrounds the electrode experience an agitation following the changes in direction of alternating electric current. This ionic agitation causes a heating around the electrode inducing in situ coagulative necrosis. The thermal damage caused by radiofrequency is dependent on both the tissue temperature achieved and the duration of heating. The goal of the procedure is to create a necrosis volume that includes the tumor and a safety margin of 1 cm around the target.

Radiofrequency ablation is usually performed under intravenous sedation or, alternatively, under general anesthesia. The procedure may be performed percutaneously, laparoscopically, or at open surgery. When a percutaneous approach is used, guidance of the placement of the electrode is more frequently performed with ultrasound.

Ablative techniques include also microwave and laser ablation and cryoablation. Their use has been described in kidney, lung, bone, breast, or adrenal tumors also.

Case 5: Pleural Drainage

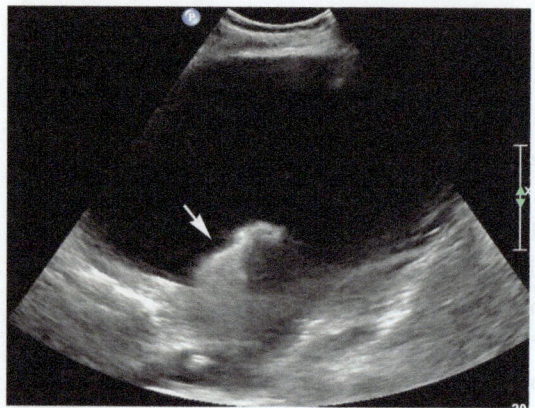

Fig. 9.5.1

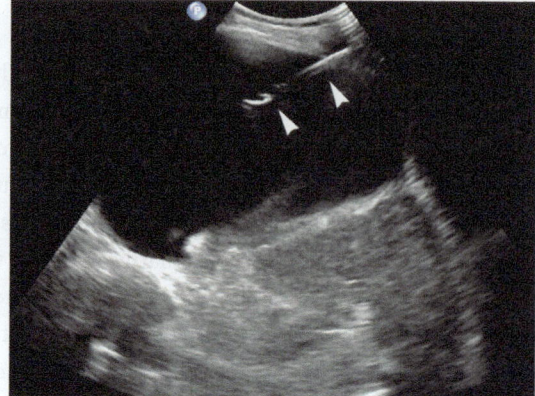

Fig. 9.5.2

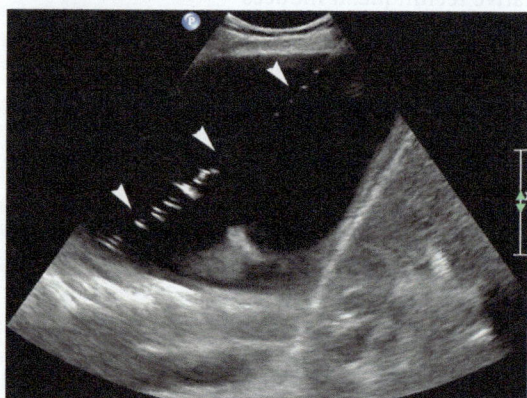

Fig. 9.5.3

A thoracic radiography (not shown) obtained in a 63-year-old male patient with heart disease and dyspnea demonstrated a severe left pleural effusion. Thoracic ultrasound (Fig. 9.5.1) showed a huge amount of fluid in the pleural space. In the image, an echogenic band (*arrow*) corresponding to the collapsed lung can also be observed. With the diagnosis of a massive pleural effusion, pleural drainage was performed with ultrasound guidance (Fig. 9.5.2), inserting a catheter (*arrowheads*) through the thoracic wall. At the end of the procedure (Fig. 9.5.3), the catheter (*arrowheads*) appears located in the interior of the effusion, allowing the fluid to be drained.

The evacuation of a pleural effusion or pleurocentesis can be done without image guidance. However, the pleurocentesis performed without image guidance can sometimes fail: when the fluid is very dense or when the body habitus of the patient or the thickness of the pleura makes it impossible to reach the pleural cavity with conventional needles. Ultrasound guidance allows performing the evacuation of the pleural effusion with reliability and avoiding directing the puncture needle to areas in which no effusion exists.

The pleurocentesis can be performed for diagnostic or therapeutic purposes. When performed for diagnostic purposes, it is enough to introduce a needle in the pleural cavity and to aspirate the fluid needed for the analysis. If treatment of the effusion is the aim, it is advisable to place a pleural drainage catheter when dealing with large effusions that cause dyspnea, parapneumonic effusions, or haemorrhagic effusions. This placement is performed more easily and precisely using ultrasound guidance. In patients with complicated parapneumonic effusion or empyema, the use of catheters, even of small bores, has a high rate of success and permits avoiding surgery in most of the cases.

The procedure can be done with the patient seated or prone. In order to select the puncture point, the place where the pleural fluid is more abundant should be searched with the ultrasound. Tip: select the puncture point in an intercostal space in which fluid can be seen above and below it. Doppler US can be useful to confirm that the intercostal artery is not in the path of the catheter.

To perform the procedure, the transducer should be aligned with the intercostal space and the needle or the catheter inserted, with continuous ultrasound monitoring, following the plane of the image from one of the sides of the transducer. When the fluid is fibrinous, hemorrhagic, or has a high density, the evacuation can be difficult. In these cases, intrapleural fibrinolytics can be used. It is essential to connect the catheter to a system to avoid the entrance of air in the pleura, such as water seal system or one-way valve, e.g. Heimlich valve.

Case 6: Treatment of Shoulder Calcific Tendinitis

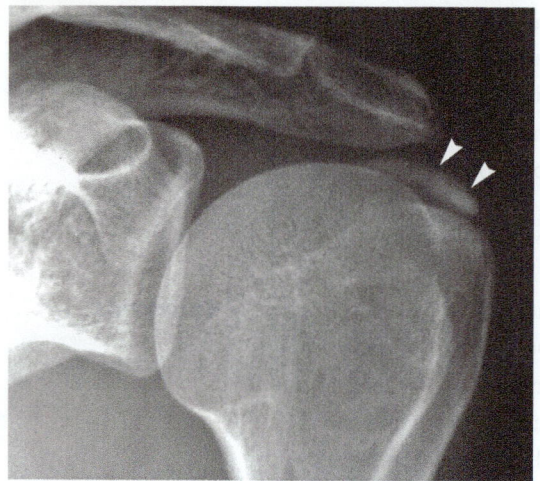

Fig. 9.6.1

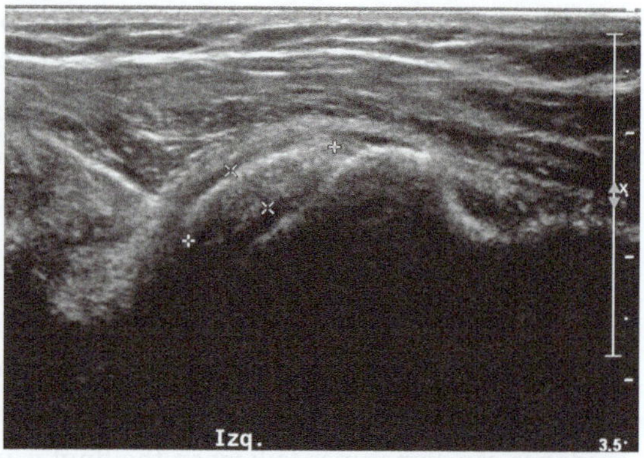

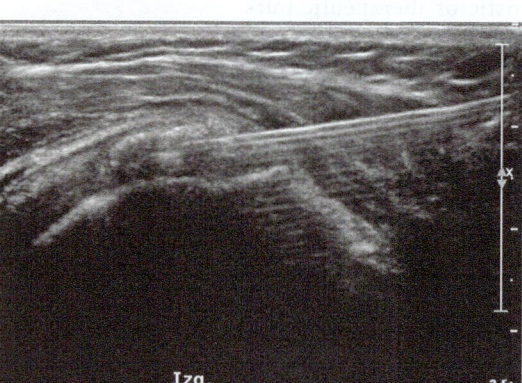

Fig. 9.6.2

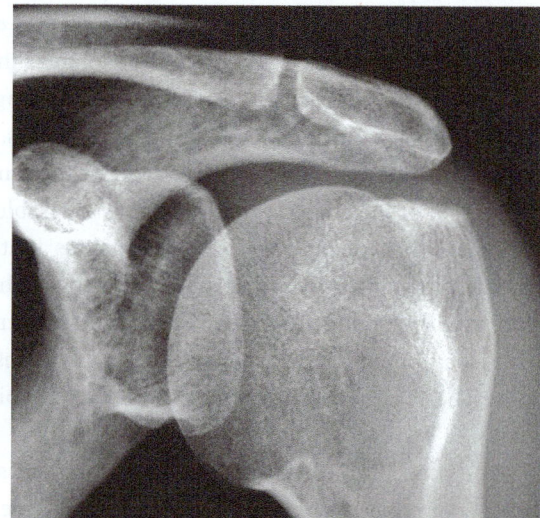

Fig. 9.6.3

Fig. 9.6.4

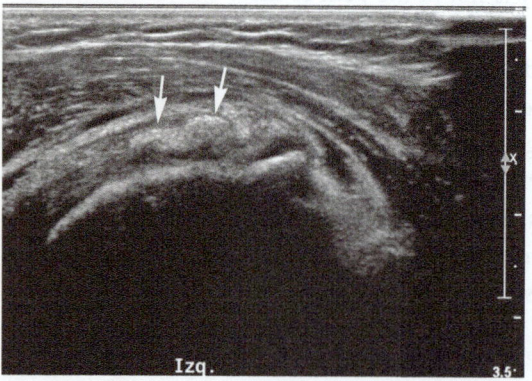

Fig. 9.6.5

In a 48-year-old female, with pain in her left shoulder, the shoulder X-ray (Fig. 9.6.1) demonstrated a long calcification (*arrowheads*) between the acromion and the head of the humerus. An ultrasound (Fig. 9.6.2) confirmed the presence of a calcification (between the *marks*) in the left supraspinatus tendon.

Case Presentation and Imaging Findings

With the diagnosis of calcific tendinitis, percutaneous treatment was indicated. Figure 9.6.3 shows the needle used for the treatment with its tip inside the calcification. In the follow-up performed 2 months later, the patient was asymptomatic, and in the radiograph (Fig. 9.6.4), the calcification had disappeared. The ultrasound performed (Fig. 9.6.5) demonstrated only a linear echogenic scar (*arrows*), with no acoustic shadowing, in the place where the calcification had been located.

Calcific tendinitis is the deposit of calcium hydroxyapatite in the tendons. This disease is much more frequent in the rotator cuff of the shoulder, being the supraspinatus the most frequently tendon involved. Often, it is asymptomatic, having been described in 7.5–20 % of the asymptomatic adults. However, in 50 % of those patients that present calcific tendinitis, these deposits become symptomatic causing acute or chronic pain that can be very intense and highly disabling. Calcific tendinitis is the cause of 7 % of the cases of a painful shoulder.

Comments

Conservative treatments (NSAIDs, corticosteroids, rehabilitation) are frequently not very effective. Surgical treatment can have complications and requires a period of several months of rehabilitation. A simple and very effective alternative is the extraction of the calcifications by ultrasound-guided percutaneous "washing."

To perform this treatment, the calcification is punctured under continuous ultrasound guidance, inserting a 20-G needle up to the calcification, following the direction of the tendon fibers. After anesthetizing the pathway and the subacromial-subdeltoid bursa, the needle is introduced in the calcification. Once the tip is inside the calcification, it is "washed" by injecting and aspirating fluid in it. When aspired, the injected fluid draws the calcium with it to the syringe, eliminating it from the tendon.

Nearly all the patients experience an immediate improvement in their symptoms. In 20 % of the cases, it is necessary to perform a second treatment because of some remaining calcium. One year after the treatment, 91 % of the patients report full or near-complete improvement, and the calcifications totally or almost totally disappear in 89 %. It is usual to find linear echogenic scars in the treated area on 1-year ultrasound follow-up. A similar technique can be used to treat calcifying tendinitis in other locations.

Case 7: Percutaneous Treatment of Paralabral Cyst

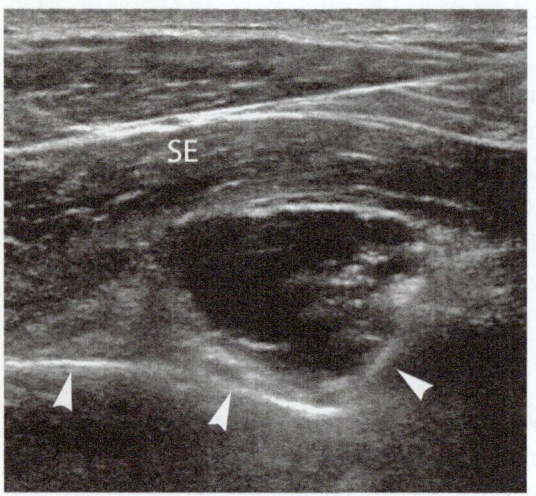

Fig. 9.7.1

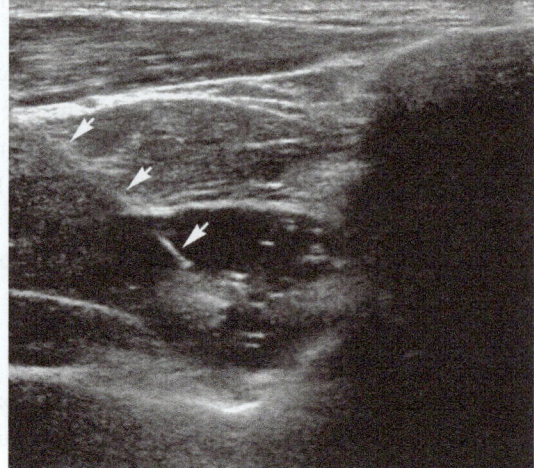

Fig. 9.7.2

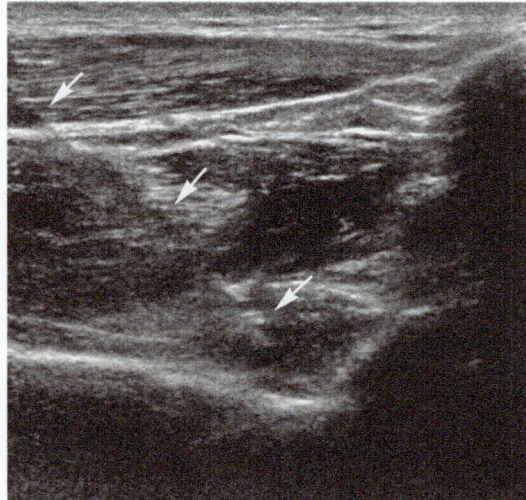

Fig. 9.7.3

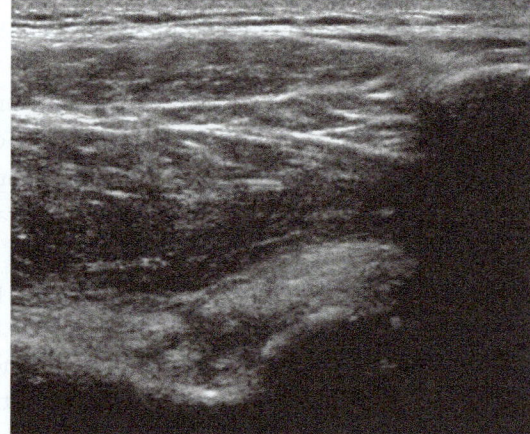

Fig. 9.7.4

A 31-year-old male presented with pain in his right shoulder. The pain increased with movements and when lying on his shoulder. An ultrasound exam was performed (Fig. 9.7.1) in which an anechoic lesion was observed in the supraspinous fossa, between the supraspinous muscle (*SE*) and the surface of the scapula (*arrowheads*). The lesion was located adjacent to the scapular glenoid. The image was characteristic of a paralabral cyst of the shoulder.

Treatment of the lesion was performed (Figs. 9.7.2 and 9.7.3) by inserting with ultrasound guidance a 14-G needle (*arrows*) in the interior of the cyst and fully aspirating its content (Fig. 9.7.3). A gelatinous, very dense fluid was obtained. The procedure ended by injecting absolute ethanol in the empty cyst in order to achieve its sclerosis. A volume of ethanol equivalent to a third of the aspirated volume was injected and withdrawn after 1 h. In the follow-up, 1 year later (Fig. 9.7.4), the cyst no longer existed, and the patient was asymptomatic.

Paralabral cysts of the shoulder are secondary manifestations of intra-articular pathology, such as the lesions of the superior labrum (SLAP tear), that allows the synovial liquid escape from the articulation to the cystic cavity. They are the equivalent of ganglia in the shoulder. Ganglia are cystic lesions that consist of collections of dense, mucinous liquid, located in the proximity of joints. They are more frequent in the upper limb. The etiology is not clear, although it has been hypothesized that they are the consequence of trauma or irritation in synovial cells located in the transition area between the synovial cells and the articular capsule.

When ganglia and paralabral cysts cause symptoms due to the compression of adjacent structures (pain, limitation of mobility, paresthesias), they need to be treated. Surgery has recurrence rates of up to 34 %. Puncturing these lesions with ultrasound guidance can improve the symptoms and frequently make them disappear. The results of the percutaneous treatment are similar to those of the surgical treatment. However, the possibility of recurrence is significant. In this case, the treatment can be repeated. As the content of the ganglia is extremely dense, gelatinous, large-bore needles should be used to treat them.

Although discussed, to avoid recurrences, the injection of corticosteroids in the lesion is advisable. Different corticosteroids can be used, especially methylprednisolone and triamcinolone. We have also used absolute alcohol with good results, filling the cavity with alcohol and removing it 1 h later.

Case 8: Percutaneous Treatment of Pseudoaneurysms

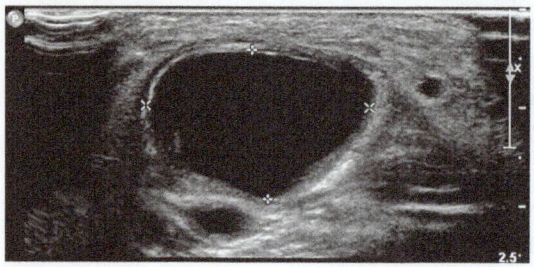

Fig. 9.8.1

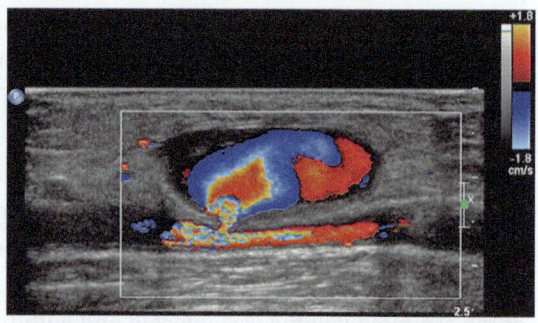

Fig. 9.8.2

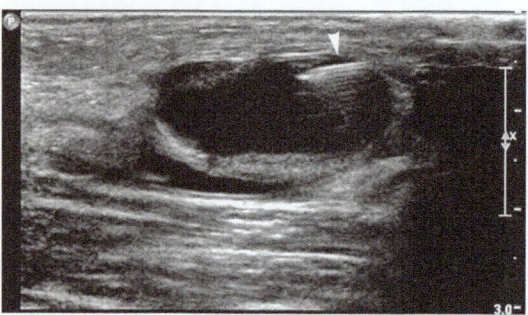

Fig. 9.8.3

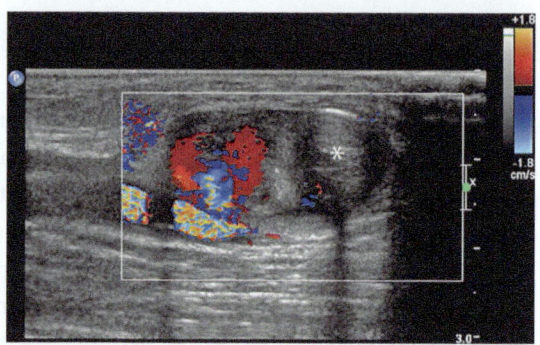

Fig. 9.8.4

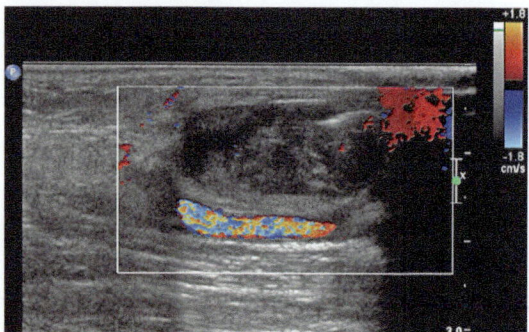

Fig. 9.8.5

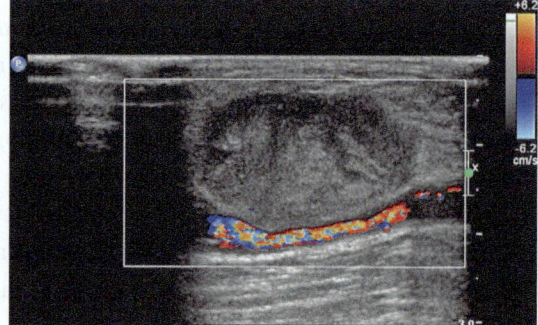

Fig. 9.8.6

A coronary arteriography was performed to a 62-year-old male patient through the brachial artery. One day after the procedure, the patient noticed the formation of a lump in the place of the puncture that presented thrill upon palpation. With the suspicion of a pseudoaneurysm, an ultrasound exam was performed confirming the existence of an anechoic cavity (Fig. 9.8.1) adjacent to the brachial artery. The Doppler ultrasound (Fig. 9.8.2) showed that the cavity had a strong color signal with alternating "to-and-fro" flow, confirming the diagnosis. Also, a communication with the brachial artery through a narrow neck was demonstrated. Percutaneous treatment was indicated. A needle (*arrowhead*) was inserted in the pseudoaneurysm with ultrasound guidance (Fig. 9.8.3). Then, human thrombin was injected inside while monitoring the formation of the thrombus (*asterisk*) using the color Doppler (Fig. 9.8.4) until the pseudoaneurysm was completely thrombosed (Figs. 9.8.5 and 9.8.6). In the 24-h follow-up, no recurrence of the pseudoaneurysm was observed.

Case Presentation and Imaging Findings

Most pseudoaneurysms have an iatrogenic origin and appear as complications after diagnostic or therapeutic angiographic procedures. They are the result of the repermeabilization of a hematoma formed at the entry point to the artery after catheterization. For this reason, the great majority are located in the femoral artery. References to the treatment of pseudoaneurysms in other locations, and especially in the upper limb, are infrequent. However, pseudoaneurysms in the upper limbs, mainly in the brachial artery, have been described, especially after cardiac catheterization.

Comments

The typical appearance on ultrasound is an anechogenic cavity, communicated with the vessel of origin through a narrow neck and with a strong "to-and-fro" flow in the color Doppler exam which has been referred to as a "yin-yang" flow.

The traditional treatment of the pseudoaneurysms has been surgery. Other techniques have also been used, such as compression guided by ultrasound and endovascular occlusion using coils or stents. However, after the technique of the percutaneous injection of thrombin within the aneurysm was introduced, it has become first choice technique in the treatment of this complication. The thrombin, injected directly into the pseudoaneurysm, manages to thrombose it in a few seconds, definitively solving the problem most of times.

Ultrasound guidance is indicated for this procedure because it allows continuous monitoring of the position of the needle and the formation of the thrombus during the injection.

Percutaneous injection of thrombin is highly effective, with a success rate of 97.2 %. It is also easy to perform, does not produce discomfort for the patient, and its complications are rare. Only some isolated cases of distal thrombosis, usually self-limited, have been described. To avoid the thrombosis of the distal vessels, it is recommended to inject the thrombin in the farthest point from the neck of the pseudoaneurysm. Some authors have proposed compressing the pseudoaneurysm and then injecting the thrombin while releasing the pressure on it.

Further Reading

Ai X, Qian X, Pan W, Xu J, Hu W, Terai T, Sato N, Watanabe S (2010) Ultrasound-guided percutaneous drainage may decrease the mortality of severe acute pancreatitis. J Gastroenterol 45:77–85

Amersi FF et al (2006) Long-term survival after radiofrequency ablation of complex unresectable liver tumors. Arch Surg 141:581–588

Benamore RE, Warakaulle DR, Traill ZC (2008) Imaging of pleural disease. Imaging 20:236–251

Del Cura JL (2008) Ultrasound-guided therapeutic procedures in the musculoskeletal system. Curr Probl Diagn Radiol 37:203–218

Del Cura JL, Torre E, Zabala R, Legórburu A (2007) Sonographically guided percutaneous needle lavage in calcific tendinitis of the shoulder: short- and long-term results. AJR Am J Roentgenol 189:W128–W134

Del Cura JL, Zabala R, Corta I (2010a) Intervencionismo guiado por ecografía: lo que todo radiólogo debe conocer. Radiologia 52:198–207

Del Cura JL, Zabala R, Corta I (2010b) Intervencionismo guiado por ecografía en el sistema musculoesquelético. Radiologia 52:525–533

Farin PU, Rasanen H, Jaroma H, Harju A (1996) Rotator cuff calcifications: treatment with ultrasound-guided percutaneous needle aspiration and lavage. Skeletal Radiol 25:551–554

Fernández de Larrinoa A, del Cura JL, Zabala R, Fuertes E, Bilbao F, López JI (2007) Value of ultrasound-guided core biopsy in the diagnosis of malignant lymphoma. J Clin Ultrasound 35:295–301

Kang SS, Labropoulos N, Mansour A, Baker WH (1998) Percutaneous ultrasound guided thrombin injection: a new method for treating postcatheterization femoral pseudoaneurysms. J Vasc Surg 27:1032–1038

Kim OH, Kim WS, Kim MJ, Jung JY, Suh JH (2000) US in the diagnosis of pediatric chest diseases. Radiographics 20:653–671

Krueger K, Zaehringer M (2005) Postcatheterization pseudoaneurysm: results of us-guided percutaneous thrombin injection in 240 patients. Radiology 236:1104–1110

Lencioni R et al (2009) Percutaneous image-guided radiofrequency ablation of liver tumors. Abdom Imaging 34:547–556

Liau CS, Ho FM, Chen MF, Lee YT (1997) Treatment of iatrogenic femoral artery pseudoaneurysm with percutaneous thrombin injection. J Vasc Surg 26:18–23

Livraghi T, Goldberg SN, Lazzaroni S, Meloni F, Solbiati L, Gazelle GS (1999) Small hepatocellular carcinoma: treatment with radio-frequency ablation versus ethanol injection. Radiology 210:655–661

López JI, del Cura JL, Zabala R, Bilbao FJ (2005) Usefulness and limitations of ultrasound-guided core biopsy in the diagnosis of musculoskeletal tumours. APMIS 113:353–360

López JI, del Cura JL, Fernández de Larrinoa A, Gorriño O, Zabala R, Bilbao FJ (2006) Role of ultrasound-guided core biopsy in the evaluation of spleen pathology. APMIS 114:492–499

Mortelé KJ, Grishman J, Szejnfeld D, Ashley SW, Erturk SM, Banks PA et al (2009) CT-guided percutaneous catheter drainage of acute necrotizing pancreatitis: clinical experience and observations in patients with sterile and infected necrosis. AJR Am J Roentgenol 192:110–116

Rhim H et al (2004) Radiofrequency thermal ablation of abdominal tumors: lessons learned from complications. Radiographics 24:41–52

Serafini G, Sconfienza LM, Lacelli F, Silvestri E, Aliprandi A, Sardanelli F (2009) Rotator cuff calcific tendonitis: short-term and 10-year outcomes after two-needle us-guided percutaneous treatment – nonrandomized controlled trial. Radiology 252:157–164

Stang A et al (2009) A systematic review on the clinical benefit and role of radiofrequency ablation as treatment of colorectal liver metastases. Eur J Cancer 45:1748–1756

Van Santvoort HC, Besselink MG, Bakker OJ, Hofker HS, Boermeester MA, Dejong CH et al (2010) A step-up approach or open necrosectomy for necrotizing pancreatitis. N Engl J Med 362:1491–1502

Wong SL, American Society of Clinical Oncology et al (2009) Clinical evidence review on radiofrequency ablation of hepatic metastases from colorectal cancer. J Clin Oncol 28:493–508

Zerem E, Hadzic A (2007) Sonographically guided percutaneous catheter drainage versus needle aspiration in the management of pyogenic liver abscess. AJR Am J Roentgenol 189:W138–W142

GPSR Compliance

The European Union's (EU) General Product Safety Regulation (GPSR) is a set of rules that requires consumer products to be safe and our obligations to ensure this.

If you have any concerns about our products, you can contact us at: Product-Safety@springernature.com

In case our publisher is established outside the EU, the EU authorised representative is:

Springer Nature Customer Service Center GmbH
Europaplatz 3
69115 Heidelberg, Germany

Batch number: 09938888

Printed by Printforce, the Netherlands

GPSR Compliance

The European Union's (EU) General Product Safety Regulation (GPSR)
is a set of rules that requires consumer products to be safe and our
obligations to ensure this.

If you have any concerns about our products, you can contact us on
ProductSafety@springernature.com

In case Publisher is established outside the EU, the EU authorized
representative is:

Springer Nature Customer Service Center GmbH
Europaplatz 3
69115 Heidelberg, Germany

Batch number: 09636588

Printed by Printforce, the Netherlands